T0342543

Equine Neck and Back Pathology

Equine Neck and Back Pathology

Diagnosis and Treatment

Second Edition

Edited by
Frances M.D. Henson
Department of Veterinary Medicine
University of Cambridge
UK

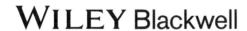

Registered Office(s)
John Wiley & Sons, Inc., 111 River Street, Hoboken, NJ 07030, USA
John Wiley & Sons Ltd, The Atrium, Southern Gate, Chichester, West Sussex, PO19 8SQ, UK

Editorial Office
9600 Garsington Road, Oxford, OX4 2DQ, UK

For details of our global editorial offices, customer services, and more information about Wiley products visit us at www.wiley.com.

Wiley also publishes its books in a variety of electronic formats and by print-on-demand. Some content that appears in standard print versions of this book may not be available in other formats.

Library of Congress Cataloging-in-Publication Data

Names: Henson, Frances M.D., editor.
Title: Equine neck and back pathology : diagnosis and treatment / edited by
    Frances M.D. Henson.
Other titles: Equine back pathology.
Description: Second edition. | Hoboken, NJ : Wiley, 2018. | Preceded by
    Equine back pathology / edited by Frances M.D. Henson. 2009. | Includes
    bibliographical references and index. |
Identifiers: LCCN 2017030342 (print) | LCCN 2017030986 (ebook) | ISBN
    9781118974506 (pdf) | ISBN 9781118974575 (epub) | ISBN 9781118974445
    (cloth)
Subjects: | MESH: Horse Diseases | Spinal Diseases–veterinary | Spinal
    Diseases–pathology | Back Pain–veterinary | Neck Pain–veterinary |
    Spine–anatomy & histology
Classification: LCC SF951 (ebook) | LCC SF951 (print) | NLM SF 951 | DDC
    636.1/0896–dc23
LC record available at https://lccn.loc.gov/2017030342

Cover images: (Background) © DavidMSchrader/Gettyimages; (Image on left) © Sarah Powell; (Images on right)
© Frances M.D. Henson
Cover design by Wiley

Set in 10/12pt WarnockPro-Regular by Thomson Digital, Noida, India
Printed and bound by CPI Group (UK) Ltd, Croydon, CR0 4YY

C9781118974445_050124

For Joan

1

The Normal Anatomy of the Neck

David Bainbridge

Introduction

The neck is a common derived characteristic of land vertebrates, not shared by their aquatic ancestors. In fish, the thoracic fin girdle, the precursor of the scapula, coracoid and clavicle, is frequently fused to the caudal aspect of the skull. In contrast, as vertebrates emerged on to the dry land, the forelimb separated from the head and the intervening vertebrae specialised to form a relatively mobile region – the neck – to allow the head to be freely steered in many directions.

With the exception of the tail, the neck remains the most mobile region of the spinal column in modern-day horses. It permits a wide range of sagittal plane flexion and extension to allow alternating periods of grazing and predator surveillance, as well as frontal plane flexion to allow the horizon to be scanned, and rotational movement to allow nuisance insects to be flicked off. Among domestic animals the equine neck is relatively long and the head relatively heavy, and so the neck has become strong, muscular and massive. This is enhanced by the fact that regular, forceful movements of this region must also occur to maintain balance when horses are running [1]. However, the length and flexible nature of the neck may also cause problems in the passage of foals through the birth canal.

In this chapter I will briefly review the anatomy of bones, joints, ligaments and muscles of the equine neck. The 'locomotor component' of the neck is a common site of pathology, and the diverse forms of neck disease reflect the sometimes complex and conflicting regional variations and functional constraints so evident in this region [2].

Unlike the abdomen and thorax, there is no coelomic cavity in the neck, yet its ventral part is taken up by a relatively small 'visceral compartment', containing the larynx, trachea, oesophagus and many important vessels, nerves and endocrine glands. However, I will not review these structures, as they do not represent an extension of the equine 'back' in the same way that the more dorsal locomotor region does.

Cervical Vertebrae 3–7

Almost all mammals, including the horse, possess seven cervical vertebrae, C1 to C7 (Figure 1.1). While C1 and C2 are extremely modified for their particular functions, C3 to C7 are more homogenous in structure. C3, C4 and C5 in particular are usually thought of as the 'typical' cervical vertebrae (Figure 1.2).

Vertebrae C3–C7 consist of an approximately cylindrical body or **centrum**, a structure present in all jawed vertebrates to resist longitudinal compression of the spinal column. The centra of the equine neck are the longest in the body, but become progressively smaller caudally. Those of C3–C7 possess a distinctively convex cranial surface, the **head**, and a correspondingly concave caudal

Equine Neck and Back Pathology: Diagnosis and Treatment, Second Edition. Edited by Frances M.D. Henson.
© 2018 John Wiley & Sons, Ltd. Published 2018 by John Wiley & Sons, Ltd.

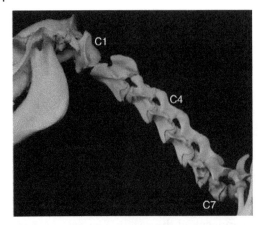

Figure 1.1 Lateral view of an articulated osteological preparation of the neck of a young horse.

surface, the **fossa**. Thus the intervertebral joints, which are far more mobile than in the trunk, may be thought of functionally as ball-and-socket joints, although their constituent parts are very structurally different from those of synovial ball-and-socket joints.

Dorsal to the centrum is the **neural arch**, formed from bilateral bony **laminae**, which surrounds and protects the spinal cord and its associated structures. The **vertebral canal** formed by successive arches is relatively wide in the neck, especially cranially, to allow the spinal cord, which is wide in this region, to flex freely. The vertebrae C3–C7 each develop from three primary centres of ossification – one in the centrum and one in each of the two laminae. Formation of cervical neural arches,

which are either statically or dynamically stenotic, is thought to be a cause of equine cervical 'wobbler syndrome' [3].

The centrum and arch are adorned with a variety of bony processes for the attachment of ligaments and muscles, and which often develop as secondary centres of ossification. These vertebral processes are a feature evolved by land vertebrates to permit complex movements in three dimensions and resist torsional forces.

a) The single dorsal midline **spinous process** is distinctively short in equine C3–C5.
b) In contrast, all equine cervical vertebrae bear a characteristically large **ventral crest**, often with a pronounced **caudal tubercle**.
c) The bilateral **transverse processes** are large but squat, and thought to incorporate vestigial ribs, sometimes yielding the name 'costotransverse processes'. In C3–6, the processes are bifid and slanted, with a cranial **ventral tubercle** and caudal **dorsal tubercle**. The transverse processes of C1–6 are perforated by a large **transverse foramen**, which conveys the vertebral artery and vein.
d) Lateral to the neural arch lie the large, irregular **articular processes**, with their smooth ovoid articular surfaces. The caudal facets are directed ventrolaterally, and the complementary cranial facets dorsomedially. Ventral to the caudal process lies a notch for passage of the laterally coursing spinal nerve.

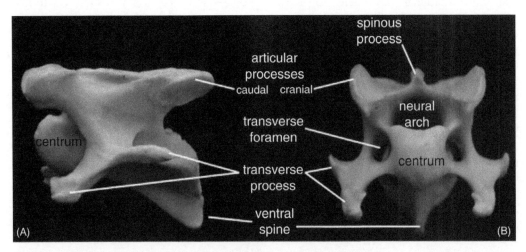

Figure 1.2 (A) Lateral view of equine C4 vertebra and (B) cranial view of C5.

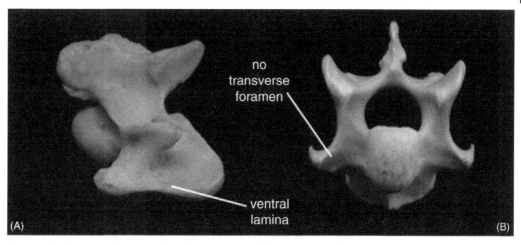

Figure 1.3 (A) Lateral view of equine C6 vertebra and (B) cranial view of C7.

The sixth cervical vertebra (Figure 1.3) differs from its cranial neighbours in that it bears pronounced paired bony sheets, the **ventral laminae**, which act as a site of attachment and force redirection of muscles, especially longus colli. In the horse these laminae are elaborated into **cranial and caudal tubercles**. C6 also possesses a longer spinous process than C3, 4 and 5 – a reflection of a gradual transition to a more 'thoracic' morphology.

This trend continues in C7 (Figure 1.3), which has an even longer spinous process, non-bifid transverse processes, and no transverse foramen – the vertebral arteries arise too far cranially to pass through C7. However, C7 does possess a caudal notch for the passage of a spinal nerve, but it should be emphasised that the nomenclature of the spinal nerves in inconsistent. Unlike the rest of the body, cervical spinal nerves emerge *cranial* to the vertebra of the same number, and the nerves emerging caudal to vertebra C7 are named C8, even though there is no corresponding C8 vertebra. Finally, the centra of C7 caudally bear unconvincing **costal facets** for the articulation of the cranial extremities of the capitula of the first ribs [4].

Atlas and Axis, C1 and C2

The anatomy of the caudal part of the axis, C2 (Figure 1.4), is similar to that of the more caudal cervical vertebrae – with centrum and neural arch formed from the same three centres of ossification, as well as the spinous process, ventral crest and tubercle, caudal articular facets and dorsal tubercle of the transverse process. However, the cranial part of the bone is markedly aberrant to allow the unique rotational, trochoid, 'head-shaking' movement of the atlanto-axial joint. Its unusual shape results from the incorporation of embryonic elements of C1.

A fourth primary centre of ossification, actually the annexed centrum of C1, forms the **dens** ('tooth') or **odontoid process** of C2. This cranially directed process is attached ventrally to the main centrum of C2 by a base formed from a further, secondary centre, which represents the cranial epiphysis of C2. The dens articulates closely with the ventral part of C1, and thus is smooth on its ventral surface, but is roughened dorsally with a midline gutter to allow attachment of stabilising ligaments. The smooth articular region of the dens is continuous with the large bilateral saddle-shaped **cranial articular surfaces**, which slide across reciprocal surfaces on C1 to allow rotation of the joint. These surfaces also develop from their own secondary ossification centres.

The axis contains a relatively large amount of trabecular bone compared to the other cervical vertebrae, and is also characterised by a large spinous process. Equine C2 is also distinctive in possessing bilateral foramina for the passage of the second pair of spinal nerves,

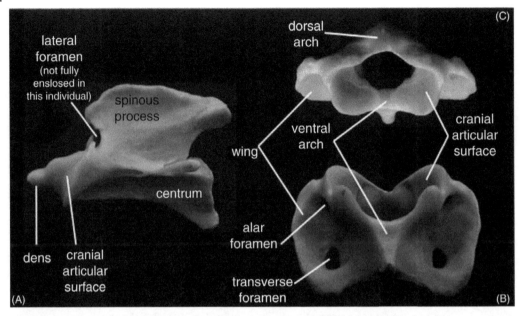

Figure 1.4 (A) Lateral view of equine C2 vertebra, and (B) ventral and (C) cranial views of C1.

which do not emerge between adjacent vertebrae, as all the more caudal spinal nerves do. In some texts these are called 'intervertebral foramina', which seems illogical, so the name **lateral foramina** is perhaps preferable.

The atlas, C1 (Figure 1.4), is the most bizarre of all the vertebrae, due to it performing specialised movements with both the skull (sagittal plane flexion and extension/'nodding'/'yes' movement) and the axis (rotation about the long axis of the spine/'shaking head'/'no' movement).

The atlas has no centrum and no neural spine, but is instead constituted by one large hollow cylinder formed by **dorsal and ventral arches** of bone. The dorsal arch is equivalent to the neural arches of other vertebrae, but the thicker ventral arch is a unique structure probably derived from paired cranial epiphyseal developmental elements. The absence of a centrum means that, unlike C2, C1 contains an unusually low proportion of trabecular bone. The caudal part of the dorsal, internal surface of the ventral arch is the smooth **fovea dentis**, which articulates with the dens of the axis, whereas the more cranial 'floor' of the atlas is much rougher.

The equine atlas is relatively large compared to that of humans, but small compared to that of

dogs. Attached laterally to the arches are the irregular **lateral masses**, which support the **caudal articular surfaces** as well as the wide, ovoid and profoundly concave **cranial articular surfaces**. Also attached laterally are the large modified transverse processes termed **wings** or **alae**. The wings, distinctively concave ventrally in the horse, form the attachment of several of the long and short muscles of the cranial neck, and also contain transverse foramina similar to those in C2–C6. The alar notches present on the cranial edge of the wings of the atlas in some species are entirely enclosed into **alar foramina** in the horse, and mark the tortuous course of the vertebral arteries [5,6]. A further, slightly medial foramen permits the entry of the artery into the vertebral canal as well as the exit of spinal nerve C1 and, as with the equivalent 'non-intervertebral' route taken by nerve C2 through the bony laminae of the axis, this is best termed the **lateral foramen**.

Joints of the Neck

The articulations between C2, 3, 4, 5, 6 and 7 are similar to those found in the trunk region. Once labelled with the somewhat confusing name 'amphiarthroses', these intervertebral joints are best considered as compound joints each comprising two completely different forms of articulation.

First, the adjacent centra are bonded together by a single **intercentral joint**, a unique form of symphysis more often called an **intervertebral disc**. Each disc is interposed between two centra and contains two parts. An outer ring, the **annulus fibrosus**, consists of multiple layers of interwoven fibrous tissue with alternating diagonally oriented collagenous fibres that resist torsion and extension of the spine. The annulus becomes less fibrous centrally. Encircled by the annulus is the **nucleus pulposus**, an unusual admixture of fibrous tissue, gel-like matrix, and swollen cells derived evolutionarily and developmentally from the notochord. Indeed, small foveae in the centra often hint at the fact that the notochord once passed all along the body, piercing through longitudinal foramina in every centrum. However, the nucleus still retains its ancestral function, which is to resist compression. Disc disease may be rare in horses, although the age-related degeneration of their intervertebral discs has been little studied [7].

The second type of intervertebral articulation is formed by the bilateral **interneural joints (also known as articular process joints, or APJs)**, synovial diarthroses between the facets on the articular processes that lie lateral to the neural arch. These joints are more mobile in the neck than in the trunk, although their joint capsules are strong and fibrous.

The C1–C2 **atlanto-axial joint** is, as mentioned previously, an unusual trochoid or pivot joint. The dens and cranial articular surfaces of C2 articulate with caudal articular surfaces and fovea dentis of C1 by means of what is, in horses, a large single synovial joint capsule – there is no disc. The congruence of the articular surfaces is poor, and the centre of rotation is maintained just above the axis of the dens by a series of ligaments, discussed later.

The C1–skull **atlanto-occipital joint** is a specialised sagittal-plane ginglymus or hinge joint. The paired convex **occipital condyles** of the bilateral exoccipital skull bones form a

good fit with the large concave cranial articular facets of the atlas, allowing rotation about a transverse axis – again, there is no disc. In all horses their joint initially consists of paired bilateral synovial spaces, although these may form a ventral interconnection in later life in some individuals [6]. Genetic congenital malformation of this joint has been reported in Arab foals [8].

Ligaments of the Neck

The equine neck ligaments represent a modification, sometimes dramatic, of the ligaments present more caudally in the spine. This is due to not only the greater mobility in the region but also the constraints of supporting the large head.

The 'yellow', interlamellar or **interarcuate ligaments**, or ligamenta flava, are sheets of elastic tissue that span the space between adjacent vertebral neural arches. They contact the epidural space medially, the neck musculature laterally, blend with nearby synovial capsules, and each contain a gap via which spinal nerves may exit the vertebral canal. In the equine neck they are unusually extensive and flexible to allow movement.

The **dorsal longitudinal ligament** runs along the dorsal surface of the centra of all the cervical vertebrae, and thus along the 'floor' of the vertebral canal. It is narrower over the body of each centrum and then fans out to a wide attachment on the dorsal edge of each intervertebral disc. Notably, the **ventral longitudinal ligament** does not extend into the cervical region in the horse.

The **interspinous ligaments** are elastic in the equine neck to permit movement, but their small size reflects the diminutive nature of the spinous processes in this species. Intertransverse ligaments are not clearly apparent in the equine neck.

The **supraspinous ligament** is greatly elaborated in the equine neck into the extensive, strong, elastic **nuchal ligament** (Figure 1.5). The function of this ligament is to support the weight of the massive head and neck, and

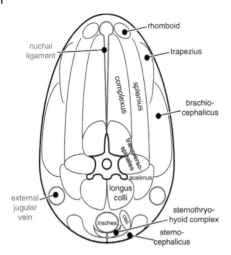

Figure 1.5 Schematic midcervical transverse section of the equine neck, showing position of muscles.

to store elastic potential energy when the head is lowered to the ground to graze, so that energy may then be retrieved to lift it. The ligament is elaborated into two parts. The **funicular part** is a strong cord connecting the withers to the nuchal region of the skull, laterally compressed at its cranial end. The funicular part is equivalent to the nuchal ligament of the dog, although in that species it terminates on the axis. The nuchal ligament is actually constituted by paired bilateral components, and through much of the length of the funicular part these are separated by an almost invisible midline fibrous seam. Cranially, there may be a slight divergence of the two sides of the ligament. The **lamellar part**, which has no equivalent in the carnivores, consists of fibres radiating from the withers and funicular part to the spinous processes of C2–C7. Some consider there to be two subdivisions of the lamellar part: a thinner caudal division inserting on C7, C6 and C5, and a thicker cranial division inserting on C4, C3 and C2. The lamellar part does not constitute a complete sheet filling the space between the funicular part and the neck vertebrae, but leaves spaces, as well as areas where the ligaments may potentially abrade the spinous processes. At these points, there are often **bursae** interposed between bone and

ligament. The most constant are those overlying C1 (**atlantal bursa**), vertebra T2 (**supraspinous bursa**), but less constant ones may also be found dorsal to C2 (**axial bursa**) and C3. These bursae may occasionally be sites of inflammation [9].

The specialised function of the C1–C2 or atlanto-axial joint has led to the development of an unusual array of ligaments. The elastic **dorsal atlanto-axial ligament** from the spinous process of C2 to the dorsal tuberosity of C1 may be seen as a localised adjunct to the nuchal ligament, whereas the more fibrous **ventral atlanto-axial ligament** presumably prevents extension of the joint. The transverse, alar and apical ligaments, which bind the dens to the atlas in the dog, are almost absent in the horse, and instead a thick **odontoid ligament**, a continuation of the dorsal longitudinal ligament, radiates cranially from the dens to attach on the cranial roughened area of the floor of the vertebral canal of the atlas. Finally, the atlanto-axial joint is also spanned by the strong **membrane tectoria**, a fibrous sheet running from the region of the dens to the internal surface of the axis, as well as the ventral rim of the foramen magnum of the skull itself.

The C1-skull or atlanto-occipital joint is also specialised. Its main ligamentar support is from the strong paired **lateral atlanto-occipital ligaments**, which pass from the wings of the atlas to the adjacent paramastoid surface of the skull. In addition the joint is enclosed by the thin **ventral atlanto-occipital membrane** and the stronger **dorsal atlanto-occipital membrane**, which contains thick fibrous strands in a cruciate arrangement [6]. Clinical access may be gained to the underlying cisterna magna of the subarachnoid space by passing a needle through this latter membrane and the underlying meninges [10].

Muscles of the Neck

Most of the mass of the neck is made up of muscles that act to move the head and neck, the hyoid apparatus, the forelimbs or a combination of these structures. These muscles may be divided into two groups – the larger dorsal **epaxial muscles**, which act to extend the spine in the sagittal plane or flex it in the frontal plane if contracted asymmetrically, and the smaller ventral **hypaxial muscles**, which usually act to flex the spine sagittally [11]. A schematic midlevel cross-section of the neck muscles is given in Figure 1.5.

Some of the more dorsally and laterally positioned muscles probably act on the forelimb more than on the neck and head, but are mentioned here because of their origins in that region. These include the cranial portions of the **trapezii** and **rhomboids,** which insert on the scapula, the **brachiocephalicus,** which inserts primarily on the humerus, and the fibrous **serratus ventralis,** which slings the weight of the body on the forelimbs. The epaxial spinal muscles become larger and elaborated in the cervical region and take up most of the upper half of the horse's neck. The **transversospinalis** group continues into the neck as the complexus and multifidus muscles, as do the complex interleavings of the **longissimus** group, reaching as far as the skull. **Splenius** is also present in the horse, originating on vertebrae T3–T5 and inserting on the transverse processes of C1, C3, C4 and C5 and the caudal aspect of the skull. There are also short, specialised muscles in the cranial neck. The extensors are **obliquus capitis cranialis** (ventral wing of atlas to caudal skull), **rectus capitis dorsalis major** (spinous process of axis to caudal skull) and **rectus capitis dorsalis minor** (dorsal atlas to caudal skull), while **obliquus capitis caudalis** (spinous process of axis to caudal skull) is well aligned to act as a rotator. This profusion of smaller muscles attached to the atlas and axis explain why these vertebrae bear such expansive bony processes.

Some of the far-ventral hypaxial muscles do not warrant much mention in a book about the 'back'. These include the **sternocephalicus**, **omohyoideus** and the **sternothyrohyoid complex**. However, there are specific, although relatively small, spinal flexors in this region. One prime neck flexor is **longus colli**, which passes from the ventral surfaces of T1–T6 to the ventral tubercles of all the cervical vertebrae, running ventral to a bursa at T1 and the ventral laminae of C6. Another is **scalenus**, which originates on the first rib and inserts on the transverse processes of C1–C7. There is also the **rectus capitis ventralis major**, from the transverse processes of T3–T5 to the ventral skull, the **rectus capitis ventralis major** from the ventral atlas to the ventral skull, and the more laterally positioned but similarly short **rectus capitis lateralis** [12].

It is unclear to what extent these muscles are sites of pathology, especially as many of them are not amenable to direct clinical examination.

References

1 Zsoldos, R.R. and Licka, T.F. The equine neck and its function during movement and locomotion. *Zoology (Jena)* 2015; **118**:364–376.

2 Stashak, E. *Adams' Lameness in Horses*, 4th edn. Philadelphia, PA: Lea and Febiger, 1976.

3 Janes, J.G., Garrett, K.S., McQuerry, K.J., et al. Comparison of magnetic resonance imaging with standing cervical radiographs for evaluation of vertebral canal stenosis in equine cervical stenotic myelopathy. *Equine Veterinary Journal* 2014; **46**:681–686.

4 Barone, R. *Anatomie Comparée des Mammifères Domestiques*, Tome 1: *Osteologie*. Lyon: Ecole Nationale Vétérinaire, 1966.

5 Share-Jones, J.T. *The Surgical Anatomy of the Horse*, London: Baillière, Tindall and Cox, 1908.

6 Barone, R. *Anatomie Comparée des Mammifères Domestiques*, Tome 2: *Arthrologie et Myologie*. Lyon: Ecole Nationale Vétérinaire, 1968.

7 Fölkel, I.M. Lumbar intervertebral disc disease (IVDD) in horses: a longitudinal ultrasonographic and

histomorphological comparison. Master Thesis, Utrecht.

8 Watson, A.G. and Mayhew, I.G. Familial congenital occipitoatlantoaxial malformation (OAAM) in the Arabian horse. *Spine* 1986; **11**:334–339.

9 García-López, J.M., Jenei, T., Chope, K. and Bubeck, K.A. Diagnosis and management of cranial and caudal nuchal bursitis in four horses. *Journal of the American Veterinary Medicine Association* 2010; **237**:823–829.

10 Johnson, P.J. and Constantinescu, G.M. Collection of cerebrospinal fluid in horses. *Equine Veterinary Education* 2000; **12**:7–12.

11 Pasquini, C., Spurgeon, T. and Pasquini, S. *Anatomy of the Domestic Animals*, 9th edn. Pilot Point: Sudz, 1995.

12 Getty, R. *Sisson and Grossmans's Anatomy of the Domestic Animals*, 5th edn. Philadelphia, PA: Saunders, 1975.

2

The Normal Anatomy of the Osseous and Soft Tissue Structures of the Back and Pelvis

Leo B. Jeffcott, Jessica A. Kidd and David Bainbridge

Introduction

In order to understand the pathological conditions that affect a horse's back and pelvis it is necessary to have an excellent working knowledge of its structure. The back and pelvis are made up of osseous structures, joints, muscles, ligaments, blood vessels and nerves, all of which can be altered or affected in disease. In this chapter the osseous and soft tissue structures of the back (i.e. the thoracolumbar spine, sacrum and pelvis) are discussed.

2.1 Normal Anatomy of the Osseous Structures

Leo B. Jeffcott

The vertebral column runs from the atlanto-occipital joint to the last coccygeal vertebra (Figure 2.1). As it passes through the body the vertebral column does not form a straight-line structure; rather it descends sharply from the atlanto-occipital joint to reach its lowest point at the cervicothoracic junction. The column then ascends gently to the caudal lumbar region and descends down, via the sacrum, to the coccygeal vertebrae (Figure 2.1). The external appearance of the horse, however, presents a different picture in the cranial thoracic region. Externally the withers (corresponding approximately to T3–T7) is the highest point of the back, even though the vertebral bodies

are ventral to most other vertebral bodies at this point. This is due to the external elevation provided by the long dorsal spinous processes (DSPs) in the withers region, which creates a contrary impression [1].

Vertebral Numbering System

The nomenclature for the classification of different vertebral segments is fairly standardised between different texts and papers, with vertebral segments traditionally counted within spinal regions from a cranial reference point. Within each region the vertebrae are numbered sequentially from cranial to caudal, e.g. T1 (first thoracic vertebra), T2 (second thoracic vertebra). However, occasionally, some authors use modified reference systems, using caudal reference points [2]. It is important to be aware of this alternative numbering system when consulting the literature in this area to avoid confusion. In this book the standard cranial reference system will be used.

Vertebral Formula

The spine of the horse is made up of cervical, thoracic, lumbar, sacral and coccygeal vertebrae (Figure 2.2). The standard vertebral formula for the horse is 7 cervical vertebrae, 18 thoracic vertebrae, 6 lumbar vertebrae, 5 sacral vertebrae and between 15 and 21

Equine Neck and Back Pathology: Diagnosis and Treatment, Second Edition. Edited by Frances M.D. Henson.
© 2018 John Wiley & Sons, Ltd. Published 2018 by John Wiley & Sons, Ltd.

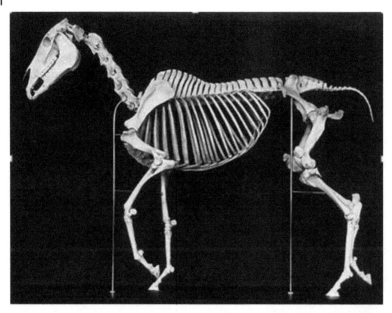

Figure 2.1 A photograph of the skeleton of the horse. The vertebral column runs from the atlanto-occipital joint to the last coccygeal vertebra. The vertebral column descends sharply from the atlanto-occipital joint to reach its lowest point at the cervicothoracic junction. The column then ascends gently to the caudal lumbar region and descends down, via the sacrum, to the coccygeal vertebrae.

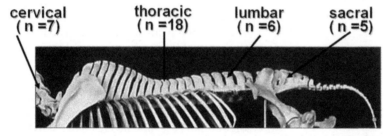

cervical (n =7)   thoracic (n =18)   lumbar (n =6)   sacral (n =5)

Figure 2.2 The bones of the vertebral column from the seventh cervical vertebra to the penultimate coccygeal vertebra. The vertebral column is divided into cervical, thoracic, lumbar, sacral and coccygeal regions. There are 7 cervical vertebrae, 18 thoracic vertebrae, 6 lumbar vertebrae, 5 sacral vertebrae and 15–21 coccygeal vertebrae in the normal horse.

Table 2.1 Average vertebral formula for the horse.

Anatomical site	Number of vertebrae
Cervical	7
Thoracic	18
Lumbar	6
Sacral	5
Coccygeal	15–21

coccygeal vertebrae [3] (Table 2.1). Although there may be some variation in the number of specific vertebrae in the axial skeleton, the total number in the formula is more constant. Anecdotally, so-called 'short-backed' horses, such as Arabians, have been reported as having fewer vertebrae than other horses [4]. More objective data on the numbers of vertebrae have come from studies investigating the numbers of vertebrae within a population, with a number of studies designed to investigate the frequency of occurrence of the standard six lumbar vertebrae. Haussler et al. [2], in a study on thoroughbred horses, showed that only 69% of horses had the expected six lumbar vertebrae. However, it has been suggested that variations in the number of vertebrae within one spinal region are compensated for by an alteration in number in an adjacent vertebral region, in many cases to give a constant overall total vertebral number. There has been no proven association between the numbers of vertebrae that a horse has and any pathological condition.

Ossification Centres and Growth Plate Closure Times

The primary ossification centres of the vertebral bodies and neural arches (i.e. those surrounding the embryonic notochord in the centrum and lateral to the neural tube in the vertebral arch) fuse shortly after birth [5], whereas the secondary separate centres of ossification do not fuse until later on in life, if at all.

Secondary centres of ossification occur in the summits of the DSPs of the cranial thoracic vertebrae (the caudal thoracic and lumbar DSPs have fibrocartilaginous caps), the extremities of the transverse processes (TPs) of the lumbar vertebrae, the epiphyses of the vertebral bodies and the ventral crest.

The age at which these secondary centres of ossification fuse to the parent bone depends on the method of estimation of growth plate closure. Postmortem and histological growth plate closure times will always report an older age of closure than radiographic surveys because radiography is a less sensitive method of identifying the presence of an open growth plate.

The secondary centres of ossification present in the summits of the DSPs of the cranial thoracic region from T2 to around T9 are reported to fuse to the parent bone between 9 and 14 years of age [3], but in many cases, in the author's experience, they never fuse to the parent bone, even in aged

horses. Thus they can be confused with fractured summits of the DSPs on radiographs if this developmental feature is not appreciated (Chapter 8).

The secondary centres of ossification at the cranial and caudal epiphyses of the vertebral bodies have reported closure times of between 3 and 3½ years of age using radiographic techniques (Chapter 8) [5]. However, gross anatomical studies suggest that the plates fully close later and asynchronously. The physes are reported to close between 4.9 and 6.7 years, with the cranial physis closing first, usually 1–2 years before the caudal physis [2]. The secondary centres of ossification of the TPs close in the first few months of life, although specific reports of this are not available.

Structure of the Thoracic and Lumbar Vertebrae

A typical thoracic vertebra is made up of a vertebral body, a vertebral arch and vertebral processes (Figure 2.3). The vertebral body provides the surface against which the intervertebral disc sits, whereas the vertebral arch provides a gap in the osseous structure through which the spinal cord runs. The vertebral processes are the sites of attachment for various ligaments and muscles and are named the DSPs, the transverse processes (TPs) and the articular processes (APs) (Figure 2.3). These processes vary subtly within each anatomical region and this variation reflects the functional and structural demands at that particular anatomical site, e.g. the length of the DSP varies from region to region, being particularly long between T3 and T7. The lumbar vertebrae, in contrast, have long TPs and medium height DSPs.

Vertebral Bodies

The vertebral bodies of the equine thoracolumbar spine (see Figure 2.3) provide support for weight-bearing and attachment sites

(A)

(B)

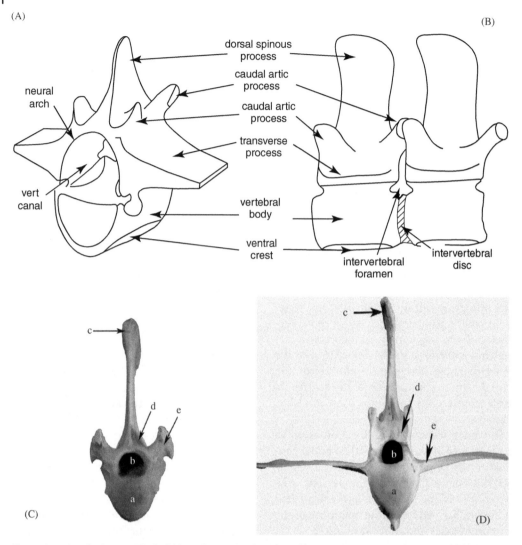

(C)

(D)

Figure 2.3 Vertebral anatomy: (a, b) line diagrams of a thoracic vertebra labelled to show the different anatomical regions of the vertebra: (a) a craniocaudal oblique diagram, (b) a lateral diagram. (c, d) Photographs of typical vertebrae: (c) thoracic vertebra, (d) lumbar vertebra; A, vertebral body; B, vertebral canal; C, dorsal spinous process; D, articular facet; E, transverse process. Note the much longer transverse processes in the lumbar vertebra compared with the thoracic vertebra.

for soft tissues and muscles. They are convex in shape cranially and concave in shape caudally. Ventrally a ridge of bone, the 'ventral crest' (Figure 2.3) is observed on approximately four to eight vertebrae (mean 5.5 ± 0.8 [2]) centred around the thoracolumbar junction.

The shape of the vertebral bodies changes from a rounded shape in the thoracic region to a dorsoventrally flattened shape in the caudal lumbar and sacral regions. It has been hypothesised that this shape change limits movement laterally between these vertebrae, but not dorsoventrally. Other anatomical variations between sites include the observation that prominent ventral body ventral crests are found in the cranial thoracic area and between T15 and L3. The ventral crest at the latter site, which can vary in the number of vertebrae involved, is believed to be the site of insertion of the crura of the diaphragm.

Intervertebral Discs

The intervertebral discs (or fibrocartilages) are positioned between adjacent vertebral bodies to form fibrocartilaginous articulations. They function to aid weight bearing, axial shock absorption and the maintenance of vertebral flexibility; they have both proprioceptive and nocioceptive fibres in the outer third of the disc. The discs are made up of a gelatinous central *nucleus pulposus* and an outer fibrous *annulus fibrosus*; this *annulus fibrosus* is designed to provide rotational stability to the intervertebral joint by being formed of concentric layers of fibres angled relative to each other.

The width of the intervertebral discs differs between anatomical sites. In one study it was demonstrated that the intervertebral discs were thicker at T1–T2 (average 5.9 mm, [6]) than elsewhere in the thoracic spine, with the average diameter of an intervertebral disc in the midthoracic region being 2.5 mm. It was also shown that the lumbosacral junction has a wider intervertebral disc compared with elsewhere in the spine (average 3.6 mm).

In the horse, relatively few clinical problems arise from intervertebral disc pathology, particularly compared with the high frequency of pathology at this site in dogs and humans. However, discospondylitis and intervertebral disc degeneration are occasionally seen. Intervertebral disc herniation is extremely rare in the horse, possibly because of the poorly developed *nucleus pulposus* and thin intervertebral disc.

Vertebral Arch

The spinal cord runs through the vertebral arch, which is made up of the dorsal part of the vertebral body ventrally, the vertebral lamina dorsally and the pedicles laterally. Dorsally in the vertebral arch the ventral laminae are connected by the ligamenta flava. The vertebral arches of the spinal vertebrae together form the continuous vertebral canal housing the spinal cord and its associated structures up to the cranial sacral region where the spinal cord terminates in the *cauda equina* (Chapter 3). The vertebral arch is relatively large compared with the diameter of the spinal cord, ensuring no compression of the cord during movements of the spinal segments in the normal spine. However, in pathological conditions narrowing of the vertebral arch can occur (i.e. if there is displaced bone secondary to a fracture or new bone formation in osteoarthritis). In these cases spinal cord compression may result in onset of neurological signs.

Intervertebral Foramina

Between the vertebral arches of each vertebra there is a small opening on either side – the intervertebral foramina (Figure 2.4). These

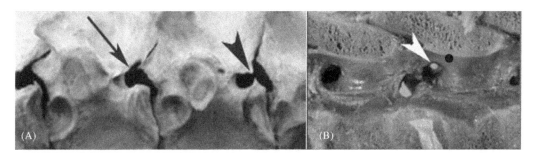

Figure 2.4 Intervertebral and lateral foramina of the thoracic spine: (A) photograph of a skeleton; (B) a cross-section from a postmortem specimen. In (A) an open intervertebral foramen is seen (black arrow) in the vertebral segment cranial to an intervertebral foramen that has spurs of bone formation protruding into it from dorsal and ventral (arrow head). In (B) this new bone formation is seen on the postmortem specimen.

intervertebral foramina are formed by ventral notches in the cranial and caudal margins of the vertebral arch. The intervertebral foramina permit soft tissue structures (nerves, blood vessels and lymphatics) to exit the bony vertebral canal at each segment.

Lateral Foramina

In addition to the intervertebral foramina that are observed on either side of the spine at each segmental junction between vertebrae, a second lateralised opening out of the bony canal is also present intermittently in some individuals. These are known as the lateral foramina. Thoracic vertebrae T11, T15 and T16 have been reported as showing the highest incidence of fully formed lateral foramina in the thoracolumbar spine [7].

The origin of the lateral foramina is not known; however, it has been proposed that they arise from the intervertebral foramina as a consequence of spur formation in the caudal ventral notch of the vertebral arch (Figure 2.4). Progressive calcification of the caudal ventral notch can occur, similar to that seen in ventral spondylitis (Chapter 13). In addition to a fully enclosed lateral foramen, there are a number of other variations in the anatomy of the caudal notch of the vertebral arch, including one or more spurs protruding into the notch [7]. It has been demonstrated that, where present, the lateral foramen contains spinal nerves and some vessels, and the presence of lateral foramina may possibly be associated with spinal nerve impingement during and subsequent to this calcification.

Sacral Foramina

In the sacrum the soft tissue structures exit the fused vertebral arches via either dorsal or ventral (pelvic) sacral foramina. The dorsal branches of the sacral spinal nerves exit via the dorsal sacral foramina. The pelvic sacral foramina communicate with the vertebral canal ventrally and contain the ventral branches of the sacral spinal nerves.

Vertebral Canal Contents

The vertebral canal contains the spinal cord and the structures surrounding the spinal cord (i.e. the cerebrospinal fluid, meninges, fat and vascular plexus). The spinal cord has segmentally paired dorsal and ventral motor roots that converge within the intervertebral foramen to form the spinal nerves (see Chapter 3).

Transitional Vertebrae

Transitional vertebrae are located between two adjacent vertebral regions and have the morphological characteristics of both these regions, i.e. they are 'hybrid' vertebrae. They occur, therefore, at the cervicothoracic, thoracolumbar or lumbosacral junction. A few studies have documented the incidence of transitional vertebrae. Haussler et al. [2] showed that 22% of their study population had thoracolumbar transitional vertebrae, none had lumbosacral transitional vertebrae and 36% had sacrococcygeal transitional vertebrae. Transitional vertebrae may exhibit their unusual morphology either through left-to-right asymmetry or via altered cranial-to-caudal graduation in the morphology. In large-scale studies of lumbosacral transitional vertebrae in humans and dogs, the morphological characteristics of the transitional vertebrae have been demonstrated to occur at the vertebral arches and transverse processes rather than at the vertebral body.

In clinical practice the most common transitional vertebra is transitional C7, which is often detected on lateromedial radiographs of the base of the spine and is characterised by having a short DSP, when it would normally have none at all.

Dorsal Spinous Processes

The DSPs project dorsally from the vertebral arch to rise above the vertebra into the epaxial musculature. The function of the DSPs is considered to be as levers for the muscular and ligamentous attachments of the vertebral column; bilateral contraction of the muscles that attach to the DSPs causes spinal extension, and unilateral contraction causes rotation.

The DSPs vary in their length, shape and angulation in different regions and will be considered anatomically from T1 running caudally. T1 has an extremely small DSP, rising approximately to twice the height of the vertebral body dorsally (Figure 2.5). This is the first elongated DSP in the vertebral column in most horses; however, occasionally an elongated DSP is seen on C7 (i.e. C7 has the properties of a transitional vertebra). Care must be taken not to automatically assume that the first obvious DSP on a lateromedial radiograph is therefore T1.

Although T1 has a small spinous process, the DSPs in the cranial thoracic vertebral region are markedly elongated in the region of T2–T8 to form the withers (Figure 2.6). The apex of the withers is formed by the DSPs of T4–T7 (Figure 2.6). As noted above, the tips of the DSP of approximately T4–T7 have separate centres of ossification. From an apex at T6

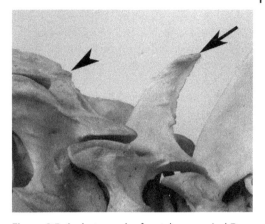

Figure 2.5 A photograph of vertebrae cervical 7 (C7) and thoracic 1 (T1). Note the elongated dorsal spinous process on T1 (arrow) compared with C7 (arrowhead).

or T7 the length of the DSP decreases down to approximately T12; the height of the DSP decreases slightly down to the anticlinal vertebra (the vertebra at which the angulation of the DSPs changes; see below, Figure 2.6) and then increases gently to the last lumbar vertebra (Figure 2.6).

The shape of the DSPs also depends on the anatomical site from which they arise. DSPs from vertebrae T1–T10 are narrow and tend to be quite straight (Figure 2.6). At T11–T16 they have a marked beak-shaped outline, wider at their base than at their apex and forming a cranial beak with a rounded caudal

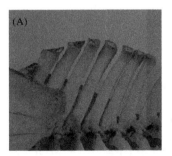
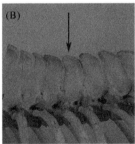
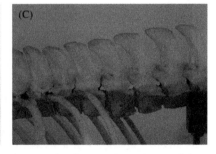

Figure 2.6 Three photographs of the vertebral column of a horse showing the shape and angulation of the dorsal spinous processes (DSPs): (A) cranial thoracic region (withers); the DSPs are markedly elongated and angle caudally. Note the separate centres of ossification in the most cranial vertebrae. In (B) the DSPs of the mid-thoracic region are seen. At this site the DSPs are shorter than in the cranial thoracic region and have a 'beak shape' at their summits. The DSPs of the more cranial vertebrae angle caudally until the 'anticlinal' vertebra (black arrow). From this point caudally the DSPs angle cranially. In (C) the DSPs of the caudal thoracic and first four lumbar vertebrae are seen. The DSPs angle cranially.

aspect at their summits. The cranial and caudal borders of the DSPs are often roughened due to new bone formation on these edges, which are the insertions of the interspinous ligaments; the dorsal summits of the DSPs are also often roughened at the sites of attachment of the supraspinous ligament (Chapter 10).

The angulation of the thoracolumbar DSPs changes from T1 caudally to the lumbosacral junction. From T1 to T14 the DSPs are angled dorsocaudally (i.e. towards the tail; Figure 2.6A). At T15, the so-called '*anticlinal vertebra*' (Figure 2.6B), the DSP is upright and then from T17 to L6 the DSPs are angled dorsocranially (towards the head) (Figure 2.6C). The anatomical reason for this alteration in DSP angulation is suggested to be due to attached soft tissue interactions. The position of the anticlinal vertebra suggests an alteration, at this anatomical site, of the soft tissue forces acting on the spine. The cranial thoracic region transmits forces from the head, neck and forelimbs, whereas the caudal thoracic and lumbosacral regions transmit forces associated with the hindlimbs; therefore the pull of the associated soft tissue structures does indeed alter either side of the anticlinal vertebra.

A further change in DSP angulation is observed in the sacrum, which is inclined dorsocaudally (Figure 2.7). The anatomical consequence of this alteration in angulation, without the intermediary of an anticlinal vertebra as occurs in the thoracic spine, is that a wide interspinous space is formed at the lumbosacral junction (Figure 2.7). It has been suggested that this wide interspinous space allows an increased range of motion at this site without the risk of process impingement. The wide space between L6 and S1 is a relatively consistent finding; however, in one study 36% of horses had an equally wide interspinous space between L5 and L6 [2]. This has, at the current time, little clinical relevance apart from possibly making more difficult the identification of the landmarks for cerebrospinal fluid retrieval from the lumbosacral space.

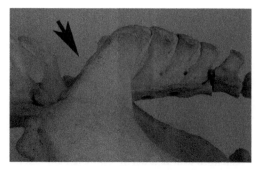

Figure 2.7 A photograph of the lumbosacral region: the wing of the ilium is seen in front of the cranial part of the sacrum. The last lumbar vertebra angles cranially and the sacrum angles caudally. The lumbosacral space is wide compared with any other interspinal space in the vertebral column (black arrow).

The distance between the summits of the DSPs varies between anatomical sites and between individuals. In most horses there is a small but clear gap between the DSP in the region T1 to T11; however, after T11 the DSPs become closer together. In some cases, post mortem or on lateromedial radiographs, the DSPs are seen to overlap with no evidence of bony contact (i.e. they are not quite in the same sagittal plane). Thus there is no bony contact and no evidence of bony remodelling. However, in many cases the close proximity of the DSPs does lead to a bony contact, remodelling and, in some cases, false joint formation. This condition is known variously as 'kissing spines' or 'overriding dorsal spinous processes' and can cause back pain (Chapter 13).

Articular Processes (Facets)

Paired articular processes (facets) arise both cranially and caudally from the vertebral arch and extend dorsally laterally. Between the cranial articular process of one vertebra and the caudal articular process of an adjacent vertebra a synovial joint is formed (i.e. a zygapophyseal joint). At each vertebral junction a pair of these joints is thus formed. The size, shape and orientation of the articular

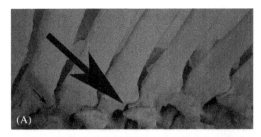

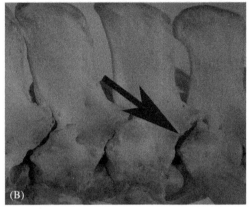

Figure 2.8 Two photographs to show the angulation of the articular facets at different regions of the vertebral column: (A) cranial thoracic vertebrae; articulations are close to horizontal (black arrows). (B) Caudal thoracic vertebrae: articulations are more vertically oriented (black arrow).

facets and hence joint surface differ within the vertebral column. In the cervical region and T1 the articular surfaces are large and lie at 45° to the horizontal. At T2 there is a transition from a 45° angle to a horizontal positioning of the articular facets. In the remainder of the thoracic region until about T16 (in 11 of 21 horses [6]), the articular surfaces continue

to lie approximately horizontal with the cranial articular surfaces facing dorsally and the caudal articular surfaces facing ventrally (Figure 2.8A). The morphology of the articular facets is, however, not always symmetrical; one study reported that 83% of horses had asymmetrical facets [2]. At T16 and then into the lumbar region the articular surface orientation changes from horizontal to vertical (Figure 2.8B). In addition to the change in orientation of the articular facets, changes are also seen in the actual shape of the processes. In the thoracic region the facets are relatively flat; from T16 onwards their articular surfaces change such that the cranial articular surfaces are dorsally concave and the caudal articular surfaces ventrally convex. The alteration in the angulation and shape of the articular processes may reflect the movements of the different parts of the spine; in the thoracic vertebral region vertebral motion is mostly rotation and lateral flexion. In the lumbosacral region motion it is mainly dorsoventral.

It has been proposed, based on the morphology of the articular facets, that the equine thoracolumbar spine can be divided into four regions: the first thoracic intervertebral joint (T1–T2), the cranial and midthoracic region (T2–T16), the caudal thoracic and lumbar region (T16–L6), and the lumbosacral joint (L6–S1) [6]. Studies on the amount and type of movement at each of these sites have indicated that each of these four sites does have a characteristic movement [8] and thus a structure–function relationship at these sites is likely (Table 2.2).

Table 2.2 The relative amounts of movement in the joint complexes of the four regions of the equine thoracolumbar spine and the structure of the articular facets at each site.

Region	Angle of articular facets	Shape of articular facets	Flexion and extension	Axial rotation	Lateral bending
T1–T2	45°	Flat	++	+	+
T2–T16	Horizontal	Flat	+	+++	+++
T16–L6	Vertical	Concavity	+	+	+
L6–S1	Vertical	Small, flat	++++	+	+

Adapted from Townsend et al. [8] and Townsend and Leach [6].

Transverse Processes

The TPs exit the vertebrae at right angles to the direction of travel of the spinal cord and protrude out into the soft tissues of the back. Their function seems to be as lever arms to provide support to the vertebral column, and permit movement of the column via the muscles and ligaments that attach to them. Thus the TPs serve to maintain posture and permit rotation and lateral flexion. TPs alter in length at different sites within the vertebral column. In the cranial thoracic vertebral region the TPs are short and blunt in the thoracic region. In the lumbar region the TPs are markedly elongated and flattened horizontally. These TPs provide attachment sites for a number of muscles, including iliopsoas.

The TPs have articulations with a number of different osseous structures, again dependent on site. In the thoracic region the TPs articulate with the ribs at the costotransverse articulations. In the lumbar region the horse is unusual in that there are intertransverse synovial articulations between the TPs of the last two or three lumbar vertebrae and the lumbosacral articulation [6,9]. The latter articulation has the largest surface area, with more cranial articulations being smaller. These intertransverse articulations usually occur as paired structures at any given anatomical site; however, asymmetrical distributions of these articulations have been reported (9% [9] and 14% [2]). The number is not constant between horses and it has been suggested that the number of lumbar vertebrae dictates the number of intertransverse articulations (i.e. horses with six lumbar vertebrae have an extra articulation [10]). The genus *Equus* and the rhinoceroses are the only mammals with this particular anatomical feature.

In addition to intertransverse articulations found in all horses, intertransverse ankylosis has also been a relatively common finding [6,11], with Smythe [12] reporting its occurrence in 50% of horses. The relationship between intertransverse ankylosis and back pain has not been proved in the horse.

Lumbosacral Junction

The lumbosacral junction is the articulation between the last lumbar vertebra and the sacrum. As discussed above, in most individuals, the DSPs of the lumbar vertebrae point cranially, whereas the sacral DSPs point caudally, giving an 'open' lumbosacral space (i.e. a large gap between DSPs dorsal to the bony roof of the vertebral arch). In some cases a large open interspinous space is also noted between L5 and L6.

Sacrum

The sacrum of the horse is a triangular structure with slightly convex dorsal and concave ventral surfaces. In most horses it is made up of five vertebrae that become fused by the age of 5 years (Figure 2.9). The sacral vertebrae have two secondary centres of ossification, which can be visualised radiographically after birth: the cranial and caudal sacral internal physes. The cranial physis closes at 5.4 ± 1.5 years, the caudal one at 5.0 ± 1.5 years [2].

In the sacrum the spinal cord passes through the vertebral canal, which is formed from the fused vertebral arches. The spinal nerves exit the sacrum via dorsal and ventral sacral foramina – the sacral version of the thoracic and lumbar intervertebral foramina as discussed above. The sacral spinal nerves and the lumbar spinal nerves form the lumbosacral plexus.

Sacroiliac Joint

The vertebral column articulates with the pelvis at the bilateral sacroiliac joints (Chapter 15). It is at this site that the propulsive forces of the hindlimb are transferred to the vertebral column. The sacroiliac joint is actually a highly specialised point of contact, essentially between two flat bony surfaces. The point of contact is a synovial joint with unusual histological characteristics. Most

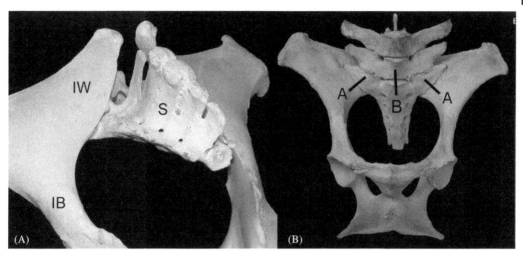

Figure 2.9 Photographs to show the sacroiliac region. (A) Caudocranial oblique view of a postmortem specimen of ilial wing (IW) and the sacrum (S). (B) A ventral view of the sacroiliac articulation, where (A) shows the wings of the sacrum, (B) the last lumbar vertebra. Note the flat articulation of the sacrum upon the ilial wing.

synovial joints in the body are formed between two hyaline cartilage surfaces; in the sacroiliac region the joint is formed between a hyaline cartilage surface (sacral surface) and a fibro-cartilage surface (ilial surface) [13].

Unlike other important synovial joints in the body the sacroiliac joint does not have the advantage of osseous contouring to aid the maintenance of joint integrity, as is found, for example, in ball-and-socket joints. Therefore, in order to provide biomechanical stability to the meeting of two flat surfaces, the horse uses three strong sacroiliac ligaments: the dorsal sacroiliac, ventral sacroiliac and interosseous sacral ligaments. These ligaments are discussed in detail later on in this chapter.

Articulations of the Vertebral Column

Haussler [10] points out that an often overlooked aspect of the vertebral column is the large number of articulations present. He considered that the vertebral column was unique because of the potential for the presence of two types of articulation at each vertebral segment: a synovial articulation between the articular processes and a fibro-cartilaginous articulation at the intervertebral disc. The exact number of articulations at each anatomical site varies (Table 2.3).

The Pelvis

The bony pelvis of the horse is made up of the os coxae, the sacrum and the first two or three coccygeal vertebrae. The os coxae has three parts – the ilium (*os ilii*), the ischium (*os ischii*) and the pubis (*os pubis*) – which meet at the acetabulum (i.e. the cavity into which the head of the femur fits and articulates) (see Figure 2.9). The three parts of the *os coxae* are present in the developing fetus but become fused by 1 year of age. The growth plate closure times of the pelvis are detailed in Table 2.4.

The Ilium

The ilium, the largest of the three bones, can be subdivided into different structural and functional areas (see Figure 2.9). The largest and widest part of the bone is the ilial wing, the

Table 2.3 The number of articulations at different anatomical regions of the spine.

Anatomical site	Number of articulations	Articular surfaces
Thoracic vertebrae	12	2 intervertebral discs 4 synovial intervertebral discs 4 costovertebral discs 2 costotransverse processes
Cranial lumbar vertebrae	6	2 intervertebral discs 4 synovial intervertebral discs
Caudal lumbar vertebrae	10	2 intervertebral discs 4 synovial intervertebral discs 4 synovial intertransverse processes
Sacral vertebrae	0	Fused; no articulations

most dorsal part of the ilium is the *tuber sacrale*, the most ventral and lateral part of the ilium is the *tuber coxae* and the most medial part is the ischiatic spine.

The ilial wing itself has two surfaces: the gluteal (outer) and the pelvic (inner) surfaces. The surface of the ilium has a number of modifications of structural importance. The gluteal line is found running from the *tuber coxae* to the middle of the medial border. The middle and deep gluteal muscles attach here. The ilium is also modified to allow the passage of important vessels and nerves to cross its surface. The iliolumbar artery crosses the lateral border of the ilium, the iliacofemoral artery also crosses the lateral border more ventrally, just above the psoas tubercle (site of attachment of *psoas minor*), and the sciatic nerve runs over the

medial surface of the bone at the greater sciatic notch.

The *tuber sacrale* is the highest point of the skeleton in most horses. At this point the ilial wing curves upwards and caudally and, at the summit, the *tuber sacrale* is roughened to provide the attachment for the dorsal sacro-iliac ligament.

The *tuber coxae* is the most lateral part of the pelvis and forms the 'point of the hip'. The *tuber coxae* is the elongated lateral angle of the pelvis, narrow in the middle of the angle and enlarged at either end.

The ischiatic spine is smooth medially and roughened laterally and is attached to the wing of the ilium by the ilial shaft. Medially there are grooves for the obturator vessels and nerve.

The Ischium

The ischium forms the caudal part of the ventral floor of the pelvis (Figure 2.9). When in situ it is approximately horizontal in the body and has two surfaces: the pelvic (interior) surface and the ventral (exterior) surface. The paired *tuber ischii* are the most caudal part of the ischium. These are triangular structures that are palpable either side of the tail.

The Pubis

The pubis forms the anterior part of the ventral floor of the bony pelvis (Figure 2.9).

Table 2.4 The growth plate closure times of the equine pelvis.

Anatomical site	Growth plate closure time (years)
Tuber sacrale	5.8 ± 1.2
Tuber coxae	5.8 ± 1.5
Ischial tuberosity	5.2 ± 1.4
Pubic symphysis	5.7 ± 1.4

Of note are the reported anatomical differences between the sexes in the anatomy of the pubis. In the stallion the pelvic surface (interior) is convex, whereas in the mare the pelvic surface is smooth and concave. Also the medial angle of the pubis (where the two pubic bones meet at the cranial end of the pubic symphysis) is much thinner in mares than it is in stallions.

Obturator Foramen

The obturator foramen is an oval hole in the pelvis, situated between the pubis and ischium, with its margin grooved for the obturator nerve and vessels.

Coccygeal Vertebrae

The number of coccygeal vertebrae ranges from 15 to 21. The first coccygeal vertebra is separate from the sacrum in most horses but can become fused to the sacrum in older horses.

The coccygeal vertebrae have a number of modifications compared with the thoracic and lumbar vertebrae. Notably both the cranial and caudal surfaces of the vertebral bodies are convex. The articulations between the bodies are therefore mediated via a thick intervertebral disc. The coccygeal vertebrae have TPs but these steadily decrease in size towards the last coccygeal vertebra. Other anatomical features of note are that the DSPs of the first two coccygeal vertebrae are bifid (as is occasionally seen in the sacrum) and that DSPs are essentially absent from the rest of the vertebrae. The coccygeal vertebrae have articular processes; small cranial APs with expanded extremities are usually found down to coccygeal Cy7 but caudal APs are usually absent.

The vertebral canal gradually peters out in the coccygeal region. From a point beyond Cy3–Cy6 the neural processes do not meet and the canal is merely an open groove, which itself stops at approximately Cy8. From Cy8 onwards the vertebrae are cylindrical with no vertebral arches.

2.2 Normal Anatomy of the Soft Tissue Structures of the Back

Jessica A. Kidd

Introduction

The soft tissue structures of the equine back are myriad. Put simply, the soft tissue structures can be grouped into their types, i.e. muscles, ligaments and other, miscellaneous, soft tissue structures (e.g. fascia). In order to provide a comprehensive reference point for these structures, the names, origins, insertions and functions of these structures are listed alphabetically in Table 2.5. Additional information about selected structures is discussed in the text below.

Musculature

There are numerous muscles in the equine thoracolumbar region, which can be classified according to a number of different schemes. The intrinsic back muscles attach only to the axial skeleton and originate from the vertebrae, ribs or fascia. One of the simplest classification schemes is, therefore, to divide the muscles into two groups, depending on where they are positioned relative to the transverse processes (TPs) of the vertebrae, i.e. into epaxial or hypaxial muscle groups. Epaxial muscles are those that are dorsal to the TPs whereas hypaxial muscles are ventral to the TPs (Figure 2.10). The epaxial muscles function to extend the spine but can also create lateral movement when contracted unilaterally. The hypaxial muscles function to flex the spine and can also induce lateral movements (Figures 2.11 to 2.13).

Epaxial Musculature

Within the epaxial muscle group, there are nine pairs of muscles in the thoracolumbar area. These pairs of muscles can be divided into three layers [3].

Table 2.5 Soft tissue structures of the back.

Structure	Other names	Latin/Greek origin/derivation	Function	Origin	Insertion
Muscles					
Iliacus	With psoas collectively called iliopsoas	Pertaining to region of the ilium; Latin *ilium* = flank and iliac bone. Originally, as small intestines are largely supported by this bone, and old term for small intestines was ilia (plural of ilium)	Stabilises vertebral column when hindlimb is fixed	Sacroiliac surface of ilium, wing of sacrum and psoas minor tendon	With psoas major on lesser trochanter of the femur
Iliocostalis thoracis	Iliocostal muscle, thoracic portion; longissimus costarum	From ilium (see iliacus) to ribs (costa/costae); middle English, from Latin *thorax*, breastplate, chest, from Greek	Stabilises thoracic vertebrae; extends spine; lateral flexion	Transverse processes of lumbar vertebrae, and fascial sheet which separates iliocostal muscles from longissimus. (Fascial sheet is also known as 'Bogorozky's tendon')	Caudal border of ribs 1–15; deeper tendinous insertions on cranial aspect of ribs 4–18 and to transverse process of C7
Iliocostalis lumborum		Latin *lumbus* = loin	Stabilises lumbar vertebrae and ribs; extends spine; lateral flexion	Iliac crest	Caudal border of rib 18 and transverse process of middle lumbar vertebrae
Interspinal	Interspinales		Supports ventroflexion	Spinous processes of caudal cervical, thoracic and L1–L3	Adjacent spinous processes
Intertransverse	Intertransversarii; intertransversales	Latin *transversus*, from past participle of *transvertere* = to turn across	Assists coordinated movement of vertebral column; stabilises vertebral column; lateral flexion if contracted unilaterally	Mamillary processes of lumbar and thoracic vertebrae	Transverse processes of lumbar and thoracic vertebrae
Latissimus dorsi		Latin *Latissimus* = superlative of *latus* meaning wide; *dorsi* = back	Suspends forelimbs from neck and trunk; retracts leg; draws trunk cranially when leg fixed	Thoracolumbar fascia and supraspinous ligament of thoracic and lumbar vertebrae	Medial aspect of the proximal humerus

Muscle	Synonyms/notes	Etymology	Action	Origin	Insertion
Longissimus thoracis and lumborum	Longissimus dorsi; erector spinae muscles	Latin *Longissimus* = superlative form of *longus*; "the longest"	Extends and stabilises thoracic and lumbar spine; supports rider and saddle; lateral flexion when not contracted bilaterally; controls stiffness of back at the walk	Spinous processes of the sacral, lumbar and thoracic vertebrae; ventral ilium; thoracolumbar fascia	Articular, mamillary and transverse processes of thoracic vertebrae and proximal ribs
Multifidus	Part of transversospinalis group; multifidus is transversospinalis group in thoracolumbar region; multifidus dorsi; juxtavertebral muscle; multifidous	Latin = many	Extends spine; stabilises and rotates vertebral column; proprioception of spine; coordination of long muscles	Numerous overlapping segments; lateral sacrum, lumbar articular processes and thoracic transverse processes	Spinous process of preceding vertebrae from C7 to S2
Omotransversarius		Greek *omo* = shoulder	Suspends forelimbs from neck and thorax	Shoulder fascia	Transverse processes of C2–C4
Psoas major	With iliacus collectively called iliopsoas	Greek *psoas* = muscle of loin; *major*, comparative of *magnus* = great	Flexes hip joint; if hindlimb is fixed, flexes lower back at sacroiliac articulations	Ventral vertebrae of T16–T18, transverse processes of L1–L6	With iliacus on lesser trochanter of femur
Psoas minor	With iliacus collectively called iliopsoas	Late Latin *minor* = lesser	Flexes hip joint; if hindlimb is fixed, flexes lower back at sacroiliac articulations	Ventral vertebrae of T16–L6	Pelvic inlet on psoas minor tubercle of ilium
Quadratus lumborum		Latin *quadratus* = a square in shape. Latin *lumbus* = the loin	Weak stabiliser of lumbar vertebrae	Proximoventral surface of ribs 17 and 18 and lumbar transverse processes	Ventral sacrum and sacroiliac ligaments
Rectus abdominis		Latin *rectus* = straight	Flexes thoracolumbar spine	Lateral costal cartilages T4–T9	Prepubic tendon and head of femur via accessory ligament
Rhomboideus		Greek *rhombus* = lozenge, *eidos* = resemblance	Draws scapula dorsally and cranially, elevates neck; suspends forelimbs from neck and thorax	Spinous processes of T2–T7 via dorsoscapular ligament	Medial surface of scapular cartilage
Serratus dorsalis cranialis	Serratus dorsalis anterior		Used in inspiration; encases iliocostalis	Thoracolumbar fascia and dorsoscapular ligament	Lateral surface of rib 5 or 6 to rib 11 or 12

(continued)

Table 2.5 (*Continued*)

Structure	Other names	Latin/Greek origin/derivation	Function	Origin	Insertion
Serratus dorsalis caudalis	Serratus dorsalis posterior		Used in expiration; encases iliocostalis	Thoracolumbar fascia	Lateral surface of ribs 11 or 12–18
Serratus ventralis	Serrate muscle; serrate face is another name for medial scapula	Latin *serratus* = notched from *serra* = saw	Suspends neck and thorax from forelimbs	First seven ribs	Medial scapula
Spinal	Spinalis thoracis		Extends and fixes spine	Spinous processes of lumbar and last six thoracic vertebrae	Spinous process of T1–T6/7 and C3–C7
Transverse spinal muscles	Transversospinales			Spinous process	Transverse process of adjacent vertebra
Trapezius		Latin, from Greek *trapeza* = table because of shape formed by muscles	Suspends forelimbs from neck and thorax; elevates scapula	Supraspinous ligament of T3–T10	Dorsal portion of spine of scapula
Ligaments		Latin *ligamentum* = ligament; from *ligare* = to bind			
Costotransverse ligament			Stabilises thoracic vertebrae and ribs	Ribs	Transverse processes
Costovertebral ligament			Stabilises thoracic vertebrae and ribs	Ribs	Vertebral body
Dorsal longitudinal ligament	Ligamentum longitudinale dorsales		Supports intervertebral discs; vertebral stability	Spans length of vertebral column along floor of vertebral canal	
Interspinous ligament	Ligamenta interspinalis		Stabilises spinous processes; prevents vertebrae sliding dorsally	Spinous process	Adjacent spinous process
Intertransverse ligament	Ligamenta intertransversaria		Limits lateral flexibility and rotation	Lumbar transverse processes	Transverse process of adjacent vertebra
Ligamentum flavum	Interarcuate ligaments	Latin = yellow ligament	Supports weight of trunk	Fills interarcuate spaces	

Nuchal ligament (laminar portion)	Lamina nuchae	Latin *nucha* = the back of the neck	Supports weight of trunk	Dorsal portion of nuchal ligament and spinous processes of T2 and T3	C2–C7
Short spinal ligament			Runs between individual vertebrae to protect the spinal cord	Vertebra	Adjacent vertebra
Supraspinous ligament			Stability of thoracolumbar vertebrae	Caudal continuation of nuchal ligament; in caudal thoracic region it fuses with lumbodorsal fascia and tendinous insertions of latissimus dorsi	With lumbodorsal fascia and tendinous insertions of latissimus dorsi, attaches to periosteum of caudal thoracic and lumbar vertebrae and interspinous ligament
Ventral longitudinal ligament	Ligamentum longitudinale ventralis		Vertebral stability	Spans length of vertebral column on ventral aspect of vertebrae	
Fascia and other soft tissue structures					
Supraspinous bursa	Supraspinal subligamentous bursa		Cushions nuchal ligament as it passes over tallest thoracic spinous process		
Thoracolumbar fascia	Lumbar dorsal fascia		Attachment site for multiple muscles	Attaches to thoracolumbar spinous processes	Also attaches to cranial ilial wing
Dorsoscapular ligament			Limits dorsal movement of scapula; shock absorber for shoulder region	Part of the thoracolumbar fascia; supraspinous ligament over the highest spines of the withers	Deep surface of rhomboideus muscle. Many branches that insert on deep scapula alternating with branches of serratus ventralis

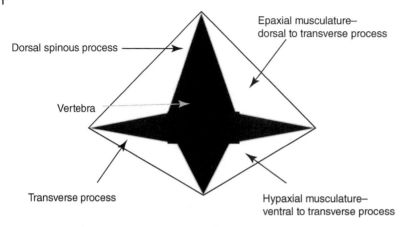

Epaxial musculature–
dorsal to transverse process

Dorsal spinous process

Vertebra

Transverse process

Hypaxial musculature–
ventral to transverse process

Figure 2.10 Schematic cross-section through the spine at the level of T12 to show relative positions of epaxial and hypaxial musculature.

First Layer

- *Trapezius thoracalis*
- *Latissimus dorsi.*

These two muscles are extremely superficial. *Trapezius thoracalis* originates from the supraspinous ligament between T3 and T7 and inserts on the scapular spine. Running

just under the skin and fascia, *trapezius thoracalis* acts to elevate the shoulder. *Latissimus dorsi*, so called because it is the widest muscle of the back, has a broad origin in the

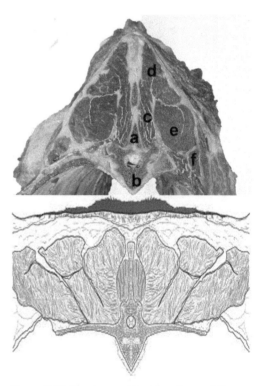

Figure 2.11 The cross-sectional anatomy of thoracic vertebra 1. A postmortem section B line diagram: A = dorsal spinous process, b = vertebral body, c = *longissimus dorsi*, d = *longissimus dorsi (spinalis)*, e = *multifidus*, f = *ilio costarum*. (For a colour version of this figure, see the colour plate section.)

Figure 2.12 The cross-sectional anatomy of thoracic vertebra 7. A postmortem section B line diagram: a = dorsal spinous process, b = vertebral body, c = *multifidus*, d = *longissimus dorsi (spinalis)*, e = *longissimus dorsi*, f = *ilio costalis*. (For a colour version of this figure, see the colour plate section.)

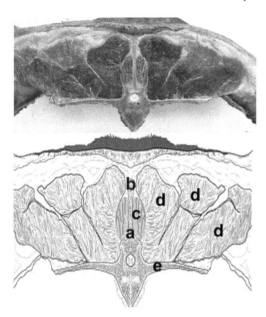

Figure 2.13 The cross-sectional anatomy of lumbar vertebra 2. A postmortem section B line diagram: a = dorsal spinous process, b = supraspinous ligament, c = *multifidus*, d = *longissimus dorsi*, e = transverse process. (*For a colour version of this figure, see the colour plate section.*)

thoracolumbar fascia and from the ribs. Caudally it tapers into the lumbar region. It inserts on to the tendon of *teres major* and other related cervical muscles, and functions to aid neck extension via its cervical attachments.

Second Layer

- *Rhomboideus thoracalis*
- *Serratus dorsalis anterior*
- *Serratus dorsalis posterior.*

These three muscles form the next layer of the back. *Rhomboideus thoracalis* originates from the dorsal spinous processes (DSPs) between T2 and T7 and inserts on the medial aspect of the cartilage of the scapula. Similar to *trapezius thoracalis*, *rhomboideus thoracalis* acts on the scapula; in this instance it draws the scapula upwards and forwards. *Serratus dorsalis anterior* and *posterior* are thin muscles that lie under *rhomboideus, serratus ventralis* and *latissimus dorsi*. The *serratus dorsalis* muscles originate from the lumbodorsal fascia and dorsoscapular ligament and insert on the

ribs. *Serratus dorsalis* anterior inserts from ribs 5–6 to 11–12, functioning to draw the ribs forwards and outwards as an aid to the inspiratory phase of respiration. In contrast, *serratus dorsalis posterior* inserts on the last seven or eight ribs and functions to draw these ribs backwards, assisting expiration.

Third Layer

- *Longissimus costarum (iliocostalis)*
- *Longissimus dorsi*
- *Multifidus dorsi*
- *Intertransversales lumborum.*

The *longissimus costarum* muscle (or *iliocostalis* as it is commonly known) is a long thin muscle consisting of a series of overlapping segments or fascicles. This muscle is the most lateral of the large group of epaxial muscles made up of the *longissimus costarum* and *dorsi* muscles and the *spinalis* muscles. *Longissimus costarum* is the flattest muscle in the back and originates from the deep layer of the lumbodorsal fascia back to L3–L4 and the anterior borders of the last 15 ribs. Each segment spans several vertebrae with the muscle fibres oriented cranioventrally. The muscle lies next to *longissimus dorsi*, dorsal to the angle of the ribs. The short lumbar portion of *longissimus costarum* is not distinct but instead fuses with the lumbar portion of *longissimus dorsi*. *Longissimus costarum* inserts on the posterior border of the ribs and the TPs of the last cervical vertebrae. Its action, when contracting bilaterally, is to assist in expiration by depressing and retracting the ribs. However, when *longissimus costarum* contracts unilaterally, it has been proposed that it may participate in lateral movement of the spine.

Longissimus dorsi is the largest and longest muscle in the body, running from the sacrum and ilium in the pelvis to C7. It is the major muscle of the back, arranged segmentally with multiple individual attachments. *Longissimus dorsi* fills the space between the TPs and DSPs of the vertebrae. It is thickest in the lumbar region where it is covered in thoracolumbar fascia, and narrows in the thoracic region. It originates from the ilium, DSPs of S1–S3, DSPs of the lumbar and thoracic vertebrae, and the supraspinous ligament. It inserts on the TPs and articular processes of the lumbar vertebrae, TPs of the thoracic vertebrae, TPs and DSPs of C4–C7, and lateral surfaces of the ribs (except the first rib). The *spinalis* muscles sit dorsomedially on the *longissimus dorsi* muscles and are adjacent to the dorsal aspect of the spinous processes. In most diagrammatic representations and text, they are considered to be part of *longissimus dorsi* and they certainly function as such.

Longissimus dorsi is the main extensor of the back and loins of the horse. In addition, via its costal attachments, it helps in expiration. As with *longissimus costarum*, unilateral contraction may assist in lateral movement of the spine. *Longissimus dorsi* also raises the hindlimbs for bucking and the forelimbs for rearing. It has its greatest extension during the swing phase of the hindlimb stride and is used to transmit energy from the hindlimbs to the back during this phase. In well-muscled horses, this muscle can extend above the tops of the dorsal spinous processes; this results in a groove running down the midline of the back.

Multifidus dorsi is the most medial epaxial muscle and is located adjacent to the DSPs. *Multifidus dorsi* is part of the transversospinalis group; in the thoracolumbar region it is the entirety of this group. It is made up of numerous overlapping segments that extend from the lumbar to the cervical regions. *Multifidus dorsi* originates from the lateral part of the sacrum, articular processes of the lumbar vertebrae and TPs of the thoracic vertebrae, and inserts on the DSPs of S1 and S2, lumbar and thoracic vertebrae and C7. The action of *multifidus dorsi* is to extend the back – acting unilaterally it flexes the spine laterally.

The *intertransversales lumborum* muscles are thin, muscular and tendinous structures that occupy the TPs of L1–L5. They therefore originate and insert on the TPs and function to assist the flexion of the loins laterally or, conversely, to hold the region in a fixed posture.

The muscles described above complement the long muscles of the back. There are numerous short muscles that are responsible for fine movement of segments of the back, as well as proprioception and proprioceptive correction. It is worth noting that opinion is divided over the presence of the intertransverse muscles in the thoracic and lumbar spine: some anatomists state that the intertransverse muscles are present in the thoracic and lumbar spine, whereas other texts state that the intertransverse muscles occur only in the cervical and tail regions. They are included in Table 2.5 for completeness and not as any definitive statement of their existence.

Hypaxial Musculature

- *Psoas major*
- *Psoas minor*
- *Iliacus*
- *Quadratus lumborum.*

Psoas major originates from the ventral surface of the TPs of the lumbar vertebrae and the last two ribs. It inserts on the trochanter minor of the femur and functions to flex the hip joint and rotate the proximal hindlimb outwards. *Psoas minor* originates from the bodies of T15–T18, L1 to L4–L5 and the vertebral ends of ribs 16–17. It inserts on the *psoas* tubercle of the ilium in the pelvis and acts to flex the pelvis relative to the loins and move it laterally if contracted unilaterally. *Iliacus* originates from the ventral surface of the ilium lateral to the iliopectineal line, the ventral sacroiliac ligament, the wing of the sacrum and the tendon of psoas minor. It inserts, with *psoas major*, on the trochanter minor of the femur and acts similarly to flex the hip joint and rotate the proximal hindlimb outwards. Finally, in this group, *quadratus lumborum* originates from the last two ribs and the TPs of the lumbar vertebrae, and inserts on the ventral surface of the sacrum and the ventral sacroiliac ligament. The action of *quadratus lumborum* is to hold the last two ribs fixed and, acting unilaterally, to produce lateral flexion of the loins.

Ligaments

The ligamentous structures of the thoraco-lumbar region of the equine back can be divided into long and short ligaments.

Long Ligaments

- *Supraspinous ligament*
- *Dorsal longitudinal ligament*
- *Ventral longitudinal ligament.*

The supraspinous ligament (SSL) is the thoracolumbar continuation of the nuchal ligament of the neck. Compared with the nuchal ligament, the SSL is much narrower. The reason for this decrease in thickness and hence strength has been hypothesised to be because, unlike the nuchal ligament, the SSL does not function to support the head and, therefore, does not need to be as strong as the nuchal ligament. The laminar ligament, or sheet-like portion of the nuchal ligament, runs from the cervical region and attaches to the dorsal processes of C2 to T2–T3.

The function of the SSL is to stabilise the thoracolumbar vertebrae and their associated spinous processes. Its dimensions alter as they pass through the body: the SSL is wider and has more elastic properties in the cranial and mid-thoracic spine than in the rest of the thoracolumbar spine; it is also stronger in the cranial thoracic portion. In the caudal thoracic region, the SSL fuses with the lumbodorsal fascia (see below) and the tendinous insertions of *latissimus dorsi*. Collectively these insert on the periosteum of the proximal spinous processes of the caudal thoracic and lumbar vertebrae and the interspinous ligament. The lumbar portion of the SSL is thicker and denser than the thoracic portion and is absent between the last lumbar and the first sacral vertebrae.

The dorsal longitudinal ligament runs along the floor of the vertebral canal from C2 to the sacrum and attaches to each intervertebral disc, whereas the ventral longitudinal ligament runs along the ventral aspect of the vertebrae to the sacrum and also attaches to each intervertebral disc.

Short Ligaments

- *Interspinous ligament*
- *Ligamentum flavum*
- *Costovertebral ligament*
- *Costotransverse ligament.*

Multiple short ligaments make up a complex mechanism for stabilisation of the thoracolumbar vertebrae. The interspinous ligament (ISL) runs between adjacent DSPs and dorsally fuses with the SSL whereas its ventral fibres attach to the ligamentum flavum. The ISL, similar to the SSL, also stabilises the thoracolumbar vertebrae and their DSPs and is elastic in the thoracic spine. The *ligamentum flavum* sits in the spaces between the vertebral laminae. It is primarily elastic, which ensures that, when the spine is completely extended, it does not impinge on the dorsal aspect of the vertebral canal. Finally, the costovertebral ligaments attach vertebral bodies to ribs whereas the costotransverse ligaments attach TPs to ribs; both function to stabilise the thoracic vertebrae and ribs. The intertransverse ligaments are only in the lumbar region and link adjacent TPs to limit lateral flexibility.

Miscellaneous Soft Tissue Structures

- *Supraspinous bursa*
- *Thoracolumbar fascia*
- *Dorsoscapular ligament.*

The supraspinous bursa is always present in horses and is situated between the SSL and the highest DSP of the withers, usually T6. Other bursae are sporadically recorded in this region on the summits of the DSPs.

The thoracolumbar fascia (TLF) is a part of the deep fascia of the trunk and has a number of components. It is the attachment site for many muscles and courses between the thoracolumbar DSPs and the cranial aspect of the ilial wing. Part of the TLF forms an aponeurosis with *latissimus dorsi* and the caudal portion of *serratus dorsalis caudalis*. Caudally it becomes the gluteal fascia and cranioventrally it merges with the axillary fascia.

Cranially it also becomes the *spinocostotransversal fascia* in the shoulder region, where it forms three layers. The superficial layer attaches to *serratus ventralis*. The middle layer surrounds and separates *longissimus dorsi* and *longissimus costarum*.

The dorsoscapular ligament, part of the TLF, originates in the SSL over the highest DSP of the withers, at which point it is mostly fibrous. It courses ventrally deep to *rhomboideus thoracalis*, attaching to the deep surface of this muscle, at which point it is mainly elastic. It has multiple branches that interdigitate with portions of *serratus ventralis* and insert on the medial aspect of the scapula. It functions as a shock absorber for the shoulder as well as restricting the range of dorsal movement of the scapula. Finally, the superficial fascia of the trunk includes the cutaneous trunci muscle and fans into the TLF and attaches to the DSPs.

2.3 Normal Anatomy of the Soft Tissue Structures of the Pelvis

David Bainbridge

Introduction

Over hundreds of millions of years, the pelvis of land vertebrates has evolved in concert with nearby structures to perform a variety of functions. The pelvis/sacrum/cranial tail complex is the musculoskeletal unit which:

- Transfers supportive and propulsive forces from the hindlimb to the trunk
- Is itself a portion of the spinal column
- Serves as the point of attachment of many spinal, abdominal and hindlimb muscles
- Contains within it major components of the alimentary, urinary, reproductive, vascular, lymphatic and nervous systems.

While conforming to the basic mammalian plan, the equine pelvis shows specialisations for the natural way of life of the species. The horse is thought to have evolved to survive on pasture of an unpredictable and frequently extremely low quality, leading to a large abdominal mass, which has in turn meant that the soft tissues of the pelvis have become extremely strong and fibrous to support the weight. Some other adaptations are often termed 'cursorial specialisations', although they probably reflect a need to walk and graze efficiently for long periods, interspersed with only occasional bursts of speed to evade predators; for example, hindlimb movement is more restricted to the sagittal plane in horses than in any other major domestic species. Also, the hindlimb muscle mass is unusually concentrated at the proximal end in horses to reduce the moment of inertia of the swinging limb – by loss of distal muscle mass and the proximal 'creep' of muscle origins [14]. Presumably also related to the need to escape predators is the fact that the equine birth process is relatively rapid; to allow this the birth canal is wide and straight compared with that of some other large ungulates.

In this chapter the non-osseous locomotor structures of the pelvis are reviewed [3,15–17]. The author has divided them into three groups:

1) The sacroiliac joint: the main route of transfer of compressive forces from hindlimb to trunk is considered, along with other structures that support its function.
2) The diverse structures that form the dorsolateral and caudal walls of the pelvic cavity – limb muscles, ligaments, the pelvic diaphragm, and the structures of the anal and perineal regions.
3) The complex network of thick connective tissue that strengthens the ventral aspect of the pelvis.

Sacroiliac Joint

The sacroiliac joint is essentially a synovial joint, although the synovial component is considerably augmented by additional connective tissue. The nomenclature of some structures can vary confusingly between written sources [18].

The synovial joint is formed between the roughened articular surfaces of the medial ilium and the modified transverse processes, or wing, of the sacrum. The equine iliac wing runs obliquely between its two distinct prominences, the ventrolateral *tuber coxae* and the dorsomedial *tuber sacrale*. The joint is formed closer to the latter prominence and the joint space is angled at approximately 30° to the horizontal. The irregularities of the bony facets on the sacrum and ilium are complementary and both surfaces are lined with a thin layer of articular cartilage. In life the articular surfaces are separated by a narrow cleft filled with fluid secreted by the encircling synovial membrane. The joint is surrounded by a tight fibrous capsule, but much of the strength of the joint itself is conferred by strong bands of connecting tissue that span the joint space [19].

The synovial joint is surrounded by the strong ventral sacroiliac ligament (Figure 2.14), a series of fibres radiating from around the articular circumference of the sacrum to insert on the ventromedial aspects of the *tuber sacrale* and iliac wing. The ligament is strongest dorsally and serves to reduce rotational and sliding movements of the joint.

Even more substantial is the dorsal sacroiliac ligament, which consists of two dissimilar parts (Figure 2.15). The first is the cord-like 'funicular' portion, which passes in a caudocranial direction from the neural spines of the sacral vertebrae to the tuber sacrale. The relationship of this portion to the adjacent lumbodorsal fascia (or thoracolumbar fascia) can differ between individual horses – being lateral in some and ventral in others. The second part of the ligament is the 'membranous part', a triangular sheet fanning out ventrocaudally from the lateral sacrum (and medial tuber sacrale) to blend with the lateral surface of the sacrosciatic ligament (discussed later). This second portion is also occasionally called the 'lateral sacroiliac ligament'.

The movements of the joint are dramatically restricted by this ligament support and it is assumed that it undergoes only small sliding (planar), pivoting (trochoid) and impact-absorbing movements. These movements are so small as to be almost impossible to measure *in vivo*, although *in vivo* a tiny pivoting movement of $0.8 \pm 0.5°$ has been reported, which occurs alongside a much larger movement at the lumbosacral joint [20,21].

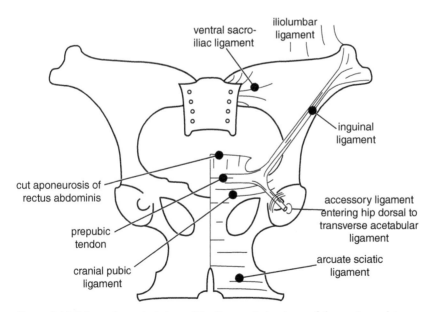

Figure 2.14 Schematic ventral view of the ligament structures of the equine pelvis.

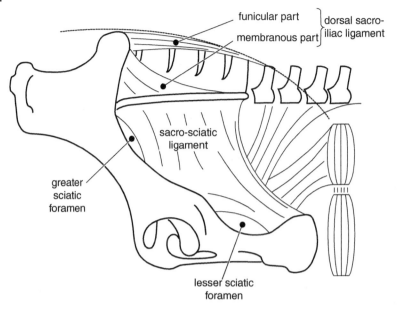

Figure 2.15 Schematic lateral view of the ligament structures of the equine pelvis.

An additional degree of stabilisation is conferred by the iliolumbar ligament (see Figure 2.14). This sheet of thick connective tissue is a lateral extension of the intertransverse ligament, which lies between all the lumbar vertebrae. These broad triangular ligaments widen caudally until they insert on the wing of the ilium, ventral to the origin of the *longissimus* musculature. Thus, they indirectly bridge the junction between the pelvis and vertebral column and resist extreme tension on either side of that junction – possibly as an adaptation to rearing.

The Dorsolateral and Caudal Walls

With the exception of the necks and wings of the *ilia* and the cranial tail, the pelvic cavity is not bounded dorsolaterally or caudally by bone. Instead, a variety of soft tissue structures perform this role, including the pelvic diaphragm and perineal structures. There are considerable differences between their configuration in the horse and that in other domestic species. To complicate matters further, human anatomical terminology is often

unhelpful here – horses do not have a muscular 'pelvic floor'; they have a 'coccygeus' muscle but no coccyx and their '*levator ani*' muscle does not 'lift the anus'. The relevant structures are described in order from superficial to deep [22].

This area is covered by thick fasciae. The *gluteal fasciae* are the caudal continuation of the lumbodorsal fascia and cover the prominent buttock region of the horse. The main points of attachment of the fasciae are the *tubera sacrale* and *coxae*, the neural spines of the sacral vertebrae and the sacrosciatic ligaments. Their function is thought to be to provide general mechanical support to the region and to constrain the movements of underlying muscles within 'fascial tunnels'. Thus, the gluteal fasciae send off a series of intermuscular septa between the *middle gluteal, biceps femoris, semitendinosus* and *semimembranosus* muscles. Although in the most part separated from the true 'pelvic diaphragm' by the muscles of the hip region, these fasciae are important in allowing those muscles to maintain tone that supports the soft tissue boundaries of the pelvic cavity. From the *gluteal fasciae* and dorsal sacroiliac

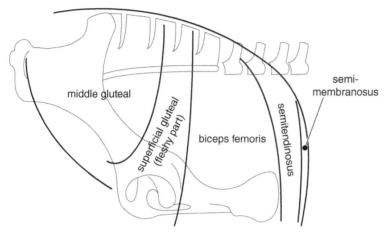

Figure 2.16 Schematic lateral view of the outlines of the rump muscles covering the equine pelvic region.

ligament arise the tail fasciae, which, although simply surrounding the cranial tail muscula-ture, are tightly adherent caudal to the anus [2].

Several skeletal muscles (Figure 2.16) are important in indirectly maintaining the integrity of the walls of the pelvis, by exerting pressure on the ligamentar sheets deep to them. However, they can also confound veter-inary attempts to image the structures beneath. The important muscles include the following:

- The middle gluteal muscle is extensive in the horse and supports much of the cranial part of the underlying sacrosciatic ligament. Its origin on the concavity of the lateral iliac wing is supplemented by attachments on the gluteal fasciae, the lateral surfaces of the sacrosciatic and sacroiliac ligaments, and via an aponeurosis as far cranially as the first lumbar vertebra. The relative enlargement of this muscle has also been proposed to be an adaptation for rearing.
- The equine superficial gluteal muscle orig-inates more proximally that that of other domestic species, from the gluteal fasciae and the *tuber coxae*. It effectively fills a shallow depression between the middle glu-teal and *biceps femoris* muscles.
- *Biceps femoris* has additional proximal ori-gins, or 'long heads', which lie caudal to the middle gluteal muscle. As well as its origin on the sciatic tuberosity, it has attachments on the gluteal and tail fasciae and the

sacrosciatic and sacroiliac ligaments. Thus, it covers the lateral aspect of the middle region of the sacrosciatic ligament in this species.

- The equine *semitendinosus* muscle also sup-plements its attachments with more proxi-mal origins on the transverse processes of the first two caudal vertebrae and the tail fasciae. Thus, this muscle, readily delineated in the standing animal, completes the triad that confers additional lateral support on the dorsolateral pelvic wall.
- The *semimembranosus* muscle is more on the caudal aspect of the limb, but it too has extensive proximal origins, in this case on the caudal sacrosciatic ligament. Its origins, and its bulk in horses, mean that the left and right *semimembranosus* muscles bulge towards each other on either side of the anus, covering the sciatic tuberosities and ischiorectal fossae in a way that is quite unlike the arrangement in carnivores and ruminants.
- A final muscle that deserves brief mention is *sacrocaudalis ventralis*, the most ventral muscle of the tail which, covered by the tail fasciae, forms the dorsal boundary of the caudal pelvic cavity.

Deep to the rump and thigh muscles lies the sacrosciatic ligament (Figure 2.15), also known as the sacrotuberous ligament. The development of this ligament appears to be related to absolute species body size – small species lack it. In dogs it is a taut cord passing from the sacrum to the sciatic tuberosity; in horses and cattle it is very extensive. The dorsal attachment of the equine sacrosciatic ligament runs along the lateral aspect of the sacrum and the transverse processes of the first two caudal vertebrae, where it blends with the fibres of the membranous part of the dorsal sacroiliac ligament. From here the sheet-like ligament courses caudoventrolaterally to attach along the dorsal edge of the iliac neck and ischium. The free caudal edge of the ligament is strengthened by a strong 'funicular' component, which inserts on the dorsal aspect of the sciatic tuberosity and is further supported by the long head of semimembranosus. Thus, the left and right sacrosciatic ligaments may be compared with a tent over the pelvic cavity, suspended from the 'ridge pole' of the sacral and caudal vertebrae, and 'tethered down' ventrally to the pelvis. Each ligament is fenestrated at two points: the greater sciatic foramen lies in the dorsocaudal concavity of the iliac neck and allows passage of the sciatic nerve; the lesser sciatic foramen lies caudal to the sciatic spine and permits passage of the internal obturator muscle. The tautness of the sacrosciatic ligaments (and indeed the sacroiliac ligaments) is under hormonal control – they become laxer before birth, although this is less clinically evident in horses than cattle due to the presence of thick overlying muscles.

The caudal part of the sacrosciatic ligament overlies the pelvic diaphragm (the internal surface of the cranial part is lined only by peritoneum). Important features of this region include the following:

- Interposed between the ligament and the diaphragm, and bounded ventrally by the ischium, is a fat-filled space called the ischiorectal fossa, although in this species this cannot be palpated lateral to the anus because it is overlain by *semimembranosus*.
- The coccygeus muscle is the only convincing 'diaphragm' muscle in the horse, resembling another 'ridge tent' nestling inside the

caudal part of the larger, fibrous sacrosciatic ligaments. It originates on the caudoventral part of the internal surface of that ligament, and its fibres course caudodorsomedially to insert via two leaves of tendon on the first four tail vertebrae and the tail fasciae. Thus, the muscle serves to enclose the caudal parts of the pelvic viscera and to flex the tail.

- Whereas *levator ani* of the carnivores inserts primarily on the tail and supplements the action of coccygeus, the same muscle in the horse inserts mainly on the circumference of the external anal sphincter in a complex manner. It originates on the sciatic spine and nearby regions of the sacrosciatic ligament. Thus, it does not provide such complete enclosure for the pelvic contents and acts mainly to resist eversion and prolapse of the anus.

The caudal wall of the pelvis (Figure 2.17) is bounded by a series of structures related to the termination of the gastrointestinal and reproductive tracts. The anus and the vulva or bulb of the penis are suspended from the tail in the pelvic outlet. They are bounded dorsolaterally by the free edges of the sacrosciatic ligament and the pelvic diaphragm. In horses, considerable lateral support is also given by *semimembranosus*. In mares, the *rima vulvae* often hangs ventrally so that much of it is ventral to the sciatic arch of the pelvis; indeed, it is considered good conformation for it to do so, because it may reduce the incidence of ascending genital infections. The following are the structures that make up the caudal wall of the pelvis:

- The anal sphincters are suspended from the caudal fascia dorsally and themselves suspend from the perineal fascia ventrally. The striated external sphincter blends with the fibres of *levator ani*, retractor muscles (see below) and especially the *constrictor vulvae* of the female. The smaller, smooth muscle, internal sphincter lies cranial to the external sphincter and represents a terminal thickening of the wall of the rectum. Further cranially lies *rectococcygeus*, a band of rectal smooth

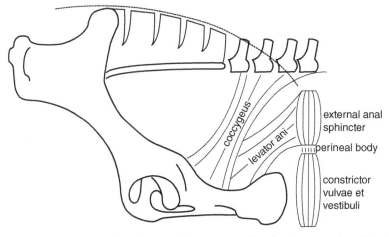

Figure 2.17 Schematic lateral view of the equine pelvic diaphragm and caudal pelvic region.

muscle that extends to the ventral surfaces of the fourth and fifth caudal vertebrae, thus suspending the rectum from the vertebral column.

- The *constrictores vulvae* and *vestibuli* are well-developed oval rings of muscle that act to constrict the respective portions of the female urogenital opening. The more caudal of the two, the *constrictor vulvae*, blends its fibres extensively with those of the external anal sphincter. The *constrictor vestibuli* is intermixed with the fibres of the retractor muscle.
- The *retractor penis/clitoridis muscles* course ventrally from the caudal vertebrae, run deep to the *levator ani* and fuse in the midline ventral to the anus. Further fibres continue ventrally to insert on the penis or to blend with the fibres of the constrictor muscles of the female.
- The perineal body is a fibrous and muscular node between the anus and vulva or bulb of the penis. It contains a complex arrangement of connective tissue and intermixed strands of all the striated muscles mentioned above. It is of clinical relevance due to its importance in the conformation of mares and its propensity for laceration during dystocia.

The innermost layer of the pelvic wall is the thick pelvic fascia, which lines the inner surface of the above structures. Cranially, in the pelvic cavity, this is supplemented by the peritoneal reflections, which protrude into the pelvis from the abdominal cavity.

The Ventral Fibrous Structures

The major components of the ventral boundary of the pelvis are, of course, the *pubes* and *ischia*. In foals these bones are fused in the midline by a symphysis, although this ossifies relatively rapidly in horses, with the cranial part mineralising first. Once a synostosis has formed, what little movement existed at the joint is lost. The bony floor of the pelvis is augmented by a series of interconnected fibrous structures both dorsally and ventrally, although it is the ventral structures that predominate. Some of these have other functions unrelated to the integrity of the pelvis, but all are now considered, in a cranial-to-caudal order (Figure 12.14).

The inguinal ligament is the free caudal margin of the external abdominal oblique muscle, which is largely tendinous in this region. It runs caudoventromedially from the *tuber coxae* to the iliopubic eminence where it blends with the prepubic tendon. The ligament spans the cranioventral concavity of the neck of the ilium and thus bounds a D-shaped opening, the femoral canal, which conveys the femoral artery, vein and nerve, iliopsoas and the deep inguinal lymph nodes.

The prepubic tendon is a complex structure, especially in the large ungulates [23]. Although often described rather like a ligament running between the right and left iliopubic eminences, it actually represents the blended tendons of *rectus abdominis, pectinei, graciles*, and even the *external* and *internal abdominal oblique* muscles, via its connection with the inguinal ligament. Cranially, it is also continuous with *tunica flava* and *linea alba* of the abdomen. Its caudal relations are also complex; it blends into the pelvic symphysis, gives rise to the accessory ligaments of the hip and is really the most cranial part of the extensive sheet of fibrous material that covers the ventral aspect of the pelvis. Thus, the prepubic tendon of the horse is one of the most important nexuses of connective tissue in the entire body.

Among the major domestic species, the accessory ligament of the hip is unique to equids. Arising from the caudal aspect of the prepubic tendon, this ligament runs caudolaterally to enter the hip joint via the ventral notch in the acetabulum. To do this, it passes dorsal ('deep') to the transverse acetabular ligament to insert on the fovea of the head of the femur. The accessory ligaments reduce the ability of horses to abduct their hips, presumably to minimise inefficient mediolateral movements of the hindlimb. Some abduction is still allowed, however, partly because the ligaments insert close to the point of rotation of the hip joints, rendering them less effective than

might be expected. There is some evidence that the accessory ligament may represent a bizarre additional head of the contralateral pectineus muscle.

Caudal to the prepubic tendon, the ventral connective tissue is profuse and strong and occasionally denoted by specific terms:

- The taut transverse band ventral to the pubes is the cranial pubic ligament.
- The curved fibres running along the sciatic arch at the caudal-most part of the bony pelvic floor are the arcuate sciatic ligament.
- These ventral structures are continuous with, and support, the mammary fascia.
- The obturator foramen is almost entirely closed by the obturator membrane although in life this is covered by the laterally directed fibres of the internal obturator (dorsally) and external obturator (ventrally) muscles. A small hole in the cranial membrane permits passage of the obturator nerve. Unlike some ungulates, horses do not have an obvious bony notch through which this nerve passes.

In conclusion, it can be seen that the soft tissues of the equine pelvis are a heterogeneous collection of structures with a variety of functions. Some are dedicated to supporting the structure of the pelvis or sacroiliac joints, whereas others have more varied functions to enclose the pelvic viscera, move the tail, hindlimb or abdomen, or constrain the movement of those parts of the body. Also, the equine pelvis can be seen to exhibit specialisations related to the equine way of life – high body mass, continual walking and grazing, and a speedy birth process.

References

1 Jeffcott, L.B. and Dalin, G. Natural rigidity of the horse's backbone. *Equine Veterinary Journal* 1980; **12**:101–108.

2 Haussler, K.K., Stover, S.M. and Willits, N.H. Developmental variation in lumbosacropelvic anatomy of Thoroughbred racehorses. *American Journal of Veterinary Research* 1997; **58**:1083–1087.

3 Getty, R. (ed.) *Sisson and Grossman's The Anatomy of Domestic Animals*, 5th edn. Philadelphia, PA: *W. B.* Saunders, 1975.

4 Dyce, K.M., Sack, W.O. and Wensing, C.J.G. *Textbook of Veterinary Anatomy*, 3rd edn. Philadelphia, PA: Saunders, 2002.

5 Jeffcott, L.B. Radiographic examination of the equine vertebral column. *Veterinary Radiology* 1979; **20**:135–139.

6 Townsend, H.G.G. and Leach, D.H. Relationship of intervertebral joint morphology and mobility in the equine thoracolumbar spine. *Equine Veterinary Journal* 1984; **16**:461–466.

7 Gloobe, H. Lateral foramina in the equine thoracolumbar vertebral column: An anatomical study. *Equine Veterinary Journal* 1984; **16**:469–470.

8 Townsend, H.G.G., Leach, D.H. and Fretz, P.B. Kinematics of the equine thoracolumbar spine. *Equine Veterinary Journal* 1983; **15**:117–122.

9 Stecher, R.M. Lateral facets and lateral joints in the lumbar spine of the horse. A descriptive and statistical study. *American Journal of Veterinary Research* 1962; **23**:939–947.

10 Haussler, K.K. Osseous spinal pathology. *Veterinary Clinics of North America: Equine Practice* 1999; **15**(1):103–111.

11 Townsend, H.G.G., Leach, D.H., Doige, C.E. and Kirkaldy-Willis, W.H. Relationship between spinal biomechanics and pathological changes in the equine thoracolumbar spine. *Equine Veterinary Journal* 1986; **18**:107–112.

12 Smythe, R.H. Ankylosis of the equine spine: pathologic or biologic? *Modern Veterinary Practice* 1962; **43**:50–51.

13 Dalin, G. and Jeffcott, L.B. Sacroiliac joint of the horse. 1. Gross morphology. *Anatomia, Histologia, Embryologia* 1986; **15**:80–94.

14 Barone, R. *Anatomie Comparée des Mammifères Domestiques*. Lyon: Ecole Nationale Vétérinaire, 1968.

15 Stashak, E. *Adams' Lameness in Horses*, 4th edn. Philadelphia, PA: Lea & Febiger, 1976.

16 Pasquini, C., Spurgeon, T. and Pasquini, S. (1995) *Anatomy of the Domestic Animals*, 9th edn. Pilot Point: Sudz, 1995.

17 Share-Jones, J.T. *The Surgical Anatomy of the Horse*. London: Baillière, Tindall and Cox, 1908.

18 Tomlinson, J.E., Sage, A.M. and Turner, T.A. Ultrasonographic abnormalities detected in the sacroiliac area in twenty cases of upper hindlimb lameness. *Equine Veterinary Journal* 2003; **35**:48–54.

19 Erichsen, C., Berger, M. and Eksell, P. The scintigraphic anatomy of the equine sacroiliac joint. *Veterinary Radiology and Ultrasound* 2002; **43**:287–292.

20 Degueurce, C., Chateau, H. and Denoix, J.-M. *In vitro* assessment of movements of the sacroiliac joint in the horse. *Equine Veterinary Journal* 2004; **36**:694–698.

21 Engeli, E., Yeager, A.E., Erb, H.N. and Haussler, KK. *Ultrasonographic technique and normal anatomic features of the sacroiliac region in horses. Veterinary Radiology and Ultrasound 2006*; **47**:391–403.

22 Tomlinson, J.E., Sage, A.M., Turner, T.A. and Feeney, D.A. Detailed ultrasonographic mapping of the pelvis in clinically normal horses and ponies. *American Journal of Veterinary Research* 2001; **62**:1768–1775.

23 Habel, R.E. and Budras, K.D. Anatomy of the prepubic tendon in the horse, cow, sheep, goat, and dog. *American Journal of Veterinary Research* 1992; **53**:2183–2195.

3

The Normal Anatomy of the Nervous System

Constanze Fintl

Introduction

A working knowledge of normal neuro-anatomical features is important in order to understand and interpret abnormal clinical findings. This chapter describes the main features of the distribution and function of the central and peripheral nerves of the equine neck, back and pelvis. The reader is advised to consult specialised anatomical texts for a more detailed description of these [1,2,3].

The Spinal Cord Segments

A discussed in Chapter 2, the equine spinal cord consists of 8 cervical, 18 thoracic, 6 lumbar, 5 sacral and 5 or 6 caudal segments [4]. However, the positioning of the spinal cord segments and the corresponding vertebrae are not perfectly matched. During embryonic development, the vertebral and neural components develop closely and during the initial stages the spinal cord fills the entire vertebral canal [5]. However, at the latter stages of foetal development, the vertebral column begins to grow in length relatively faster than the spinal cord [4,5]. The consequence of this is that, in the adult horse, the first three sacral spinal cord segments are over the vertebral body of L6 while the last two sacral and the first few caudal segments are over the body of S1 and cranial part of S2 [4,6]. Thus the spinal cord containing the last three to four caudal segments ends at S2 [1,6].

The spinal cord segments also vary in their relative size with the larger segments supplying the peripheral nerves to the appendages. For the forelimbs these include parts of segments C6–T1 whilst for the pelvic limbs parts of L4–S1 are involved [1,7]. These enlarged segmental regions form the cervicothoracic and lumbosacral intumescences respectively. Caudal to the lumbosacral intumescence, the spinal cord tapers gradually into an elongated cone, the *conus medullaris*, which is finally reduced to a uniform strand of glial and ependymal cells, the terminal filament (*filum terminale*). The terminal filament continues caudally where it soon becomes enveloped by dura mater to form the spinal dura mater filament (caudal ligament) [8]. The caudal ligament is joined by sacral and caudal spinal nerves that stream caudally through the vertebral canal to exit at their respective intervertebral foramina. The *conus medullaris*, the caudal ligament as well as the long spinal nerves that run caudally through this distal part of the vertebral canal together constitute the *cauda equina*.

The Spinal Nerves

Anatomical Distribution

From each spinal cord segment, paired spinal nerves emerge through the vertebral

Equine Neck and Back Pathology: Diagnosis and Treatment, Second Edition. Edited by Frances M.D. Henson.
© 2018 John Wiley & Sons, Ltd. Published 2018 by John Wiley & Sons, Ltd.

foraminae. This means that the horse typically has 42 paired spinal nerves [3].

The majority of the cervical spinal nerves arising from a particular spinal cord segment emerge through the vertebral foramen cranial to the corresponding vertebrae. The exceptions to this are the first and last cervical spinal nerves, which emerge through the lateral vertebral foramina in the arch of the atlas and caudal to the 7th cervical vertebrae (and therefore cranial to the first thoracic vertebrae) respectively. The spinal nerves from the thoracic and lumbar segments exit through the intervertebral foramen caudal to the corresponding vertebrae.

The sacral vertebrae have a slightly different arrangement because of the fusion of the vertebrae (Chapter 2). Therefore, rather than having intervertebral foraminae, the sacrum has dorsal and pelvic foraminae. This means that after the spinal nerves have formed within the sacral vertebral canal, they divide into dorsal and ventral branches before exiting through the dorsal and pelvic foramina respectively [6]. Finally, the caudal nerves emerge through lateral vertebral foraminae caudal to the corresponding vertebrae.

Because the spinal nerves always travel to the intervertebral foramina formed by the corresponding vertebrae, the spinal root length reflects the location of the spinal cord segment relative to its numerical vertebra. This is particularly evident in the caudal part of the spinal cord where the spinal nerves from the last segments travel a considerable distance to exit at their respective foraminae.

The Composition of the Spinal Nerve

On both sides of each spinal cord segment, varying numbers of dorsal and ventral nerve rootlets emerge and fuse to form the dorsal and ventral roots respectively (Figure 3.1). Contained within the dorsal root of each spinal cord segment, and hence within the vertebral canal, is the spinal ganglion, previously referred to as the dorsal root ganglion [1,9]. The dorsal and ventral roots then join to form

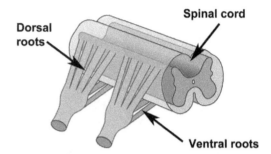

Figure 3.1 A schematic drawing illustrating the dorsal and ventral rootlets of a spinal nerve. *Source:* Adapted from [9].

the paired segmental spinal nerves as they exit the intervertebral foramen.

After emerging through the intervertebral foramen, the spinal nerve soon divides into (typically) four main branches. These include the main dorsal and ventral branches as well as a communicating and a variable meningeal branch (Figure 3.2). The dorsal branches innervate the epaxial tissues while the ventral branches innervate the hypaxial tissues, including the limbs [1]. Both branches are of a mixed composition containing both motor and sensory neurones. Prior to describing further features of these branches, a brief review of the sensory and motor systems follows.

The Sensory (Afferent) System

Sensory information arising from the neck, back and pelvis, and indeed of blood vessels and viscera of the body cavities, is mediated through the general somatic afferent, the general proprioceptive functional systems and the general visceral afferent systems respectively. The classification of these different groups is based on the site of the origin of the impulse [1].

The General Somatic Afferent System

General somatic afferent (GSA) activity arises through input from peripheral receptor

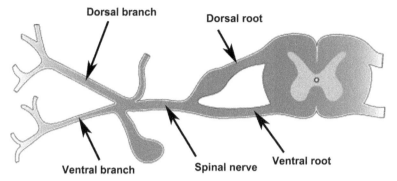

Figure 3.2 A schematic diagram to illustrate the distribution of the branches of the lumbar spinal nerves in the horse. *Source*: Blythe 1999. Reproduced with permission of Elsevier.

organs which are specialised to mediate the sensations of pain, pressure, touch and temperature. The cell body of these unipolar neurones is located in the spinal ganglion while the axon continues proximally through the dorsal root. The axon subsequently divides into branches coursing cranially and caudally through the adjacent two or three spinal segments forming a pathway referred to as the dorsolateral fasciculus [1]. Connections from these branches enter the dorsal grey column at several points over the segments covered by a particular neurone.

The General Visceral Afferent System

General visceral afferent (GVA) neurones have their receptor structors located within the internal viscera of the body. Their cell bodies are also located in the spinal ganglion but, unlike the GSA system, the axons of the GVA neurones of the abdominal cavity travel to the spinal cord in nerves that contain neurones from the sympathetic and parasympathetic general visceral efferent (GVE) systems. Once in the spinal cord, the axons terminate on neuronal cell bodies located in the dorsal grey column.

It is likely that the pathway for conscious projection of both GSA and GVA neurones follow a similar course through a multisynaptic system involving the thalamus with further projections to the cerebral cortex [1].

The General Proprioceptive Pathway

The general proprioceptive pathway (GP) provides important information to the animal regarding the position of the body in relation to the world around. This information, when analysed with information from the eyes and the vestibular system, provides the basis of maintaining posture and a base from which movements can be made – either a simple segmental reflex action or more complex reflex and conscious responses. The receptor organs (muscle spindles, Golgi tendon organs, etc.) for this system relay information through afferent neurones that join the particular spinal nerves. As for the GSA and GVA systems, the cell body of the GP neurone is located in the spinal ganglion. From the spinal ganglion, the axon continues in the dorsal root to enter the dorsal grey column of the spinal cord where it may synapse directly on alpha motor neurones (general somatic efferent neurones) to complete a reflex arc whereas others indirectly complete a reflex arc by synapsing on one or more interneurons [1].

Other pathways relay both conscious and unconscious proprioceptive information from the body to the brain. Conscious proprioception is relayed to the cerebral cortex via the dorsal funiculus in the spinal cord in the *fasciculus gracilis* while unconscious proprioception is relayed to the cerebellum through the spinocerebellar tracts of the lateral funiculus of the spinal cord [1].

The Motor System

The efferent motor system is classified on the basis of where the motor neuron terminates. As their names imply, the general somatic efferent (GSE) system innervates voluntary striated muscles while the general visceral efferent (GVE) system innervates involuntary smooth muscles of the visceral structures, blood vessels and glands. However, both systems consist of lower motor neurones (LMN) that connect the central nervous system (CNS) with the muscle to be innervated [1].

The General Somatic Efferent System

The cell bodies of the LMN are topographically organised in the ventral grey horn of the spinal cord. The GSE neurones innervating the axial musculature populate the medial portion of the column while those innervating the appendicular musculature are located laterally and cause the lateral bulge of the ventral grey column that is evident at the cervicothoracic and lumbosacral intumescences respectively [4]. From the neuronal cell body located in the ventral grey column, the axon of GSE neurones courses through the white matter through the ventral root and joins the spinal nerve on course to its final destination to a skeletal muscle as part of a specific peripheral nerve. A motor neuron and all of the muscle fibers it innervates constitute a motor unit.

The General Visceral Efferent System

In contrast to the GSE system, general visceral efferent (GVE) lower motor neurones represent involuntary effector responses as part of the autonomic nervous system. It is composed of two neurones interposed between the CNS and the organ, vessel or gland innervated where the first cell body is located in the grey matter of the CNS and its axon courses through a spinal nerve to a peripheral ganglion [1]. This neuron synapses with a second (postganglionic) peripheral motor neuron, which subsequently terminates in the structure to be innervated.

Spinal Nerve Distribution

As described above, the spinal nerve carrying motor, sensory as well as autonomic neurones emerges through the intervertebral foramen where it soon divides into four major branches. The two main branches of the spinal nerve, the dorsal and ventral branches, generally subdivide into medial and lateral branches before giving rise to numerous smaller branches (Figures 3.3 and 3.4) [9]. Both the dorsal and ventral branches are mixed, providing sensory and motor innervation. The following summary is based on that described in the anatomical text by Sisson [3] and describes the distribution of these branches and their predominant function. The reader is advised to consult anatomic textbooks such the one mentioned for a more detailed description.

The Dorsal Branches

Soon after separating off the main spinal nerve, this branch courses in a dorsal direction before it divides into lateral and medial branches. These branches supply the epaxial muscles and skin near the dorsal midline [9,10,11], providing motor and sensory functions respectively.

In the horse, the distribution and location of the dorsal branches in the cervical region generally follow those of the rest of the body although there are some minor variations between the different cervical branches. The dorsal branches of the first cervical vertebra emerge through the lateral vertebral foramen of the atlas and then pass dorsolaterally between the *obliqui capiti craniales* and the *recti capitis dorsales* muscles supplying these as well as the skin of the poll. The branches of the second and third vertebrae follow a similar course, ascending between the *semispinalis capitis* and the nuchal ligament and the *intertransversarii cervicis* muscles respectively before ramifying to supply these as well as relaying sensory information from the skin and the poll. The fourth and fifth cervical dorsal spinal branches also follow a

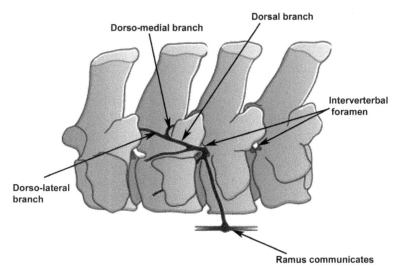

Figure 3.3 A schematic diagram of the divisions of a typical spinal nerve. *Source*: Adapted from [9].

similar pattern of distribution and innervation. Communicating twigs unite the dorsal branches with each other and those of the third and sixth nerves to form the dorsal cervical plexus. The final three dorsal spinal branches (C6–C8) again follow a dorsal path, providing both sensory and motor information. Branches from the last two of these (C7 and C8) ascend between the *longissimus cervicis* and *multifidus* muscles, giving off branches to these as well as others including *rhomboideus cervicis*.

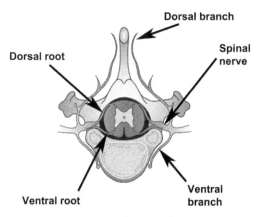

Figure 3.4 A schematic drawing of a cross-section through a vertebra illustrating the anatomy of the spinal nerve outflow. *Source*: Adapted from [9].

An understanding of the normal distribution and composition of these dorsal spinal branches is important in order to understand any abnormal responses revealed during the neurological examination. Rooney [12] described two cervical reflexes involving the dorsal branches, which are of clinical relevance. The first of these involves sensory information relayed by the dorsal branches of the cranial cervical segments (C1–C3) when the skin in this region is tapped with a blunt instrument. This results in a twitching of the ear due to a connection between the GSA neurones of that region, ascending tracts of the spinal cord and medulla to the facial nucleus, and finally GSE neurones through the facial muscles to the auricular nerves. This reflex does not, however, involve the ventral branches of the corresponding spinal nerves.

In contrast, the second reflex described by Rooney [12] involves both dorsal and ventral spinal branches. This reflex, which is a caudal local cervical reflex (caudal to C3–C4), will respond to tapping by local muscle contraction. Once again, GSA neurones from the dorsal branches relay the input and the GSE system through the ventral spinal branches initiates a local muscle contraction as well as a more generalised cervical muscle response caused by contraction of the *cutaneous colli* muscle [12].

Another interesting and clinical relevant aspect involving the cervical dorsal spinal branches relates to that of the GP pathways. In a study it was demonstrated that the local anaesthetic block of the first three cervical dorsal branches in macaque monkeys and baboons resulted in clinical signs of peripheral vestibular disease [13]. A similar clinical syndrome of symmetrical peripheral vestibular signs has been experimentally reproduced in ponies [14]. It is reasonable to assume that the neuronal pathways will be similar between the horse and the primates and that a connection exists between the GP neurones located in the proximal cervical area and the vestibular nerves. It also explains why trauma to this region may result in symptoms similar to those seen in peripheral vestibular disease.

The distribution of the dorsal spinal branches in the thoracic and lumbar areas in principle follows that of the cervical branches. The thoracic branches emerge caudal to the *levatores costarum* muscles and divide into lateral and medial branches [10]. From these, the dorsolateral branches pass laterally under the *longissimus thoracicus* and *longissimus lumborum* muscles to surface between the *longissimus* muscles and *iliocostalis thoracis* and *lumborum* muscles providing cutaneous sensory innervation of the thoracic dorsolateral spinous areas [6,10].

In the lumbar and cranial pelvic areas the lateral branches provide cutaneous sensory innervation of the dorsum as well as the areas overlying the superficial gluteal muscles and are collectively called the cranial clunial nerves. The medial clunial nerves are formed from the dorsolateral branches of the sacral nerves and supply the skin from the dorsum, laterally and ventrally to include the areas overlying the *biceps femoris* muscle mass. The caudal clunial nerves, which are branches of the caudal femoral cutaneous nerve, supply the skin surrounding the ischial tuberosity

and caudal thigh areas to the stifle [11]. A branch of the pudendal nerve provides cutaneous sensory innervation of the perineal area as well as the areas overlying the *semitendinosus* muscle.

The dorsomedial branches of the spinal nerve are directed caudodorsally (Figure 3.4) deep to the *multifidus* muscles, to which they send branches [6,10]. They then continue caudodorsally to innervate the vertebral rotator muscles (in the thoracic region) and proceed to provide sensory innervation from the laminae and periosteum of the vertebral arch [6]. The terminal dorsomedial branches also supply the caudal aspect of the articular processes of its corresponding segment. In addition, branches of the same nerve terminate on the cranial aspect of the articular processes caudal to its adjacent vertebrae. This means that, for instance, the dorsomedial branch that innervates the caudal aspect of the articular process of L1 also innervates the cranial aspect of the articular process of L3.

Currently, innervation of the intervertebral disc in the horse has not been determined although in the dog it was established that the annulus fibrosus was innervated but not the nucleus pulposus [15]. In addition, each annulus was found to be innervated by nerves from the cell bodies in the spinal ganglia of two spinal nerve segments cranial and caudal to the disc in question. Clearly similar studies will need to be performed in the horse to establish the innervation of the intervertebral discs but this study will at the very least give an indication of the arrangement that may be present also in the horse. However, it is also worth emphasising that in the horse the intervertebral discs are thin and the nucleus pulposus poorly developed, which may explain why herniation is extremely rare [16].

The Ventral Branches

The ventral branch, or rami, is generally the largest of the primary four branches and supplies the skin and muscles of the ventral aspects of the body, including the limbs [10].

The first cervical nerve emerges through the lateral vertebral foramen of the atlas and the ventral branch soon descends through the alar foramen of the atlas. From there it crosses over the *longus capitis* and *rectus capitis ventralis* muscles before dividing into cranial and caudal branches that supply the *omohyoideus* and *sternothyrohyoideus* muscles respectively. The latter muscle also receives innervation from the second cervical nerve, which joins the caudal branch of C1. The ventral branch of the second cervical spinal nerve also divides to create the great auricular nerve and the transverse cervical nerve, both providing sensory innervation to the cranioventral neck and convex surface of the ear just cranial to the wing of the atlas. The third cervical ventral branch follows a similar pattern, providing motor branches to several neck muscles including *longus capitis*, *longus colli* and *brachiocephalicus*. It also contains a large cutaneous nerve whose branches provide a sensory supply to these areas. The remaining cervical ventral branches also follow this general pattern of distribution, providing innervation to both muscle and skin. The sixth nerve provides several such branches including supply to the *longus colli*, *brachiocephalicus*, *serratus ventralis cervicis* and *rhomboideus cervicis* muscles as well as sensory innervation to the corresponding skin areas. However, a smaller branch of this nerve also enters the brachial plexus. The neuronal supply to the latter is provided by the last three ventral branches, and particularly those of the seventh and eighth, which are large and go almost exclusively to supply this.

Other particular features of the distal cervical region include the phrenic nerve, which provides motor function to the diaphragm. This nerve is formed mainly by the ventral branches of the sixth and seventh cervical nerves with a smaller and inconstant contribution by the fifth nerve.

The distribution of the ventral thoracic branches, or intercostal nerves, follows a similar pattern of distribution as that described for the cervical region and is reasonably similar for all 18 of these. They are connected with the sympathetic trunk by rami communicantes. The first two ventral branches, and especially the first, are important contributors to the brachial plexus. The remaining intercostal nerves descend in the intercostal space at first between the *intercostal* muscles, but farther ventrally they become mainly subpleural. They supply the intercostal muscles and also give off large cutaneous branches supplying further muscle groups, including the pectoral muscles, *transversus abdominis, obliquus internus abdominis, rectus abdominis* and *cutaneous trunci* – to mention a few – as well as projecting branches that convey sensory information from the skin.

One connection that is routinely assessed during the neurological examination is the *cutaneous trunci* reflex (incorrectly referred to as the panniculus reflex). In this reflex, the muscle contracts in response to tapping of the lateral trunk. The sensory information is relayed to the spinal cord via segmental thoracic dorsal branches. From there the information is passed cranially in the grey matter to the C8–T1 segment of the spinal cord before connecting with efferent branches of the lateral thoracic nerve, resulting in contraction of the *cutaneous trunci* muscle [14]. A spinal cord lesion interfering with this reflex must therefore be located cranially to the area being tested. This reflex may not occur caudal to the midlumbar region [1].

Finally, the first two or three lumbar ventral branches provide innervation to the sublumbar muscles while the ventral branches of the last three lumbar and the first two sacral nerves give rise to the lumbosacral plexus. The third and the fourth ventral branches of the sacral nerves are connected with each other forming the pudendal, perineal and caudal rectal nerves.

The Meningeal Rami and Ramus Communicans

Typically, the smaller meningeal branch is the first to separate from the main spinal nerve as it emerges through the vertebral foramina. This branch returns into the spinal canal to provide motor innervation to meningeal vessels as well as sensory innervation from the dura mater [13]. However, the meningeal rami described in humans and primates [17,18] are not well characterised in the horse and were not observed during dissection by Blythe and Engel [13].

The ramus communicans carry GVA and GVE (both preganglionic and postganglionic sympathetic fibres) to and from visceral structures [1]. Dermatomal sweating is thought to be due to impingement on the vertebral sympathetic nerve (or its branches), which runs alongside the vertebral artery in the paravertebral foramina [2,14].

Innervation of the Limbs

As described above, at varying distances from the intervertebral foraminae branches of the spinal nerves intermingle to form plexuses. The somatic plexuses provide sensory and motor supply to the body wall and limbs with the two major ones being the brachial and lumbosacral (and pelvic) plexuses. Only a brief outline of these will be described below, and the reader is therefore again advised to consult anatomical texts for further details.

The Brachial Plexus

The brachial plexus is located cranial to the first rib and is usually composed of the ventral branches of the sixth, seventh and eight cervical and the first and second thoracic vertebral segmental nerves. The neurons that arise from this plexus provide sensory and motor innervation to the thoracic limbs, part of the shoulder girdle musculature as well as the lateral wall of the thorax and abdomen [11]. The branches of the brachial plexus also contain autonomic neuronal fibers from the stellate ganglion; hence it has a mixed neuronal composition.

Cutaneous sensory areas for the equine thoracic limb have been electrophysiologically mapped and areas of single nerve supply (autonomous zones) have been determined [19]. This clearly allows for a more precise lesion localisation where neurological deficits are evident.

Lumbosacral and Pelvic Plexuses

The lumbosacral plexus provides innervation for the muscles involved in pelvic limb movement as well as cutaneous sensation of the same region [1]. It is generally composed of spinal nerves arising from the fourth lumbar to, and including, the second sacral segments, although the contribution of the latter to the sciatic nerve varies. Unlike in the thoracic limb, electrophysiologically mapped cutaneous areas and autonomous zones have not yet been described in the pelvic limb and assessment of the individual nerve supply is therefore based on the topographical anatomy of the individual peripheral nerves [20,21] (Figure 3.5).

The pelvic plexus (or caudal lumbosacral plexus) is composed of ventral branches from the first to the third sacral segments and innervates the muscles and skin of the perineal region [1].

Both lumbosacral and pelvic plexuses give rise to many important peripheral nerves, each of which usually contains nerve fibres derived from more than one spinal segment. The exact origin of each of the peripheral nerves is difficult to be absolutely precise about, not least because of some individual variation. However, an outline of the origin of the peripheral nerves is shown in Figure 3.6.

Summary

In summary, it is reasonable to assume that the equine central and peripheral neuronal topography and functional distribution to the cervical and thoracolumbar region is broadly

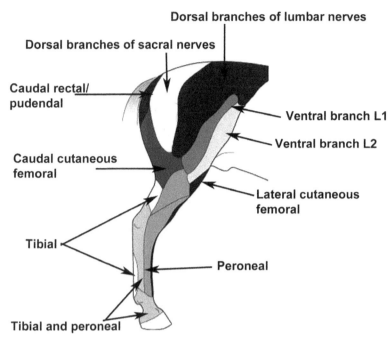

Figure 3.5 A schematic drawing to show the cutaneous innervation of the lateral surface of the pelvic limb. *Source*: Adapted from [10].

similar to other mammalian species. It is therefore also sensible to use previously published texts as a basis for interpretation of clinical findings. However, there is still a need for further detailed anatomical studies to be performed in the horse in order to accurately map and determine these important structures.

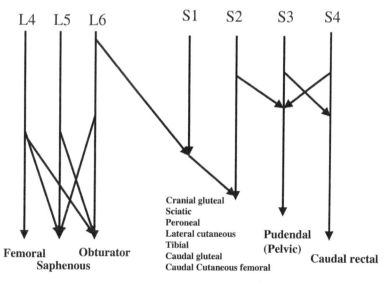

Figure 3.6 A line diagram to show an approximation of the origin of the nerves that innervate the pelvis and hindlegs from the lumbosacral plexus.

References

1 de Lahunta, A., Glass, E. and Kent, M. Chapter 21: The neurologic examination. In: *Veterinary Neuroanatomy and Clinical Neurology*. St Louis, MO: Elsevier Saunders, 2015, pp. 525–540.

2 Thomson, C. and Hahn, C.N. Chapter 12: The autonomic nervous system. In: *Veterinary Neuroanatomy – A Clinical Approach*. St Louis, MO: Elsevier Saunders, 2012, pp. 113–124.

3 Sisson, S. (1910)*The Anatomy of the Domestic Animals*, 2nd edn. Philadelphia, PA and London: W.B. Saunders Company, 1910, pp. 760–834.

4 Dellmann, H.D. and McClure, R.C. Chapter 24: Equine nervous system. In: Getty, R. (ed.), *Sisson and Grossman's The Anatomy of the Domestic Animals*, Vol. 1, 5th edn. Philadelphia, PA: W.B. Saunders Company, 1975, pp. 633–664.

5 Sinowatz, F. Nervensystem. In: Rüsse, I. and Sinowatz, F. (eds), *Lehrbuch der Embryologie der Haustiere*, 1st edn. Berlin *and* Hamburg, Germany: Verlag Paul Parey, 1991, pp. 247–286.

6 Blythe, L.L. and Engel, H.N. Neuroanatomy and neurological examination. *Veterinary Clinics of North America* 1999; **15**(1),71–85.

7 Fletcher, T.F. Lumbosacral plexus and pelvic myotomes of the dog. *American Journal of Veterinary Research* 1970; **31**,35–41.

8 Fletcher, T.F. Chapter 16: Spinal cord and, eninges. In: Evans, H.E. and de Lahunta, A. (eds), *Miller's Anatomy of the Dog*, 4th edn. St Louis, MO: Saunders Elsevier, 2013, pp. 589–611.

9 Evans, H.E. and de Lahunta, A. Chapter 17: The spinal nerves. In: Evans H.E. and de Lahunta A. (eds.), *Miller's Anatomy of the Dog*, 4th edn. St Louis, MO: Saunders Elsevier, 2013, pp. 611–658.

10 Ghoshal, N.G. Chapter 24: Spinal Nerves. In: Getty, R. (ed.), *Sisson and Grossman's The Anatomy of the Domestic Animals*, Vol. 1,5th edn. Philadelphia, PA: W.B. Saunders Company, 1975, pp. 665–688.

11 König HE,. Liebich H-G and Červeny C. (2009)Chapter 14: Peripheral nervous system. In: König HE and Liebich H-G (eds), *Veterinary Anatomy of Domestic Mammals*, pp. 522–556. (Schattauer GmbH, Stuttgart, Germany).

12 Rooney, J.R. Two cervical reflexes in the horse. *JAVMA* 1973; **162**:117–118.

13 Cohen, L.A. Role of eye and neck proprioceptive mechanisms in body orientation and motor coordination. *Journal of Neurophysiology* 1961; **24**:1–11.

14 Mayhew, I.G. The healthy spinal cord. *AAEP Proceedings* 1999; **45**:56–66.

15 Forsythe, W.B. and Ghosal, N.G. Innervation of the canine thoracolumbar vertebral column. *Anatomy Records* 1984; **208**:57–63.

16 Jeffcott, L.B. Chapter 1: The normal anatomy of the osseous structures of the back and pelvis. In: Henson, F.M.D. (ed.), *Equine Back Pathology: Diagnosis and Treatment*, 1st edn. Chichester, West Sussex: Wiley-Blackwell, 2009, pp. 3–16.

17 Stillwell, D.L. Jr. The nerve supply of the vertebral column and its associated structures in the monkey. *Anatomy Records* 1956; **125**:139–169.

18 Kumar, S. and Davies, P.R. Lumbar vertebral innervation and intraabdominal pressure. *Journal of Anatomy* 1973; **114**:47–53.

19 Blythe, L.L. and Kitchell, R.L. Electrophysiologic studies of the thoracic limb of the horse. *American Journal of Veterinary Research* 1982; **43**:1511–1524.

20 Grau, H. Die Lautinnervation an den Gliedmassen des Pferdes. *Arc Wochenschreib Pract Tierheilk* 1935; **69**:96–116.

21 Blythe, L.L. Neurologic examination of the horse. *Veterinary Clinics of North America* 1987; **3**(7),255–281.

4

Kinematics
Rene van Weeren

Introduction

Kinematics is a subdiscipline of mechanics that studies the motions of objects without taking into account the forces that generate this motion. When considering the equine back, one should realise that the back is a segmental, complex structure made up of a large number of separate, but intricately linked rigid bodies, which are the vertebrae. The motion of the thoracolumbar vertebral column is the sum of motions of the individual vertebrae, which are, however, severely restricted in their movement through numerous anatomical constraints such as muscles, ligaments, intervertebral joints and the presence of ribs. In the same way that kinematics of individual vertebrae contribute to back kinematics, back motion can be considered to be one of the constituting elements of the kinematics of the entire body, and hence of the way of moving of the individual. The question of how the back, which bridges the gap between the limbs, functions in quadrupedal locomotion has intrigued scientists for millennia and is an active area of research and discussion today.

In this chapter first an overview is given of the various biomechanical concepts that have been presented as good models for the quadrupedal back. Then, kinematics of the equine back is discussed based on *ex vivo* and *in vivo* research. After that studies are discussed that have applied newly acquired knowledge on equine back kinematics to answer clinical or equestrian questions. The chapter concludes with a brief evaluation of the importance of equine back kinematics in a general sense, and some ideas on the possible use of data on back kinematics for the management of equine health and performance in the future.

Historical Perspective

A scientific interest in the equine gait has existed since horses became an integral part of society and good orthopaedic health was vital for the satisfactory fulfilment of the roles the animal had in agriculture, transport and, most important of all, the military. Technical advances allowed research in equine gait analysis to flourish from the 1870s until the outbreak of World War II, but the rapid loss of all traditional roles of the horse in society caused interest in this kind of research to wane after World War II. However, the comeback of the species as a sports and leisure animal from the mid-1960s led to what has been called the Second Golden Age of equine locomotion research [1]. This Second Golden Age was facilitated by the vast advances in motion capture technology and computational power that simultaneously occurred during this time.

During the Second Golden Age attention focused, during the first decades, principally on limb kinematics and kinetics, with studies on the back being limited to work on cadaver specimens. Only in relatively recent years has

Equine Neck and Back Pathology: Diagnosis and Treatment, Second Edition. Edited by Frances M.D. Henson.
© 2018 John Wiley & Sons, Ltd. Published 2018 by John Wiley & Sons, Ltd.

more work on the back been done in the living animal. At present, studies are emerging that use the recently acquired fundamental knowledge of equine back kinematics and newly developed, validated analysis techniques for a variety of more applied studies. These studies try to answer questions with respect to the use and mobility of the back that have importance to both veterinary surgeons and a wider equestrian audience.

Biomechanical Models of How the Equine Back Works

From Roman Times – The 'Architectural' Analogy

Mankind has been thinking about how the mammalian back could best be understood from very earliest times. The famous Roman physician Galen (129–200 AD) described the first known concept [2]. He refers to the prevailing architecture of his days and describes the quadrupedal back as 'a vaulted roof sustained by four pillars', the limbs. The spinous processes, pointing in a caudodorsal direction on the ascending part of the arch (or the anterior thoracic part of the trunk) and in a craniodorsal direction on the descending part (posterior thoracic and lumbar part), with the anticlinal (Chapter 1) vertebra at the top, would prevent the roof from collapsing.

Though well thought out, this very first concept cannot be correct because it implies a constant contact between the spinous processes, which is not the case under physiological conditions and in fact may be, if present, a cause of pathology (Chapter 13).

The Nineteenth Century – The 'Bridge' Analogy

The next concept was proposed in the middle of the nineteenth century and was again inspired by the technical advances in engineering of those days. This was a time when the railways started to span continents, crossing rivers and ravines with the help of steel bridges that were masterpieces of daring new construction technology. In the bridge concept of the equine back the limbs are the land abutments of the bridge and the gap between these is spanned by the bridge itself [3–5]. This consists of an upper ledger (the supraspinous ligament), a lower ledger (the vertebral bodies) and a number of smaller girders, pointing in either the craniodorsal or caudodorsal direction (the spinous processes and the interspinous ligaments) (Figure 4.1). The bridge concept dominated the veterinary and zoological literature for a long period and has been further elaborated in order to include the biomechanical influences of the head and the tail by using a wide variety of bridge types (Figure 4.2). Even today the model has its

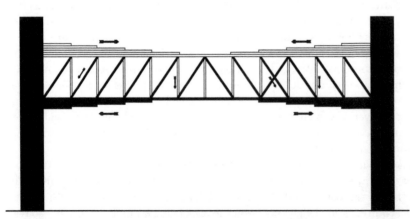

Figure 4.1 A diagram to show the bridge concept of the vertebral column as depicted by Krüger [4]. Closed arrows show compressive forces. *Source:* Adapted from [4].

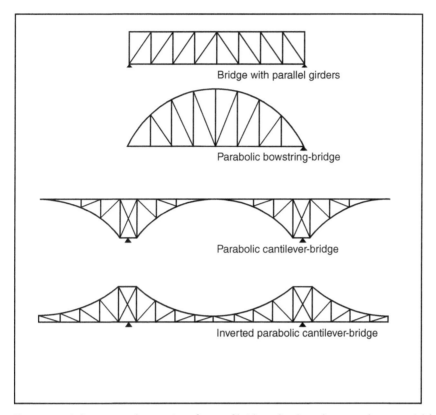

Bridge with parallel girders

Parabolic bowstring-bridge

Parabolic cantilever-bridge

Inverted parabolic cantilever-bridge

Figure 4.2 A diagram to show various forms of bridges that have been used as a model for the mammalian back. (a) Bridge with parallel girders; (b) parabolic bow-string bridge; (c) parabolic cantilever bridge; (d) inverted parabolic cantilever bridge. *Source:* Adapted from [2].

protagonists and is used in the discussions on how the equine back works. The model, however, contains an important conceptual error. The representation of the supraspinous ligament by the upper ledger and of the string of vertebral bodies by the lower ledger presumes tensional loading of the former and compressive loading of the latter, because ligamentous structures are not able to withstand compressive loads. In reality, the gravitational forces that act on bridges (and on the mammalian trunk) will cause compression in the upper ledger and tension on the lower one.

The Twenty-First Century – The 'Bow-and-String' Analogy

The current biomechanical concept of the equine back is that of the *bow and string*, in which the bow is the thoracolumbar vertebral column and the string is the 'underline' of the trunk, consisting of the linea alba, the rectus abdominis muscle and related structures. The model was first proposed by Barthez [6], but largely ignored until it was rediscovered by Slijper [2], based on his study of the positions of the spinous processes in a large number of species (Figure 4.3). It is the first concept that takes into account the entire trunk and not only the thoracolumbar vertebral column with adnexa, and presumes that there is a dynamic balance between the tension in the bow and string.

Factors that Influence the 'Bow and String'

There are many factors that influence the dynamic balance between tension in the bow and string and the ensuing intrinsic tension of the system (Figure 4.4).

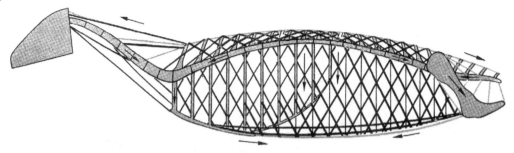

Figure 4.3 A diagram to demonstrate the 'bow-and-string' concept of the back according to Slijper [2]. The vertebral column is the bow and the ventral musculature and sternum are the string. The ribs, lateral abdominal musculature, spinous processes and ligamentous connections are additional elements. *Source:* Adapted from [7].

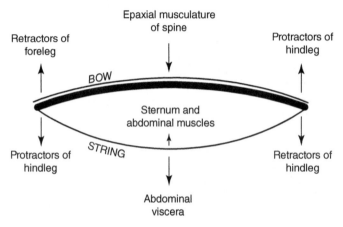

Figure 4.4 A diagram to show the factors that determine the motion of the back according to the 'bow-and-string' concept. Upward pointing arrows mean a flexing effect on the back; downward pointing arrows represent an extending effect.

- *Gravitational forces* will always act in a downward direction and hence tend to straighten the bow, i.e. extend the back or make it more hollow. Gravitational forces act on the back itself, but the gravitational pull on the large intestinal mass of the horse is a more important factor in extending the back. Pregnancy will aggravate this effect and old broodmares typically have a very hollow-backed conformation ('acquired lordosis', Chapter 14). Of course, every load on the back of the horse, including a rider, will have a similar effect.
- *Active muscular action* will also influence the dynamic equilibrium between the bow

and string. Contraction of the ventral musculature will tense the bow, i.e. flex the back or make it more arched. In contrast to the belief of many lay people, contraction of the massive epaxial musculature will have the opposite effect, as the work line of these muscles runs dorsal to the axis through the centres of the vertebral bodies. The only dorsally located muscles that have a flexing effect on the back are the psoas muscles. However, these are located between the pelvis and the ventral aspect of the lumbar and last three thoracic vertebrae [7] and will principally affect lumbosacral flexion. There is no musculature ventral to the more cranial thoracic vertebrae, which might flex this part of the spine.

- **Limb movements.** Pro- and retraction of the limbs will also affect the balance in the bow-and-string system. Protraction of the hind limbs will, through the forward position of the point of support and the anatomical connection between the gluteus medius muscle and the lumbar and sacral spinous processes through the gluteal and lumbodorsal fascia [7], flex the back or tense the bow. In a similar way, retraction of the forelimb will have the same effect. Protraction of the forelimbs and retraction of the hind limbs will have an opposite effect, i.e. produce a hollow (extended) back.
- **The head and neck.** A last, but not unimportant, factor that should be mentioned is the effect of the head and neck. Lowering the neck will tense the nuchal ligament and exert a forward rotating moment on the spinous processes of thoracic (T) vertebrae 2–6. These long spinous processes forming the basis of the withers provide a long lever arm, and traction on them in a forward direction will provoke tensing of the bow or flexion of the back. Elevation of the head will have an opposite effect.

Kinematics of the Equine Back

In order to begin to understand the kinematics of the equine back it is important to understand that the kinematics of any structure can be described as a product of 6 basic motions: three rotations and three translations.

For the equine spine the three *rotational* movements are the most important. Rotation around the dorsoventral or z-axis represents in most cases lateroflexion or lateral bending (LB), a rotation around the craniocaudal or y-axis represents axial rotation (AR) and a rotation around the axis perpendicular to the sagittal plane or x-axis represents ventrodorsal flexion–extension movements (FE) (Figure 4.5A and B). In some studies, x- and

y-axes are interchanged, which is of course only a matter of definition and does not affect outcome.

In contrast to rotational movements, *translational* movements of vertebrae with respect to each other are very limited and therefore the translations along the 3 axes represent in fact the motion of the entire body, which will not be discussed in the context of this chapter. We can, therefore, concentrate solely on the rotational movements of the spine.

Research into equine spinal kinematics has long been mainly limited to work on postmortem specimens due to the large technical problems associated with work *in vivo*. However, even in the pre-World War II era some *in vivo* work was done. Krüger [4] used two cadaver horses to examine the kinetics of the thoracolumbar column and its movements. This was achieved by manipulating long metal rods that had been inserted in holes drilled in a number of vertebrae, while the pelvis remained fixed. He determined maximal motion in dorsoventral and lateral directions, and compared the outcome with results from *in vivo* work in 3 horses. The horses were filmed from the side (lateral view) and from above (the camera had been fixed in the branches of a tree!), after marking the midline and two lines perpendicular to it, at the withers and at the pelvis, with white paint. From these experiments Krüger [4] noticed that motion *in vivo* was considerably less than the maximal ranges of motion found in the cadaver specimens. This observation was confirmed some 40 years later when Jeffcott and Dalin [8] concluded that, in comparison to other species, the natural flexibility of the horse's backbone was very limited.

A number of further studies on back flexibility have taken place. In a large study conducted at the Western College of Veterinary Medicine in Saskatoon, Townsend and co-workers [9] dissected 18 equine spines and marked them with Steinmann pins placed in the geometric centre of the ventral surface of each vertebral body, perpendicular to a plane through the long axis of the thoracolumbar spine and the transverse processes.

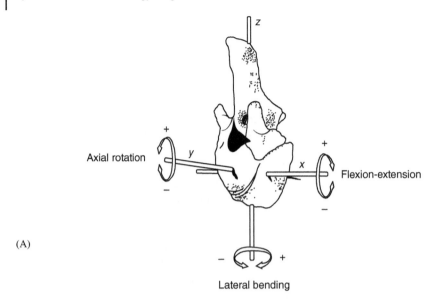

(A)

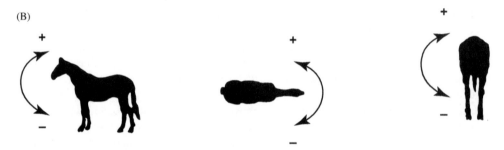

(B)

Figure 4.5 (A) A diagram to show the basic movements of the back depicted as rotations of an individual vertebra around the three axes of an orthogonal coordinate system. (B) A diagram to show the three basic movements of the equine back: flexion–extension (FE) (A), lateroflexion or lateral bending (LB) (B) and axial rotation (AR) (C).

The sacrum of each spine was fixed in a clamp and manual pressure was used to provoke FE, LB and AR, which were recorded photographically. Conditions prior to and after removal of the rib cage were compared.

In this study, dorsoventral movement (FE) was found to be maximal in the lumbosacral joint (which may be either the transition between L6 and S1 or between L5 and L6). This study demonstrated that the range of motion (ROM) at this site could attain approximately 25°, which was considerably more than in other parts of the spine where FE ROM did not exceed 4° in the area between T2 and L5/L6, and was 6–8° at the junction of T1 and T2. Lateral bending was largest at T11/T12 with 10–11° and decreased in both the cranial and caudal direction to about 4° in the cranial thoracic area and not more than 1° at the last lumbar vertebrae. Axial rotation was most prominent in the region T9–T14 (up to 5°) and decreased in the cranial (2–3°) and more so in the caudal direction (1°), with the notable exception of the lumbosacral joint (2–3°). Removal of the ribs did not affect FE or LB, but significantly increased AR in the cranial thoracic region. The regional differences in the mobility of the segments of the thoracolumbar spine could be related to anatomical peculiarities of the intervertebral joints and other anatomical or acquired structures such as the frequent fusion of the transverse processes of the last lumbar vertebrae, explaining the extreme rigidity of this part of the equine spine [10].

Denoix [11] performed a comparable, but more comprehensive, *in vitro* study on cadaver specimens. He included the influence of the position of the head and neck and paid more attention to the effect of the position of a given region of the thoracolumbar spine on the mobility of another region. In this study, FE was found to be larger in the caudal thoracic part (T14–T18) than in the rest of the spine, with the obvious exception of the lumbosacral joint. Cervical flexion provoked flexion in the thoracic spine, but also a decrease in FE range of motion in the lumbar area, which was compensated for by an increased mobility at the lumbosacral joint. In the same study, the instantaneous centres of rotation of the intervertebral joints were determined, which appeared to be situated within or near the next adjacent vertebral body. In a study focusing more on the lumbosacral and iliosacral regions, the same author applied forces on isolated pelvises in transverse, axial and dorsoventral directions to assess possible deformations of the structure generated by the forces of locomotion. In the study on the iliosacral region it was shown that the pelvis resisted high loads in the longitudinal direction (i.e. in the direction of impulse in the moving horse), but is more susceptible to forces in the other two directions, which may be substantial under conditions like taking turns at high speed on insufficiently banked tracks, rearing, etc., and might provoke damage to the pelvic and sacroiliac ligaments. The lumbosacral region was, as in preceding studies, very rigid with respect to FE, with both AR and LB being very limited as well, the latter movement being virtually impossible in the caudal lumbar area (caudal to L4) because of the formation of joints between the transverse processes. It was hypothesised that this high degree of rigidity

could lie at the base of the region's tendency to develop intervertebral ankylosis [12].

The relatively frequent diagnosis, or at least suspicion of sacroiliac pathology as a cause of poor performance or of subtle and obscure hind limb lameness (Chapter 15), has boosted the interest in the kinematics of this very inaccessible area. In an elaborate study using a number of dissected pelvises with pins placed at strategic sites and a state-of-the-art kinematic analysis system, Degueurce et al. [13] showed that the amount of nutation and counternutation (rotation of the sacrum respective to the pelvic bones in the sagittal plane) did not pass 1°, which is too small to be detected in the living horse. Goff et al. [14] confirmed this observation, but showed a larger range of motion in the transverse plane, when lateral and oblique forces were applied to the pelvis, which may give more insight into the physiological role of iliosacral mobility and might explain the relatively large importance attributed to the area in clinics (Chapter 15).

Kinematics of the Equine Back – *in vivo* Research

Whereas studies on the kinematic analysis of limb movement appeared in large numbers from the early 1970s onwards [15], *in vivo* work on back kinematics remained virtually absent for almost another 3 decades. This was primarily due to the technical difficulties involved in measuring the small movements of the equine thoracolumbar spine.

Skin Marker Based Measurement Techniques

The first attempts at measuring equine back kinematics *in vivo* all focused on FE, which is easiest to measure and is influenced least by skin displacement when using skin markers. Audigié et al. [16] used a method developed by Pourcelot et al. [17] and placed 5 skin markers in the midline over the top of the withers, the 12th and 18th thoracic vertebrae, the tuber sacrale and the sacrocaudal junction. The markers were used to measure what was called the thoracic angle, the thoracolumbar angle and the lumbosacral angle in sound trotting horses. The range of motion for all three angles was shown to be less than 4° and variability, both intraindividual and interindividual, was low. Horses extended the back during the first part of each diagonal stance phase and flexed in the last half of the stance phase. Comparing the kinematic data with electromyographic data obtained earlier [18] showed that activity of the epaxial musculature tended to limit FE motion, rather than cause it. A similar conclusion was reached by Licka et al. [19], who presumed, based on an electromyelogram (EMG) study, that the main action of the *longissimus dorsi* muscle was the stabilisation of the vertebral column against dynamic forces. Licka and Peham [20] used a kinematic analysis system and skin markers on T5, T10, T16, L3 and on the sacrum in an attempt to objectify the induction of maximal flexion using manual diagnostic tests. Flexion–extension and LB were investigated and expressed as mean transversal movement (LB) and mean vertical flexion (FE) relative to the height of the withers. Although perhaps not illogical, this measure makes comparison with most of the other literature, where back motion is expressed in degrees, difficult. In a follow-up study, in which LB and FE were induced in the standing horse under simultaneous registration of the positions of markers on the spinous processes of T5, T12, T16, L3 and S3 and EMG activity of the *Longissimus dorsi* using surface electrodes, it was concluded that T12 was the best place to take EMG recordings. The EMG on both sides of the spinous process of T12 had the highest and the EMG at the height of L3 the lowest amplitudes [21].

The same research group investigated back kinematics in walking horses on a treadmill. They found maximal LB at L3, which is further caudal than in most other studies. Flexion–extension was maximal at the sacrum. This motion reflects in fact the upward–downward motion of the pelvis as induced by the hindlimbs; it cannot be compared to the results of the *in vitro* studies as in those studies the pelvis was fixed and thoracolumbar motion was assessed relative to this fixed point.

Kinematic analysis methods using skin markers always suffer to a certain extent from the so-called *skin displacement artefact*, which is caused by the fact that the skin will not always exactly follow the motion of the underlying bone, a phenomenon that was actually noted 100 years ago [22]. Skin displacement will be of relatively minor importance for FE where the marker will directly follow the movement of the underlying spinous process, but the coupling of LB and AR during any movement of the spine out of the sagittal plane [23] indicates that the composed movements of markers under that circumstance cannot be unambiguously broken down into the lateral bending and axial rotation components. Therefore, equine spinal kinematics could never be described fully using skin marker based techniques.

Invasive Marker Measurement Techniques

The only way to overcome the problems associated with measurements using skin markers was to resort to invasive techniques in which a rigid connection is made between the vertebra and an external marker or measuring device. Haussler et al. [24] used such an approach. They implanted Steinmann pins into a number of spinous processes and connected the pins by liquid metal strain gauges, positioned according to the three axes of rotation. The technique is accurate (resolution of 0.07° in FE and about 0.5° in AR and LB), but laborious and simultaneous measuring of the motion of a substantial number of vertebrae is difficult. In their first paper Haussler et al. [24] reported a ROM of FE at the lumbosacral junction at walk of 4°. AR and LB were on the order of 1° at that site. In a follow-up paper the same technique was used to investigate segmental motion at T14–T16, L1–L3 and L6–S2 at walk, trot and canter. The largest ROM for all three rotations was found at the lumboscral junction with the largest ROM for the canter and the smallest

Figure 4.6 A diagram to show a marker device with four markers (A–D) attached via a Steinmann pin to the spinous process of a vertebra and oriented in the laboratory coordinate system (*x*, *y*, *z*). (From Faber et al. [26] with permission from the American Veterinary Medical Association.)

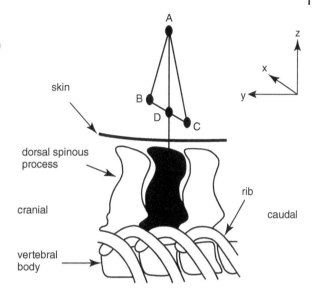

Figure 4.7 A photograph to show a horse on the treadmill with marker devices attached to Steinmann pins implanted into the spinous processes of T6, T10, T13, T17, L1, L3, L5 and S3, and both tubera coxae.

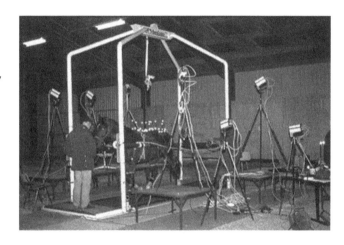

for the trot. ROM for FE, LB and AR at canter were approximately 5, 3.5 and 4.5° [25].

The approach chosen by Faber et al. [26] used a technique that also was based on the implantation of Steinmann pins into the spinous processes. Pins were placed under fluoroscopic guidance in the spinous processes of T6, T10, T13, T17, L1, L3, L5, S3 and in the tips of the coxal tubers. To this pins custom-made devices were attached carrying reflective markers that could be detected by the ProReflex®[1] kinematic analysis system (Figure 4.6). In this way, a rigid

connection was realised between the optical markers and the vertebral body and the 3-D motion of the markers therefore represented the movements of the underlying vertebrae. For data analysis, a newly developed method was used that allowed for the determination of 3-D spinal kinematics without defining a local vertebral coordinate system [27]. Measurements were performed on a treadmill at walk, trot and canter (Figure 4.7), and kinematic motion patterns of the vertebrae studied were established [26,28,29]. Motion patterns of all 3 basic rotations had a sinusoidal shape related to the stride cycle. Flexion–extension is induced

1 Qualisys Medical AB, Gotheburg, Sweden.

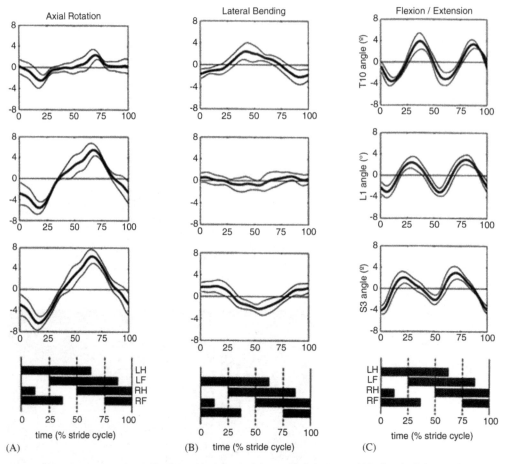

Figure 4.8 A diagram to show the mean (thick line) and standard deviation (thin lines) of the motion patterns of three vertebrae (T10, L1 and S3) of five horses walking on a treadmill at a speed of 1.6 m/s. The stride cycle is represented by the bars below (LH: left hind; RH: right hind; LF: left fore; RF: right fore). The bar is closed when the limb is in contact with the ground (stance phase). (A) Axial rotation; (B) lateral bending; (C) flexion–extension. (From Faber et al. [26] with permission from the American Veterinary Medical Association.)

by pro- and retraction of each hind limb and therefore shows two peaks for each entire stride cycle whereas LB and AR have a left and a right component, which is reflected by the positive and negative parts of a single sinus that is generated during a stride cycle (Figure 4.8). Flexion–extension motion at walk was approximately 4° at T6 and remained fairly constant at 8° for all more caudally located vertebrae. Lateral bending was maximal for the area round T10 and for the pelvic region (approximately 5°), and less in the more central region of the spine (approximately 3°). Axial rotation increased gradually from 4° at T6 to 13° for

the tuber coxae. Spinal motion is considerably less at trot than at walk. Flexion–extension ranged from 2.8 to 4.9°, LB from 1.9 to 3.6° and AR from 3.1 to 5.8° at trot [28]. At canter, maximal ranges of motion for FE, LB and AR were 15.8 ± 1.3°, 5.2 ± 0.7° and 7.8 ± 1.2° respectively [30]. The largest relative FE motion was, not surprisingly, found between L5 and S3 with 8.6°, which is, however, considerably less than the maximal values found during the *in vitro* experiments alluded to earlier, but a little more than reported by Haussler et al. [25]. Variability of spinal motion appeared to be gait-dependent and to vary per type of

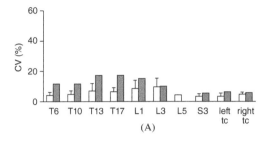

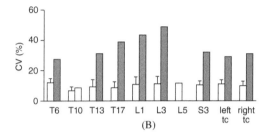

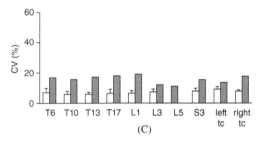

Figure 4.9 A diagram to show the within-horse (open bars) and between-horse (bars) variability at canter in (A) flexion–extension, (B) lateral bending and (C) axial rotation, expressed as a coefficient of variability (CV, as percentage of the range of motion, or ROM). *Source:* Adapted from [31].

motion (FE, LB, AR). At walk, within horse variability (WHV) was lowest at approximately 6% for AR, slightly more for FE (6–8%, but for T6 13.2%) and most for LB (7.8–18.2%). Between horse variability (BHV) was 2–3 times higher than WHV for most rotations and vertebrae, and was again higher for LB (Faber et al. [26]). At trot, LB was the most constant motion (WHV 5.7–8.2%), for FE and AR values it ranged from 5.9 to 12.9%, and with BHV 4–5 times higher than WHV [28]. At canter, WHV was lowest for FE (3.1–9.0%), followed by AR (6.3–11.6%) and LB (8.4–12.5%). Here again, BHV values were much higher (Figure 4.9) [30].

Further Modification of the Skin Marker Measurement Technique

Based on the invasively acquired data, Faber et al. [29] developed and validated a skin marker based method of assessing kinematics that could be used in clinical practice, which is obviously not possible for invasive methods. The method allows for the calculation of ranges of motion of specific vertebrae, which gives an indication of overall spinal mobility, but also for the calculation for so-called angular movement patterns (AMP's). The AMP describes the position of a given vertebra in space with respect to two other vertebrae, one on either side. For example, to calculate the flexion–extension AMP of T10, the 3-D coordinates of T6 and T13 are projected on to the y–z plane and a line (line 1) is drawn between these points. Assuming that the vertebral column is curved according to the bow-and-string concept [2] and that T10 is located midway between T6 and T13, a second line (line 2) is drawn through the projection of T10 and parallel to the first line. The degree of FE for T10 can then be calculated from the orientation of line 2, relative to the horizontal axis. For LB, a similar approach is possible with projection on the x–y plane. AR can only be calculated for the sacrum and is determined from the position of the projection of the tuber coxae markers on the x–z plane, assuming negligible motion in the iliosacral connection [29]. Another parameter that can be used to assess thoracolumbar kinematics is the intravertebral pattern symmetry. For walk and trot, which are symmetrical gaits, the pattern of the AMP during the first half of the stride should be identical to the second half. The amount of similarity, calculated as the correlation coefficient between the patterns during these first and second halves, is called the intravertebral pattern symmetry. The non-invasive skin marker based analysis method was tested for repeatability with respect to day-to-day variation by measuring the same horses on 5 consecutive days, and in 2 lab settings with different breeds of horses (Warmbloods and Standardbreds). There was a high degree of between-stride and between-day repeatability in the spatiotemporal variables and in the time-angle diagrams of the vertebrae studied. Variability between horses was considerably larger for all parameters. Between the two labs and breeds small differences were found in range of motion values. It was concluded that this method for the non-invasive analysis of equine back kinematics provided reliable and repeatable data and hence could be used in a more clinical setting [31]. This validated method has further been optimised and available as a user friendly customised programme (BacKin®1), which has been used successfully in several applications of equine back kinematics for the study of clinical and equestrian questions.

Applied Kinematics of the Equine Back

A number of different parameters have been studied using the marker-based analysis system that was developed after the invasive experiments described above. These include physiological factors that may influence back motion, the effects of therapeutic or diagnostic interventions on back movement, the effect of a saddle, the effect of various head and neck positions on back mobility, the influence of induced fore and hind limb lameness, the influence of naturally and induced occurring back pain, and the effects of chiropractic treatment.

Physiological Factors

Johnston et al. [32,33] focused on physiological factors. In a study on the effect of conformation on back movement they noticed that horses with longer strides have more FE ROM in the caudal saddle region, which was evident only at walk. A long thoracic back resulted in more LB in the lumbar area and there was a negative relationship between the curvature of the midthoracic back and LB at L1/L3 and axial rotation of the pelvis [32]. In

another study that attempted to create a database for normal kinematics of the equine back as a reference source, they measured 33 normally functioning riding horses and evaluated the effect of physiological variables. Significant differences were found with respect to use and gender with larger LB at T10 and T13 for dressage horses compared to show jumpers. Range of motion for LB was greater at T10 in mares compared to geldings, but less at L5. There was a decrease of FE ROM with increasing age [33].

Therapeutic or Diagnostic Interventions

Manual Manipulation and Rehabilitation

Faber et al. [34] used the newly developed technique to assess the effect of manual manipulation on back motion and symmetry of movement. Manual treatment of alleged back problems, according to either chiropractic, osteopathic or other principles, has become very popular in recent years, but is not uncontested. Many professionals still take a very sceptical stance and doubt whether the equine thoracolumbar spine can be manipulated at all by human muscular power. Whether or not manipulation may have some effect, it is certain that the popular belief of "realigning a vertebra" after an alleged "subluxation" is not compatible with the anatomical reality and should be discarded as a possible mechanism [35]. In this case report it was demonstrated that manual treatment indeed could affect vertebral motion patterns and their symmetry and that the effect lasted (partly) for at least 7 months [34]. The *caveat* that comes from this study is that the positive clinical effect did not seem to be directly related to the improved symmetry of movement, but was brought about by a change in trainer.

More studies on the effect of chiropractic manipulations on equine spinal kinematics using much larger numbers of horses have been performed and have confirmed that chiropractic interventions can alter back kinematics. Haussler et al. [36] showed that spinal manipulative therapy had a beneficial effect on thoracolumbar kinematics in horses in which back pain had been induced by the implantation of fixation pins. Sullivan et al. [37] used chiropractic techniques in various groups of asymptomatic horses and could show that manipulation had a more profound effect on back kinematics than massage or treatment with phenylbutazone [38]. Gómez Álvarez et al. [39] used chiropractic treatment in horses with signs of back pain and showed that the main overall effect of manipulation was a less extended thoracic back, a reduced inclination of the pelvis and improvement of the symmetry of the pelvic motion pattern. However, in this study changes in back kinematics were subtle and not all of them were still measurable at a second measurement session 3 weeks after treatment. Spinal kinematics have also been used as an outcome parameter for a study on the effect of a water treadmill exercise. In that study it was shown that there was a significant increase in axial rotation when the water was at the level of the carpus or higher and that lateral bending was significantly reduced with water levels higher than the elbow. Pelvic flexion was increased with regard to baseline at all water levels higher than the hoof [40]. Lastly, spinal kinematics have been used to assess the effects of mobilization exercises of the head and cervical region, aiming at reducing neck pain and improving rehabilitation, following regular practice in the human field [41,42].

Effect of Clinical Pathology

The diagnosis of back pain is a controversial item in itself. Haussler and Erb have introduced the algometer, a device that basically measures the pain threshold when applying pressure to certain areas of the back, as an interesting device that may help in quantifying back pain [43,44]. However, in many studies back pain is diagnosed by (repeated) palpation, which is a largely subjective procedure. Wennerstrand et al. [45] compared sound

horses with horses with back pain and found a reduction in FE and AR ROM in the symptomatic horses, with a concomitant significant decrease in stride length, which is in accordance with earlier reports [34,46]. Lateral bending was increased at T13, possibly as a kind of compensatory motion. Most of these horses suffered from kissing spines or muscle soreness. Diagnoses were made by palpation, radiography and scintigraphy, but no local blocking, was performed. The same group assessed the effect of the application of local anaesthetic blocks in the interspinous spaces (T6–L2) of asymptomatic, clinically sound horses. Local blocks resulted at walk in an increase of ROM of FE in virtually all segments of the back and of LB at T10, L3 and L5. Also lateral excursion (defined as the lateral displacement of the markers T10, T13, T17, L1, L3 and L5 in relation to the line connecting T6 and S3) increased for all segments. At trot, the effect was much less. Also the injection of sodium chloride resulted in increased mobility, though to a lesser degree. The mechanism was thought to act via an influence on proprioception of the multifidus muscle [47]. This muscle is known to play a very important role in the stabilisation of the back in humans and dysfunction of the muscle is a frequent cause of back pain [48]. Recent research suggests a similar role for this muscle in the horse [49].

The influence of lameness on back kinematics and *vice versa* has been a controversial item for a long time. In a field study Landman et al. [50] found indications of both lameness and back pain in 26% of the animals belonging to a relatively large ($N = 805$) population of patients presented for orthopaedic problems. In a presumably asymptomatic control population that consisted of horses presented for prepurchase exams ($N = 399$), concurrence of back problems and lameness was found in 5% only. Dyson [51] diagnosed concurrent forelimb and hindlimb lameness in 46% of horses with thoracolumbar or sacroiliacal pain. Though interesting, the figures give, however, no evidence about a possible causal relationship. In an attempt to learn more about cause and effect, Jeffcott et al. [52]

induced transient back pain in trotters by injecting lactic acid into the epaxial musculature. They did not see an effect on linear and temporal stride parameters (stride length, stride frequency, pro- and retraction angles); a stiffer back was noted, but thoracolumbar kinematics were not quantified.

In a similar study, the same procedure was used in Dutch Warmbloods. There were also no effects on the spatial and temporal gait characteristics, but back kinematics were clearly affected, showing a two-stage response that was attributed to an acute reaction to the painful injection and ensuing muscle stiffness in the following days [53]. From the other side, it has been shown that fore- or hindlimb lameness may alter biomechanics of the back [17,54]. Horses showed a moderate but evident lameness in these studies. The effect of very subtle forelimb lameness on back kinematics have also been studied. It appeared that a very light lameness (maximally 2/5 [55]) increased the vertebral range of motion and changed the pattern of thoracolumbar back movement in the sagittal and horizontal planes, presumably in an attempt to move the centre of gravity away from the lame side and reduce the force in the affected limb [56]. A comparable study in which a subtle lameness was induced in the hindlimbs reported hyperextension and increased ROM of the thoracolumbar back, a decreased ROM of the lumbosacral segment and rotational motion changes of the pelvis [57]. It was concluded that already a slight lameness affects back motion and might hence play a role in the pathogenesis of back problems. It should be stated that these studies have investigated the acute effect of lameness on back motion, whereas in the clinical setting chronic lameness can be presumed to have more influence. Chronic lameness is, however, much more difficult to mimic in an experimental situation.

Performance

In an in-depth longitudinal study on the effects of early training on jumping ability and on the early detection of jumping potential, Santamaría [58] used many kinematic parameters, among which kinematics of the back. It was shown that jumping technique, including the use of the back, to a large extent persisted from foal to adult age [59]. At the end of the 5-year study period, performance was judged by way of a puissance competition. Although back motion in itself was not discriminative between good and bad jumpers, the degree of hind limb retroflexion (*i.e.* backwards extending of the hind limbs relative to the back when clearing the jump) was one of the kinematic parameters that were different between the good and the bad jumpers [60].

Saddlery

De Cocq et al. [61] investigated the effect of a saddle with and without added extra weight on back kinematics. They compared 4 conditions: no tack, a girth, a saddle, and a saddle with 75 kg of lead attached to it in horses walking, trotting and cantering on a treadmill. The weighted saddle appeared to have, at all 3 gaits, an overall extending effect on the back, but ROM remained the same (Figure 4.10). At canter, the same was true for the saddle-only condition. There was a change in limb kinematics too, with forelimb retraction increasing. This observation is nice indirect evidence for the bow-and-string concept: the added weight on the back tends to extend the bow and the horse tries to counteract this influence by more retraction of the forelimbs, which has a flexing effect.

Rhodin et al. [62] and Gómez Álvarez et al. [63] studied the influence of the position of head and neck on back kinematics. The item is of interest from an equestrian viewpoint. The rules of the *Fédération Equestre Internationale* (FEI) describe the desired position of head and neck for most dressage activities as follows: 'The neck should be raised, the poll high and the head slightly in front of the vertical.' This is a position that is considerably more upright than the position the horse will assume by nature. Most classic training systems, which date back hundreds of

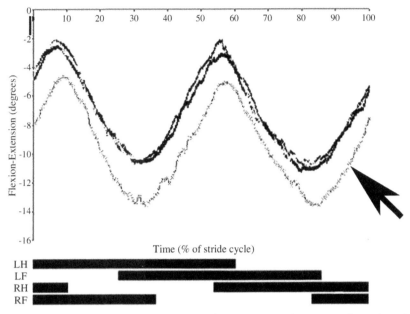

Figure 4.10 A diagram to show the range of motion (ROM) during a single stride cycle of T13 in four conditions: without a saddle, with only a tightened girth, with saddle and tightened girth, and with loaded saddle (75 kg) and tightened girth. Only the last condition (arrow) differed significantly and resulted in an overall increase in extension. However, ROM (maximal flexion minus maximal extension) remained the same. LH: left hind; RH: right hind; LF: left fore; RF: right fore. (Adapted from De Cocq et al. [61] with permission from Equine Veterinary Journal Ltd.)

years [64], use this position, or positions close to it, also during training. However, in the early 1970s it became *en vogue* in show jumping to train horses with a hyperflexed neck and a much lower and deeper position of the head, which is to a certain extent rolled up against the chest. This position was later baptised 'Rollkur' in the German literature [65]. The technique was taken over by a number of dressage riders, some of who became extremely successful, but the technique became heavily disputed because of an alleged impact on animal welfare. This has led to much debate in the lay press [66–68]. In an attempt to objectify the effect of head and neck position Rhodin et al. [69] compared the free or natural position with a higher and a lower position, effectuated by side reins, in unridden horses on a treadmill. They showed a significant reduction of FE and LB ROM of the lumbar back with the head in a high position. Also, AR was reduced. The low position, in which the head and neck were not as hyperflexed as in the 'Rollkur' position, did not differ significantly from the free position, but showed a tendency towards a restriction of movement as well. Gómez Álvarez et al. [63] studied the item more extensively as part of a large international collaborative project in which horses of Grand Prix level were measured while walking and trotting, ridden and unridden, on a treadmill with an inbuilt force plate under simultaneous motion capture by a 12-camera ProReflex[®1] system. Six head and neck positions were studied (Figure 4.11), of which head and neck position (HNP) 2 resembled the position as defined by the FEI rules, and HNP4 came as close as possible to the 'Rollkur' position. It showed that differences in head and neck positions predominantly affected the vertebral angular motion patterns in the sagittal plane (i.e. FE). The positions in which the neck was extended (HNP2, 3, 5) increased extension in the anterior thoracic region, but reduced flexion in the posterior thoracic and lumbar regions. For

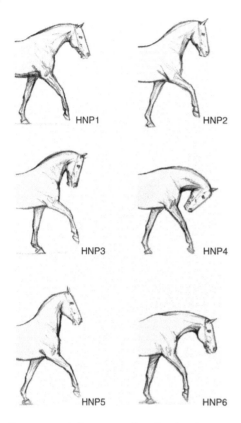

Figure 4.11 A diagram to show head and neck positions (HNPs). HNP1: control (head and neck unrestrained); HNP2: neck raised, bridge of the nose in front of the vertical; HNP3: as HNP2 with bridge of the nose behind the vertical; HNP4: head and neck lowered, nose behind the vertical; HNP5: head and neck in extreme high position; HNP6: head and neck forward downward. (From Gómez Álvarez et al. [63] with permission from Equine Veterinary Journal Ltd.)

HNP4 the pattern was opposite. Flexion–extension ROM was reduced at walk in the lumbar region in HNP2 and 5, and at trot also in HNP3. In HNP5 (extremely high head) the effect was largest and this was the only position in which intravertebral pattern symmetry was negatively affected and hindlimb protraction was reduced. In the low and deep position (HNP4) there was an overall increase in FE ROM, in both the thoracic and the lumbar area (Figure 4.12). It was concluded that a very high position of the head seems to greatly disturb normal kinematics, but that the increased mobility of the back at HNP4 lends some credibility to the statement of a number of trainers that a low position of head and neck may be a useful aid in the gymnastic training of a horse [61]. The analysis system for thoracolumbar kinematics developed by Pourcelot et al. [17] and first applied by Audigié et al. [16] was used to try to discriminate between good and bad jumpers on the basis of back kinematics. Several differences between the groups were found, among which an increased flexion of the thoracolumbar and lumbosacral junction before take-off in the bad jumpers, which might indicate a less efficient strutting action when forward movement is converted into upward movement [70]. During the airborne phase, lumboscral extension was less in the bad jumpers.

Robert et al. [71] used the same technology to analyse the effect of treadmill speed on back kinematics (and muscle activity using surface electromyography). Horses were trotted at speeds from 3.5 to 6 m/s. It was shown that the amplitude (ROM) of FE and the maximal flexion angles decreased with increasing speed, whereas the extension angles remained the same. Muscle activity increased also, confirming the view that the large trunk muscles (*M. longissimus dorsi* and *M. rectus abdominis*) act to restrict back movement, rather than actively enhancing or inducing it.

An entirely different approach was chosen by Keegan *et al.* [72]. They used skin markers in 12 normal and 12 atactic horses and analysed the data by computer-assisted fuzzy clustering techniques that were based on the calculation of signal uncertainty. It appeared that the movement of the lumbar marker (both with respect to LB and FE) was among the few markers that were able to discriminate between normal horses and horses suffering from ataxia.

Conclusions and Possible Future Developments

Much has happened in the field of back kinematics since Jeffcott spoke the following

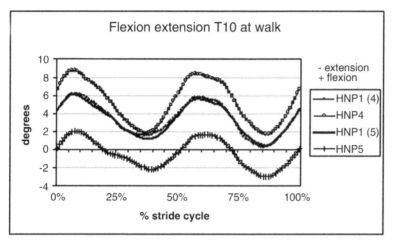

Figure 4.12 A diagram to show flexion–extension angular motion pattern (AMP) of one horse (T10 at walk). The curves represent head and neck positions 4 (HNP4) and 5 (HNP5). HNPs were compared with speed-matched trials with the head and neck in the natural position, indicated as HNP1 (4) and HNP1 (5). The stride cycle starts with the left front limb. (From Gómez Álvarez et al. [63] with permission from Equine Veterinary Journal Ltd.)

words during the 4th Sir Frederick Hobday Memorial Lecture in 1979: 'The biomechanics of the equine thoracolumbaspine have been considered to some extent, but it requires much greater study if the pathogenesis of the various thoracolumbar disorders are to be properly understood' [35]. We have since learnt much about the maximal ranges of motion of various segments of the equine thoracolumbar spine and the anatomical constraints that limit these motions through both *ex vivo* and *in vivo* research. The clinical evaluation of the motion pattern of the equine back is as difficult as it was in the 1970s, but kinematic analysis techniques have improved vastly and we are now able to document the kinematics of the equine back in a reliable and repeatable way in terms of ranges of motion and angular motion patterns of individual vertebrae, even if these values are not greater than a few cm or a couple of degrees. We should, however, recognize that the general drawbacks of kinematical analysis when used for diagnostic purposes still apply. Aberrant kinematic patterns are in most cases not very specific indicators of back pathology because there are many more possible pathological conditions than ways horses can alter their locomotion pattern. Further, there is a large grey area between normal and pathologic locomotion patterns. Because in patients almost invariably no kinematic data are available that were captured prior to the onset of the problem and individual variation in gait patterns is large, it is often impossible to draw conclusions based on a single measurement [73]. It has become clear that the item of individual variation is important, particularly in the case of thoracolumbar kinematics, especially at the walk and the canter and with respect to LB [26,30].

The measurement of back kinematics now has become a standard element of various analysis protocols for equine kinematics and back kinematics have been used very successfully to assess the effect of a number of conditions and interventions on equine motion. Because the back bridges the gap between the four extremities and back kinematics reflect, through the bow-and-string principle, what happens to the trunk, back kinematics are an excellent parameter to study the influence of any intervention on the animal as a whole. There is a need for hard, scientific data in this area, as has been demonstrated by the discussion on the use of the 'rollkur', 'overbended' or 'hyperflexed' position of the head in dressage training, which was based on emotion and prejudice rather than on scientifically proven facts. It should be realised, however, that in items where the ethical acceptability of certain practices is questioned, a more comprehensive approach is required and biomechanical data will have to be complemented by facts from entirely different disciplines.

Telling the future is a hazardous undertaking, but it takes little imagination to predict that, as in any branch of kinematics, modelling will become more important in the study of equine thoracolumbar kinematics. Preliminary studies have already been published by the group from Vienna, who presented a segmental model of the back and simulated a regional increase in stiffness to study the effect on back motion as a whole [74,75] and compared the outcome to data generated by *ex vivo* measurements on dissected spines [76]. As with any model, there is a risk that these models are going to lead a life on their own and the validation with *in vivo* acquired data remains essential. Generating good quality input data on equine back movement for these models is not very easy, and neither is the refining of the model to approach real-life conditions, given the complex structure of the back. However, more and more input data on back kinematics, force distribution under the saddle and muscle activity are becoming available, making input from more than only kinematic data in the model possible [77]. Also, developments in the modelling and animation area, partly driven by the entertainment industry, happen fast. There is little doubt that much progress will be made in the next few years. Progress in modelling of back function has not been as fast as expected over the last 10 years, which may have been due to a larger emphasis on directly applicable research, but there is little doubt this avenue will be further explored in the future.

Models may teach us more about the general reaction pattern of the equine back, but are less suitable for use in individual cases. In recent years, inertial motion unit (IMU) technology has taken a great leap. The advantage of IMUs is their easy applicability, making them very well suited for measurements outside the lab under real field conditions. Much of the work in recent years has focused on asymmetry measurements and use for lameness detection and quantification [78]. Specific use for the quantification of back motion has been limited thus far. In a study that compared (gold standard) motion capture with IMUs to quantify spinal motion, IMUs showed acceptable accuracy and good consistency for back movement. However, the small lateral bending ROM meant that changes <25% in ROM went undetected [79]. The relatively small amplitude of spinal rotations and the strong mutual influence of especially lateral bending and axial rotation may make IMU technology not the best option to capture spinal motion.

Combining data generated by the capture of back kinematics with data from other new technologies, such as saddle pressure measurement devices [80], may allow for the monitoring of subtle changes in the motion pattern of the equine athlete. Such an individualised monitoring programme, which may include other aspects of health and soundness as well, may lead to the early detection of abnormalities and hence permit timely and adequate preventive measures. In man, such an individualised approach to peculiarities of gait [81] or to the adaptation of gait to, for instance, special shoes [82] is not uncommon. Pattern recognition has been applied to horse–rider interaction as well [83]. These coaching and monitoring programmes for performance horses will never be a substitute for good horsemanship. However, they may support the good horseman in his or her decisions and they may be of help in the frequent cases of bad horsemanship, thus promoting the well-being of the horse for the benefit of the horse itself and its users.

References

1 Van Weeren, P.R. History of locomotor research. In: Back, W. and Clayton, H.M. (eds), *Equine Locomotion*, 2nd edn, pp. 1–30. London: Saunders Elsevier, 2013, pp. 1–30.

2 Slijper, E.J. Comparative biologic-anatomical investigations on the vertebral column and spinal musculature of mammals. *Proceedings of K. Ned. Acad. Wetensch.* 1946; **42**:1–128.

3 Bergmann, C. Über die Verhältnisse der Wärme-Ökonomie der Thiere zu ihrer Grösse. *Göttinger Studien* 1847; **3**:595–708.

4 Krüger, W. Über Schwingungen der Wirbelsäule – Insbesondere der Wirbelbrücke- des Pferdes Während der Bewegung. *Berl. Münchn. Tierärztl. Wschr.* 1939; **13**:129–133.

5 Zschokke, E. *Untersuchungen über das Verhältnis der Knochenbildung zur Statik und Mechanik des Vertebraten-skelettes.* Zürich: Orell Fusli, 1892.

6 Barthez, P.J. *Nouvelle Mécanique des Mouvements de l'Homme et des Animaux.* Paris: Carcassonne, 1798.

7 Koch, T. *Lehrbuch der Veterinär-Anatomie*, Bd. I: Bewegungsapparat. Jena: VEB Gustav Fischer Verlag, 1970, pp. 281–334.

8 Jeffcot, L.B. and Dalin, G. Natural rigidity of the horse's backbone. *Equine Veterinary Journal* 1980; **12**:101–108.

9 Townsend, H.G., Leach, D. and Fretz, P.B. Kinematics of the equine thoracolumbar spine. *Equine Veterinary Journal* 1983; **15**:117–122.

10 Townsend, H.G. and Leach, D. Relationship between intervertebral joint morphology and mobility in the equine thoracolumbar spine. *Equine Veterinary Journal* 1984; **16**:461–465.

11 Denoix, J.M. Kinematics of the thoracolumbar spine in the horse during dorsoventral movements: a preliminary report. In: Gillespie, J.R. and Robinson, N.E. (eds), *Proceedings of the 2nd International Conference on Equine Exercise and Physiology*, Davis, CA: ICEEP Publications, 1987, pp. 607–614.

12 Denoix, J.M. Aspects fonctionnels des régions lombo-sacrale et sacro-iliaque du cheval. *Pract. Vet. Equine* 1992; **24**:13–21.

13 Degueurce, C., Chateau, H. and Denoix, J.M. *In vitro* assessment of the sacroiliac joint in the horse. *Equine Veterinary Journal* 2004; **36**:694–698.

14 Goff, L.M., Jasiewicz, J., Jeffcott, L.B. et al. Movement between the equine ilium and sacrum: *in vivo* and *in vitro* studies. *Equine Veterinary Journal* 2006; Suppl., **36**:457–461.

15 Fredricson, I. and Drevemo, S. A new method of investigating equine locomotion. *Equine Veterinary Journal* 1971; **3**:137–140.

16 Audigié, F., Pourcelot, P., Degeurce, C., Denoix, J.M. and Geiger, D. Kinematics of the equine back: flexion-extension movements in sound trotting horses. *Equine Veterinary Journal* 1999; Suppl., **30**:210–213.

17 Pourcelot, P., Audigié, F., Degeurce, C., Denoix, J.M. and Geiger, D. Kinematics of the equine back: a method to study the thoracolumber flexion–extension movements at the trot. *Veterinary Research* 1998; **29**:519–525.

18 Tokuriki, M., Nakada, A., and Aoki, O. Electromyographic activity of trunk muscles in the horse during locomotion and synaptic connections of neurons of trunk muscles in the cat. In: *Proceedings of First (ESB) Workshop on Animal Locomotion*, Utrecht, the Netherlands, 1991, p. 36.

19 Licka, T.F., Peham, C. and Frey, A. Electromyographic activity of the longissimus dorsi muscles in horses during trotting on a treadmill. *American Journal of Veterinary Research* 2004; **65**:155–158.

20 Licka, T. and Peham, C. An objective method for evaluating the flexibility of the back of standing horses. *Equine Veterinary Journal* 1998; **30**:412–415.

21 Peham, C., Frey, A., Lickla, T. and Scheidl, M. Evaluation of the EMG activity of the long back muscle during induced back movements at stance. *Equine Veterinary Journal* 2001; Suppl., **33**:165–168.

22 Fick, R. Allgemeine Gelenk- und Muskelmechanik. In: von Bardeleben, K. (ed.), *Handbuch der Anatomie des Menschen*, Bd. 2, Abt. 1, Teil 2. Jena, 1910.

23 Denoix, J.M. Spinal biomechanics and functional anatomy. *Veterinary Clinics of North America: Equine Practice* 1999; **15**:27–60.

24 Haussler, K.K., Bertram, J.A.E., Gellman, K. and Hermanson, J.W. Dynamic analysis of *in vivo* segmental spinal motion: an instrumentation strategy. *Veterinary Comp. Orthopaedics and Traumatology* 2000; **13**:9–17.

25 Haussler, K.K., Bertram, J.E.A., Gellman, K. and Hermanson, J.W. Segmental *in vivo* vertebral kinematics at the walk, trot and canter: a preliminary study. *Equine Veterinary Journal* 2001; Suppl., **33**:160–164.

26 Faber, M.J., Schamhardt, H.C., van Weeren, P.R. et al. Basic three-dimensional kinematics of the vertebral column of horses walking on a treadmill. *American Journal of Veterinary Research* 2000; **61**:399–406.

27 Faber, M., Schamhardt, H.C. and van Weeren, P.R. Determination of 3D spinal kinematics without defining a local vertebral co-ordinate system. *Journal of Biomechanics* 1999; **32**:1355–1358.

28 Faber, M.J., Johnston, C., Schamhardt, H.C. et al. Basic three-dimensional kinematics of the vertebral column of horses trotting on a treadmill. *American Journal of Veterinary Research* 2001; **62**:757–764.

29 Faber, M.J., Schamhardt, H.C., van Weeren, P.R. and Barneveld, A. Methodology and validity of assessing kinematics of the thoracolumbar vertebral column in horses based on skin-fixated markers. *American Journal of Veterinary Research* 2001; **62**:301–306.

30 Faber, M.J., Johnston, C., Schamhardt, H.C. et al. Three-dimensional kinematics of the equine spine during canter. *Equine Veterinary Journal* 2001; Suppl., **33**,145–149.

31 Faber, M.J., Johnston, C., van Weeren, P.R. and Barneveld, A. Repeatability of back kinematics in horses during treadmill locomotion. *Equine Veterinary Journal* 2002; **34**:235–241.

32 Johnston, C., Holm, K., Faber, M. et al. Effect of conformational aspects on the movement of the equine back. *Equine Veterinary Journal* 2002; Suppl., **34**:314–318.

33 Johnston, C., Roethlisberger-Holm, K., Erichsen, C., Eksell, P. and Drevemo, S. Kinematic evaluation of the back in fully functioning riding horses. *Equine Veterinary Journal* 2004; **36**:495–498.

34 Faber, M., van Weeren, P.R., Scheepers, M. and Barneveld, A. Long-term follow-up of manipulative treatment in a horse with back problems. *Journal of Veterinary Medicine A. Physiology and Pathology in Clinical Medicine* 2003; **50**:241–245.

35 Jeffcott, L.B. Back problems in the horse – A look at past, present and future progress. *Equine Veterinary Journal* 1979; **11**:129–136.

36 Haussler, K.K., Hill, A.E., Puttlitz, C.M. and McIlwraith, C.W. Effects of vertebral mobilization and manipulation on kinematics of the thoracolumbar region. *American Journal of Veterinary Research* 2007; **68**:508–516.

37 Sullivan, K.A., Hill, A.E. and Haussler, K.K. The effects of chiropractic, massage and phenylbutazone on spinal mechanical nociceptive thresholds in horses without clinical signs. *Equine Veterinary Journal* 2008; **40**:14–20.

38 Haussler, K.K., Martin, C.E. and Hill, A.E. Efficacy of spinal manipulation and mobilisation on trunk flexibility and stiffness in horses: a randomised clinical trial. *Equine Veterinary Journal* 2010, November; Suppl., **38**:695–702.

39 Gómez Álvarez, C.B., l'Ami, J.J., Moffatt, D., Back, W. and van Weeren, P.R. Effect of chiropractic manipulations on the kinematics of back and limbs in horses with clinically diagnosed back problems. *Equine Veterinary Journal* 2008; **40**:153–159.

40 Mooij, M.J., Jans, W., den Heijer, G.J., de Pater, M. and Back, W. Biomechanical responses of the back of riding horses to water treadmill exercise. *Veterinary Journal* 2013, December; **198**(1): e120–3.

41 Clayton, H.M., Kaiser, L.J., Lavagnino, M. and Stubbs, N.C. Dynamic mobilisations in cervical flexion: Effects on intervertebral angulations. *Equine Veterinary Journal* 2010; Suppl., **38**:688–694.

42 Clayton, H.M., Kaiser, L.J., Lavagnino, M. and Stubbs, N.C. Evaluation of intersegmental vertebral motion during performance of dynamic mobilization exercises in cervical lateral bending in horses. *American Journal of Veterinary Research* 2012; **73**:1153–1159.

43 Haussler, K.K. and Erb, H.N. Mechanical nociceptive thresholds in the axial skeleton of horses. *Equine Veterinary Journal* 2006; **38**:70–75.

44 Haussler, K.K. and Erb, H.N. Pressure algometry for the detection of induced back pain in horses: A preliminary study. *Equine Veterinary Journal* 2006; **38**:76–81.

45 Wennerstrand, J., Johnston, C., Roethlisberger-Holm, K. et al. Kinematic evaluation of the back in the sport horse with back pain. *Equine Veterinary Journal* 2004; **36**:707–711.

46 Jeffcott, L.B. Disorders of the thoracolumbar spine of the horse – A survey of 443 cases. *Equine Veterinary Journal* 1980; **12**:197–210.

47 Roethlisberger Holm, K., Wennerstrand, J., Lagerquist, U., Eksell, P. and Johnston, C. Effect of local analgesia on movement of the equine back. *Equine Veterinary Journal* 2006; **38**:65–69.

48 San Juan, J.G., Yaggie, J.A., Levy, S.S. et al. Effects of pelvic stabilization on lumbar muscle activity during dynamic exercise. *Journal of Strength. Cond. Research* 2005; **19**:903–907.

49 Stubbs, N.C., Hodges, P.W. Jeffcott, L.B. et al. Functional anatomy of the caudal thoracolumbar and lumbosacral spine in the horse. *Equine Veterinary Journal* 2006; Suppl., **36**:393–399.

50 Landman, M.A.A.M., de Blaauw, J.A., van Weeren, P.R. and Hofland, L.J. Lameness prevalence in horses with back problems compared to a control population: a field study. *Veterinary Records* 2004; **155**:165–168.

51 Dyson, S. The interrelationships between back pain and lameness: A diagnostic challenge. *Proceedings of the Congress on British Equine Veterinary Association* 2005; **44**:137–138.

52 Jeffcott, L.B., Dalin, G., Drevemo, S. et al. Effect of induced back pain on gait and performance of trotting horses. *Equine Veterinary Journal* 1982; **14**:129–133.

53 Wennerstrand, J., Gómez Alvarez, C.B., Meulenbelt, R. et al. Spinal kinematics in horses with induced back pain. *Veterinary Comparative Orthopaedics and Traumatology* 2009; **22**:448–454.

54 Buchner, H., Savelberg, H., Schamhardt, H. and Barneveld, A. Head and trunk movement adaptations in horses with experimentally induced fore- or hind limb lameness. *Equine Veterinary Journal* 1996; **28**:71–76.

55 Stashak, T.S. Examination for lameness. In: Stashak, T.S. (ed.), *Adams' Lameness in Horses*, 4th edn. Baltimore, MD: Lippincott, Williams & Wilkins, 2002, p. 122.

56 Gómez Álvarez, C.B., Wennerstrand, J. Bobbert, M.F. et al. The effect of induced forelimb lameness on the thoracolumbar kinematics in riding horses. *Equine Veterinary Journal* 2007; **39**:197–201.

57 Gómez Álvarez C.B., Bobbert, M.F., Lamers, L. et al. The effect of induced hindlimb lameness on thoracolumbar kinematics during treadmill locomotion. *Equine Veterinary Journal* 2008; **40**: 147–152.

58 Santamaría, S. From foal to performer: Development of the jumping technique and the effect of early training. Thesis, Utrecht University, 2004.

59 Santamaría, S., Bobbert, M.F., Back, W., Barneveld, A. and van Weeren, P.R. Evaluation of consistency of jumping technique in horses between the ages of 6 months and 4 years. *American Journal of Veterinary Research* 2004; **65**:945–990.

60 Bobbert, M.F., Santamaría, S., van Weeren, P.R., Back, W. and Barneveld, A. Can jumping capacity of adult show jumping horses be predicted on the basis of submaximal free jumps at foal age? A longitudinal study. *Veterinary Journal* 2005; **170**:212–221.

61 De Cocq, P., van Weeren, P.R. and Back, W. Effects of girth, saddle and weight on movements of the horse. *Equine Veterinary Journal* 2004; **36**:758–763.

62 Rhodin, M., Johnston, C., Holm, K.R., Wennerstrand, J. and Drevemo, S. The influence of head and neck position on kinematics of the back in riding horses at the walk and trot. *Equine Veterinary Journal* 2005; **37**:7–11.

63 Gómez Álvarez, C.B., Rhodin, M., Bobbert, M.F. et al. The effect of head and neck position on the thoracolumbar kinematics in the unridden horse. *Equine Veterinary Journal* 2006; Suppl., **36**:445–451.

64 Decarpentry, A. *Academic Equitation.* (Translated from the 2nd revised edn of *Equitation Académique*). London: J.A. Allen & Co. Ltd, 1971.

65 Meyer, H. Rollkur. *St. Georg* 1992; **11**,70–73.

66 Balkenhol, K., Müller, H., Plewa, M. and Heuschmann, G. Zur Entfaltung kommen – Statt zur Brust genommen. *Reiter Revue* 2003; **46**(2):46–51.

67 Janssen, S. Zur Brust genommen. *Reiter Revue* 2003; **46**(2):41–45.

68 Schrijer, S. and van Weeren, P.R. Auf dem falschen Rücken ausgetragen. *Reiter Revue* 2003; **46**(7):13–15.

69 Rhodin, M., Gómez Alvarez, C.B., Byström, A. et al. The effect of different head and neck positions on the caudal back and hindlimb kinematics in the elite dressage horse at trot. *Equine Veterinary Journal* 2009; **41**:274–279.

70 Cassiat, G., Pourcelot, P., Tavernier, L. et al. Influence of individual competition level on back kinematics of horses jumping a vertical fence. *Equine Veterinary Journal* 2004; **36**:748–753.

71 Robert, C., Audigié, F., Valette, J.P., Pourcelot, P. and Denoix, J.-M. Effects of treadmill speed on the mechanics of the back in the trotting saddlehorse. *Equine Veterinary Journal* 2001; Suppl., **33**:154–159.

72 Keegan, K.G., Arafat, S., Skubic, M. et al. Detection of spinal ataxia in horses using fuzzy clustering of body position uncertainty. *Equine Veterinary Journal* 2004; **36**:712–717.

73 Van Weeren, P.R. The clinical applicability of automated gait analysis systems. *Equine Veterinary Journal* 2002; **34**:218–219.

74 Peham, C. and Schobesberger, H. Influence of the load of a rider or of a region with increased stiffness on the equine back: A modelling study. *Equine Veterinary Journal* 2004; **37**:703–705.

75 Peham, C. and Schobesberger, H. A novel method to estimate the stiffness of the equine back. *Journal of Biomechanics* 2006; **39**:2845–2849.

76 Schlacher, C., Peham, C., Licka, T. and Schobesberger, H. Determination of the stiffness of the equine spine. *Equine Veterinary Journal* 2004; **36**:699–702.

77 Groesel, M., Zsoldos, R.R., Kotschwar, A., Gfoehler, M. and Peham, C. A preliminary

model study of the equine back including activity of longissimus dorsi muscle. *Equine Veterinary Journal* 2010; Suppl., **38**:401–406.

78 Keegan, K.G., Kramer, J., Yonezawa, Y. et al. Assessment of repeatability of a wireless, inertial sensor-based lameness evaluation system for horses. *American Journal of Veterinary Research* 2011; **72**:1156–1163.

79 Warner, S.M., Koch, T.O. and Pfau, T. Inertial sensors for assessment of back movement in horses during locomotion over ground. *Equine Veterinary Journal* 2010; Suppl., **38**:417–424.

80 Von Rechenberg, B. Saddle evaluation; poor fit contributing to back problems in horses. In: Auer, J.A. and Stick, J.A. (eds), *Equine Surgery*, 3rd edn. St Louis, MO: Saunders, 2006, pp. 963–971.

81 Schöllhorn, W.I., Nigg, B.M., Stefanshyn, D. and Liu, W. Identification of individual walking patterns using time discrete and time continuous data sets. *Gait Posture* 2002; **15**:180–186.

82 Nigg, B.M., Khan, A., Fisher, V. and Stefanshyn, D. Effect of shoe insert construction on foot and leg movement. *Medical Science and Sport Exercise* 1998; **30**:550–555.

83 Schöllhorn, W.I., Peham, C., Licka, T.F. and Scheidl, M. A pattern recognition approach for the quantification of horse and rider interactions. *Equine Veterinary Journal* 2006; Suppl., **36**:400–405.

5

Neurological Examination of the Back and Pelvis

Constanze Fintl

Introduction

A general neurological assessment, including that of the back and pelvis, is usually performed while doing the routine physical examination. Further evaluation may be necessary if the clinician is alerted to apparent neurological deficits or if a lesion must be ruled out as part of a clinical investigation. In some cases of back or pelvic pathology, gait abnormalities or neurological deficits similar to those seen in neurological cases are detected. Therefore a sound knowledge of the neurological examination of the horse and some of the normal variations that can be expected is very important. Although this chapter is predominantly concerned with the examination of the back and pelvis, it is important that these findings are not interpreted in isolation but included in the overall neurological evaluation of the horse. The primary aim of the neurological examination is to determine if a neurological abnormality exists, and if so to localise the lesion(s) anatomically. Once the lesion(s) has been localised, a list of differential diagnoses can be generated and further diagnostic tests targeted. The following description of a neurological examination is based on that described by Mayhew [1].

History

A systematic approach is essential to any clinical investigation and a natural starting point is to obtain a full history containing relevant information such as age, breed and use of the animal. An attempt should be made to establish the time of onset, duration of the problem and progression of the perceived abnormality, and obviously whether there is any history of trauma. Vaccination history may also be of relevance, particularly if more than one animal is affected or new arrivals have recently been introduced into a yard. A number of important infectious diseases of horses are recognised to cause neurological deficits; these include equine herpesvirus type 1 (EHV 1), West Nile virus and equine protozoal myeloencephalitis (EPM). The latter (EPM) should be considered a differential diagnosis in those parts of the world where it is found, particularly if asymmetric focal or multifocal neurologic deficits are evident.

Examination at Rest

Once a thorough history has been obtained, the neurological examination begins with observing the horse at rest. This includes assessing any changes in behaviour or demeanour such as circling, head turning (head and neck turned to one side) or head pressing, which may indicate forebrain disease. Similarly, any evidence of postural deficits should be assessed. The neurological examination then continues by assessing simple and complex reflex pathways, testing both

Equine Neck and Back Pathology: Diagnosis and Treatment, Second Edition. Edited by Frances M.D. Henson.
© 2018 John Wiley & Sons, Ltd. Published 2018 by John Wiley & Sons, Ltd.

afferent sensory and efferent motor fibres that will help the examiner localise the anatomical site of any lesion(s).

Palpation

Palpation assessing evidence of localised pain, muscle wastage and asymmetry, as well as feeling for areas of focal sweating or areas of reduced skin sensitivity, should be performed next. Hypalgesia and analgesia of cutaneous areas of the skin are good indications of a primary neurological lesion [2]. In contrast, although increased sensitivity or pain may be indicative of a primary neurological lesion, it is more likely to result from inflammation at the level of pain receptors in peripheral tissues, such as muscles, ligaments and joints [1,2].

Sweating

Areas of localised sweating may also be of help when attempting to determine the anatomical site of a lesion and hence any such abnormalities should be carefully documented in terms of the precise anatomical location. Ipsilateral sweating caudal to the lesion indicates involvement of descending sympathetic tracts in the spinal cord while lesions involving specific pre- or postganglionic peripheral sympathetic fibres (second- or third-order neurons) cause well-demarcated dermatomal areas of sweating at the level of the lesion [1].

Cranial Nerve Assessment

Cranial nerve function is evaluated by assessing functional afferent and efferent pathways such as the pupillary right reflex and menace response rather than examining each one of these nerves individually. The reader is referred to specialised neurological texts [1,3,4] for details on performing a full examination of these. Table 5.1 summarises the different cranial nerves and their main function(s).

Reflex and Function Tests

After assessing if there is evidence of forebrain or cranial nerve abnormalities, an evaluation of the neck, forelimbs, trunk, hindlimbs, tail and anus should be performed. Evaluation of reflex arcs in these anatomical areas, some

Table 5.1 Summary of cranial nerves and their main function(s).

Cranial nerve	Cranial nerve function	Sensory (S), motor (M) and/or autonomic (A) function
I Olfactory	Olfaction	S
II Optic	Vision	S
III Occulomotor	Medial movement of globe, constricts pupil	M/A
IV Trochlear	Ventrolateral rotation of globe	M
V Trigeminal	Mastication, facial sensation	S/M
VI Abducens	Lateral rotation of globe, retracts eyeball	M
VII Facial	Muscles of facial expression	S/M/A
VIII Vestibulocochlear	Hearing, balance	S
IX Glossopharyngeal	Taste, swallowing	S/M/A
X Vagus	Laryngeal muscles, swallowing	S/M/A
XI Accessory	Innervates trapezius, brachiocephalicus (sternocephalicus)	M
XII Hypoglossal	Moves tongue	M

of which also involve higher centres, is an important part of the neurological examination and can be very useful in localising a lesion to a certain area of the central or peripheral nervous systems. They include cervical (and cervicothoracic) spinal cord reflexes such as the cervicofacial and local cervical reflexes. A third reflex, the thoracolaryngeal test ('slap test'), has also been described [5].

Cervicofacial and Local Cervical Reflexes

The exact anatomical pathways for the cervicofacial and local cervical reflexes are not precisely determined but it is hypothesised that they may involve sensory afferents and motor efferents of the particular local cervical spinal nerves as well as the facial nucleus in the medulla [1,6,7]. These reflex pathways are assessed by tapping the neck with a blunt instrument, which should result in contraction of facial muscles (seen as a lower lip curl of withdrawal) and the *cutaneous colli* respectively. Suppression of the latter two reflexes may suggest a lesion, or lesions, at any of these points, although it is worth noting that individual variability in the degree of response to this test exists so some caution in interpretation is warranted. Some very stoical horses will show very little response to stimulation.

Cutaneous, i.e. somatic afferent, sensation is best assessed using a so-called 'two-step' test described by Bailey and Kitchell [8]. In this test a fold of skin is grasped between a pair of artery forceps and once the horse has adjusted to this, a short, sharp squeeze should be performed in order to elicit a response.

Thoracolaryngeal Reflex ('Slap Test')

The 'slap test' was originally described as an aid to assess the function of the vagal or recurrent laryngeal nerves as well as the cervicothoracic spinal cord [5]. However, a more recent publication showed that the positive predictive value of the 'slap test' is low [9] and should be used with caution.

The reflex test is performed by slapping the skin just caudal to the dorsal part of the scapula with a flattened hand, whilst the other hand is used to palpate the contralateral dorsal and lateral laryngeal musculature over the muscular processes of the arytenoid cartilage. In normal horses the response to the slap is to briefly adduct the contralateral arytenoid cartilage, which can be felt as a gentle flutter under the fingers. In some cases it is difficult to palpate the response and endoscopy may be necessary to visualise the arytenoids during the test.

The laryngeal adductor reflex tests both afferent and efferent pathways. The afferent pathway is via the sensory receptors of somatic sensation and pain that send nerve fibres to the spinal cord. These fibres ascend to the medulla, where they send branches to the vagal nuclei as they ascend towards the somatosensory cortex and pain recognition areas. The efferent pathway is through the vagal nerve, which descends to the cranial thorax, and then the laryngeal branch ascends back to the larynx in the recurrent laryngeal nerve. Damage to any part of this pathway can lead to failure of the horse to respond to the laryngeal adductor reflex.

Thoracic Limbs and Trunk Reflexes

Examination of the thoracic limbs and the trunk also involves assessing reflex pathways. Cutaneous areas for the equine thoracic limbs have been electrophysiologically mapped and areas of single nerve supply (autonomous zones) have been determined [10]; hence sensory deficits of this region may sometimes be precisely located.

Tapping the side of the trunk should elicit contraction of the *cutaneous trunci* muscle (incorrectly referred to as the 'panniculus reflex'). This reflex relies on sensory information travelling to the spinal cord through thoracospinal nerves where the impulse is continued cranially to the C8–T1 segment of the spinal cord. This segment is the principal supply of the lateral thoracic nerve, of which stimulation results in contraction of the *cutaneous trunci* muscle. A spinal cord lesion interfering with this reflex must therefore be located cranially to the area being tested. This reflex may not occur caudal to the midlumbar region and again there may be individual differences in the degree of response to this test [3].

Back and Pelvis

Further assessment of the back and pelvis is performed by assessing the vertebra prominens reflex [11]. Pinching and pressing down on the thoracolumbar or lumbosacral paravertebral muscles causes a normal animal to extend (i.e. dorsiflex or dip) the thoracolumbar vertebral column, but should not result in hyperextension and buckling of the pelvic limbs unless there is abnormal weakness present. Pressure applied at the lumbosacral junction elicits the same reflex but with more obvious tilting up of the pelvis with enhancement of the supporting reaction in the hind limbs. If pressure is applied over the croup there is flexion of the lumbosacral joint as well as other limb joints. The afferent limb of this reflex must be through the dorsal branches of the sacral nerves but the efferent limb is not known [11]. In clinical cases, failure to move the back appropriately in response to stimulation may be due to a neurological problem, but is usually considered to be due to pain secondary to primary back pathology.

The ability of the horse to laterally flex the thoracic and lumbar vertebral column can be assessed by firmly stroking the skin overlying the *longissimus dorsi* musculature with a blunt instrument. Contraction of this muscle should result in lateral flexion [12]. Failure to do so may indicate a neurological deficit, particularly if severe muscle atrophy is present. However, as described above, reluctance to laterally flex the vertebral column is usually considered to be due to primary back pathology. Lesions affecting thoracolumbar grey matter cause muscle atrophy and asymmetric myelopathies may result in scoliosis of the thoracolumbar vertebral column with initially

the concave side opposite the site of the lesion [1].

Unlike in the thoracic limb, electrophysiologically mapped cutaneous areas and autonomous zones have not yet been described in the pelvic limb and assessment of the individual nerve supply is based on the topographical anatomy of the individual peripheral nerves [13,14], as depicted in Chapter 4.

Perineal Reflexes and Tail Tone

Having neurologically evaluated the thoracolumbar areas the clinician should next focus on the sacral region. Tail tone should be examined first. A normal tail hangs in a relaxed fashion. However, when handled or grasped, usually a horse will clamp the tail down. Horses with reduced or absent tail tone have a 'floppy' tail, although vast individual variation in the degree of tone and how easily the tail can be manipulated can make interpretation difficult. In addition to tail tone, anal tone should be evaluated. Anal tone is considered to be the degree of tightness with which the external anal sphincter is closed. A brisk stimulus should typically result in contraction of the anal sphincter muscle and clamping down of the tail [1]. A loss of tone in the tail implicates a lesion involving the caudal nerves or spinal cord segments, while a loss of anal tone implicates a sacral nerve or spinal cord segment lesion [3].

Finally, the perineal reflex should be tested, which assesses both sacral and caudal segments and nerves. Stimulation of this area should therefore result in both contraction of the anal sphincter and clamping of the tail [1,3]. It is also important to evaluate if the horse is able to perceive the sensation centrally, and not just performing a segmental reflex action in order to differentiate sensory and motor deficits if the reflex response is reduced or absent. This can be achieved by observing the head of the horse whilst stimulation occurs to see if it turns to the stimulus or shows other signs of perceiving the stimulus such as a laying back of the ears.

Examination of Posture and Gaits

Evaluation of posture and gait is an essential part of the neurological examination in order to determine which limbs are affected but also to assess if any abnormalities present could be caused by lameness. Neurological gait abnormalities will reveal signs of paresis (weakness) and/or ataxia (abnormalities of proprioception. Paresis may involve flexor or extensor muscle groups. Ataxia can be characterised as having components of hypermetria (high striding) or hypometria (spasicity). These abnormalities of gait may be associated with brainstem, cerebellar, spinal cord, lower motor neuron (LMN) or peripheral neuromuscular lesion(s) [1].

Although the following discussion will focus on evaluating the posture and gait of the pelvic limbs it is again important to emphasise that these findings must be incorporated in the overall neurological assessment. As part of this assessment it is clearly essential to also evaluate the posture and gait of the thoracic limbs, although this discussion is based on the assumption of no detectable abnormalities of these.

Evaluation of Weakness

The examination should begin with assessment of the gait when the horse is walked in hand. Evidence of flexor weakness may be evident if the horse has a low arc of foot flight, stumbles easily, or scuffing of its toes.

Extensor weakness may be evident if the horse is easily pulled to the side while standing still or walking, buckling on a limb when turning and trembling of the muscles to the limb(s). Extensor weakness may be caused by lesions affecting descending upper motor neuron (UMN) tracts, ventral grey matter or peripheral nerves to the main extensor muscles. If extensor weakness is only evident while walking it is suggestive of a UMN lesion. This is further supported by the finding that if a tail pull is performed with the horse standing still, the extensor reflex is indeed exacerbated. This occurs as the UMN is no longer able to dampen down this reflex. No evidence of weakness during this test also suggests that the LMN as well as peripheral nerves and neuromuscular end plates are all intact. In contrast, if there are lesions present in the latter, it is usually easy to pull the horse to the side both while walking and while standing still. If only one limb is affected it is reasonable to assume that the horse has a peripheral nerve (LMN) or muscle lesion in that limb [1], although it must be recognised that this assumption does not apply in cases of EPM. Stumbling, a low foot flight and/or dragging of the toe may be indicative of flexor weakness, particularly while turning.

In addition to the tail pull test there are other clinical tests described to ascertain weakness. Subtle signs of weakness in both pelvic and thoracic limbs may be exacerbated by pulling on the tail and head collar concurrently while circling the horse, while thoracic limb weakness may be further assessed by performing a hopping test.

Evaluation of Ataxia

When evaluating possible signs of ataxia it is important to carefully evaluate the horse at rest as well as during movement. The normal horse will stand 'four square' and will not position its limbs in unusual positions without correcting this quickly. Next the horse should be evaluated at walk and the stride length should be assessed for asymmetry or irregularity. This is best performed with the examiner walking parallel with the horse. The gait should also be evaluated for signs of hypermetria (high striding) or hypometria (spasticity) or a combination of these (dysmetria). Subtle signs may be made more evident if the horse is made to suddenly stop or back up as well as by making these manoeuvres from trot. When backing the ataxic horse careful attention to the pattern of limb movements should be noted – a normal horse will back with a diagonal gait, whilst an ataxic horse will often struggle to back up or will pace. Additionally, making the horse perform more complicated tasks such as walking up and down slopes with the head elevated will alter the visual, vestibular and proprioceptive input and may exacerbate deficits in conscious proprioception. Making the horse circle tightly around the handler may also exacerbate signs of ataxia. Horses with pelvic limb ataxia will typically pivot on the inner foot while the outer limb may display a wide swinging motion – 'circumduction'.

Another test that is routinely performed to assess proprioceptive deficits in the horse is the placing of limbs in abnormal positions. These positions include, for example, placing the foot out to the side of the horse or underneath the horse, and assessing if and how long it may take for the horse to correct itself to a normal weight-bearing position. However, whilst this can be a useful test it may not always produce consistent and reliable results. It may be of more use to observe how long the horse takes to correct the position of its limbs following a sudden stop from a trot or from backing up, and the way in which a horse stands in the stable can often give very useful information on whether a proprioceptive deficit exists.

Proprioception can also be evaluated dynamically. Walking horses up and down curbs or steps may give additional information on whether proprioceptive deficits exist. However, the results of this test are also often influenced by the temperament of the horse. Furthermore, an animal that is distracted or simply not concentrating may appear excessively clumsy while a horse with neurological deficits may be particularly careful when placing its limbs and so may not make any deficit more evident.

If proprioceptive deficits only involve pelvic limbs, the neurological lesion must be located caudal to T2 [3]. However, in the case of mild cervical spinal cord lesions, particularly when very chronic, signs of weakness and ataxia may only be evident in the pelvic limbs and in these cases it may be safer to conclude that the horse has a lesion between C1 and S3 [15].

The tests described may have to be repeated in order to reveal more subtle abnormalities that may not have been apparent during the initial examination.

Depending on the suggested anatomic site of the lesion(s) further diagnostic procedures may be performed, such as radiography, scintigraphy, ultrasonography and electromyography, that may help the clinician reach a diagnosis to aid treatment and prognosis.

References

1 Mayhew, I.G. Chapter 2: Neurological evaluation. In: *Large Animal Neurology*. Chichester, West Sussex: John Wiley & Sons Ltd, 2009, pp. 11–47.

2 Blythe, L.L. and Engel, H.N. Neuroanatomy and neurological examination. *Veterinary Clinics of North America* 1999; 15(1):71–85.

3 de Lahunta, A., Glass, E. and Kent, M. Chapter 21: The neurologic examination. In: *Veterinary Neuroanatomy and Clinical Neurology*. St Louis, MO: Elsevier Saunders, 2015, pp. 525–539.

4 Thomson, C. and Hahn, C.N. *Clinical veterinary neuroanatomy. A clinical approach*, Saunders Elsevier, 2012.

5 Greet, T.R.C., Jeffcott, L.B. and Whitwell, K.E. The slap test for laryngeal adductory function in horses with suspected spinal cord damage. *Equine Veterinary Journal* 1980; 12:127–131.

6 Mayhew, I.G. The equine spinal cord in health and disease. In: *Proceedings of the 45th American Association of Equine Practitioners*, Albuquerque, NM, 1999, pp. 56–66.

7 Rooney, J.R. Two cervical reflexes in the horse. *Journal of the American Veterinary Medical Association* 1973; 162:117–118.

8 Bailey, C.S. and Kitchell, R.L. Cutaneous sensory testing in the dog. *Journal of*

Veterinary Internal Medicine 1987; **1**:128–135.

9 Newton-Clarke, M.J., Divers, T.J., Delahunta, A. and Mohammed, H.O. Evaluation of the thoraco-laryngeal reflex ('slap test') as an aid to the diagnosis of cervical spinal cord and brainstem disease in the horse. *Equine Veterinary Journal* 2010; **26**:358–361.

10 Blythe, L.L. and Kitchell, R.L. Electrophysiologic studies of the thoracic limb of the horse. *American Journal of Veterinary Research* 1982; **43**:1511–1524.

11 Rooney, J.R. Chapter 2: Examination. In: *Clinical Neurology of the Horse*. Kennett Square, PA: KNA Press Inc., 1971, pp. 20–36.

12 Jeffcott, L.B. The examination of a horse with a potential back problem. In: *Proceedings of the 31st American Association of Equine Practitioners*, Toronto, Canada, 1985, pp. 271–284.

13 Grau, H. Die Lautinnervation an den Gliedmassen des Pferdes. *Arc Wochenschreib Pract Tierheilk* 1935; **69**:96–116.

14 Blythe, L.L. Neurologic examination of the horse. *Veterinary Clinics of North America* 1987, **3**(7):255–281.

15 Mayhew, I.G. The diseased spinal cord. In: *Proceedings of the 45th American Association of Equine Practitioners*, Albuquerque, NM, 1999, pp. 67–85.

6

Clinical Examination
Graham A. Munroe

Examination of the Neck

Introduction

Neck-related problems appear to be increasing in incidence and they are particularly common in Warmblood-based sport horses and pleasure horses. Some of this is due to better recognition and diagnosis of the problems but there may be other factors at work including: the ever-increasing size and weight of individuals affecting head and neck size; the continued high incidence of osteochondrosis in various synovial joints, including the synovial intervertebral articular or facet joints; the exponential rise of dressage and intense school work in the daily lives of Sport horses and horses used for pleasure; the continued demand for horses to work in an outline often leading to over bend of the neck through various types of tack; and the possibility of new types of problems or different manifestations previously unknown.

The presentation to owners, riders or trainers can vary enormously but can include poor or deteriorating performance; gait abnormalities particularly affecting the hindlimbs with lack of impulsion, weakness and toe dragging; possible lameness or shortening of the stride of the forelimbs; abnormal head and/or neck carriage; inadequate bending or stiffness of the neck, or axial skeleton as a whole; and a neck and head that may be stuck/fixed in an abnormal low position. The overall presentation may also be confused by other concurrent orthopaedic problems of the axial and/or appendicular skeleton, mouth pain, lack of ability in the rider, poor schooling of the horse, and in young horses (which are commonly affected with neck problems) poor muscling, lack of skeletal maturity, and behavioural issues.

Presentations of Neck Pathology

The wide variety of clinical signs that neck cases may present with makes the differential diagnosis of each case sometimes obscure and always difficult. In general, they can be split into 3 separate entities that may overlap in individual cases to a varying extent. In equine clinical practice probably the most common presentations are neck pain, changes in neck position and/or head carriage. More commonly recognised in referral practice are neurological signs, most obvious in the hind limbs, but often low grade and subtle in presentation. The final presentations are obscure forelimb lamenesses, which can be uni- or bilateral and very difficult to localise and definitively diagnose.

Clinical History

The clinical history in neck cases can vary enormously and on some occasions does not always initially suggest a problem in this area. A clear history of neck trauma may be present following falls while exercising, jumping or rearing up, collisions with solid objects or another horse, and pulling backwards when

Equine Neck and Back Pathology: Diagnosis and Treatment, Second Edition. Edited by Frances M.D. Henson.
© 2018 John Wiley & Sons, Ltd. Published 2018 by John Wiley & Sons, Ltd.

restrained or tied up. Animals may also be found with a sudden onset of neck pain or abnormal neck posture without any known trauma. A less obvious problem involving the neck may present as changes in head and neck carriage, resistance to working on the bit and a lack of bend in the neck and body. Many of these cases are not simply neck related but may be examples of compensation in the horse for a forelimb lameness or even back pain. In both circumstances the horse will hold the head/neck away from the painful side and appears to the rider not willing to bend towards that side. Quite commonly horses with neck problems will present with subtle hindlimb gait abnormalities due to mild neurological signs. The rider may feel the horse is weak or lacking power from the hindquarters, have a rather variable and odd hindlimb action on occasions and drags its toe, leading to increased wear at the toe of the shoe. The owner/rider may feel the horse is lazy and not trying, unfit or poorly schooled. This is particularly a problem in the young horse where there is no history of previous performance. Some of these horses are poorly muscled behind the saddle, and in the hind limbs generally, and the assumption is that this is the cause of the problem rather than a reflection of abnormal neurological control of the hindlimbs. Some of these cases are wrongly suggested to have back, pelvic or hindlimb lameness and many are treated initially by non-veterinarians without a proper diagnosis. This process may continue for months or even years without any veterinary input. If the horse does eventually reach veterinary care the subtle gait changes are not always identified as being of a neurological origin. Some of these cases may have concurrent orthopaedic problems which complicates the definitive diagnostic process and can make it very time consuming and expensive. Finally, the horse may present with a forelimb lameness or shortening of its stride, which is persistent and cannot be localised to any part of the limb. Some of these cases are eventually diagnosed as lower neck problems after a detailed workup.

Working on the bit may also be a problem in horses with mouth pain and dental problems. A thorough oral and dental examination is warranted if the history or clinical signs suggest this as a differential or where the horse has not had such an examination in the last 6 months.

Clinical Examination of the Neck at Rest

The horse should be examined on a flat hard surface, either in a well-illuminated large box or stall, or preferably outside in clear daylight. The horse should be inspected from all sides, from a distance, with the animal standing squarely and the axial skeleton in a straight line from the head to the tail. The resting head and neck posture, position and their conformation should be assessed and noted. The neck conformation will to some extent affect the carriage of the neck and head. Horses that are thick through the jaw (large mandible) may find it more difficult to flex the poll and work on the bit. The neck may appear short, normal or long in proportion to the rest of the axial skeleton. The shape of the neck is partially conformational and also affected by the way the horse is worked. A ewe-neck conformation, where the ventral strap muscles are abnormally well developed, is associated with horses that carry their head and neck high up, and somewhat extended. Horses that are continually worked with excessive flexion in the neck, often with the continual use of mechanical aids, may develop an over-bent, rather 'cresty' appearance. The same 'cresty' (dorsal convexity of the caudal neck) appearance is seen in stallions and many pony breeds, in the latter often associated with excessive weight and abnormal fat deposits associated with equine metabolic syndrome. The horse should be able to stand comfortably with the head at the level of the withers and in line with the midline of the back and pelvis. Persistent deviations from this are abnormal.

The musculature of the neck should also be assessed from both left and right sides and from underneath. Areas of muscle atrophy, which may be uni- or bilateral, suggest disuse because of pain, neurological lower motor neuron dysfunction, or left- or right-handedness. The latter is common and presents as the horse having a preference to bending to the left or right with subsequent increased use of the muscles and resultant asymmetry, including those in the neck (especially dorsocranially), on that side. Thin and/or poorly muscled horses may have more prominent caudal cervical vertebrae and associated dorsocaudal neck concavity. In some cases there may be compensatory overdevelopment of certain muscle groups in response to dysfunction elsewhere in the neck. Patchy sweating or localised changes in the coat (possibly caused by intermittent sweating) anywhere in the neck should be noted as these can be caused by neurological deficits at various levels (see Chapter 5).

At this point it is useful to palpate the entire neck to confirm areas of muscle loss or hypertrophy, as well as detecting any heat, pain, swelling and muscle tension or fasciculation. It would be usual to start with firm, but superficial, palpation and then go on to deeper techniques at a later stage. The author would normally start in the cranial neck, at the poll, and progress down each side to the base of the neck in front of the shoulder. Each side is palpated separately from its own side and then both sides together by standing in front of the horse. The latter allows direct comparison of each side and is particularly useful if there are unilateral changes. A specific methodical regimen of palpation is used each time to cover the caudal skull and occipitut, the throat lash region and guttural pouch, the atlas and axis vertebrae, the *ligamentum nuchae* and crest of the neck, the bodies of the neck cervical vertebrae, the jugular groove and vein, the entire muscle mass dorsal to the vertebral bodies right down to the scapula, the trachea, and the main strap muscles such as the *brachiocephalicus* and *sternomandibularis* (Chapter 2).

Following palpation, neck movement tests are undertaken, usually with the aid of a food stimulus, such as a carrot or small bowl of food (Figure 6.1). A normal horse should be very flexible in its neck, with a full range of equal movement on both sides, and up and down, and with no evidence of pain or physical restriction. Lateral flexion is usually carried out first and both sides should be compared several times. A normal horse should be able to reach its flank just caudal to its elbow with ease on both sides when being offered food at this point. A horse with a neck problem may

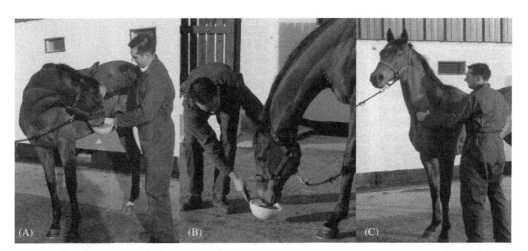

Figure 6.1 Photographs to demonstrate the assessment of neck mobility using a small bowl of feed. The neck should be palpated on both sides and assessed for symmetry, swelling, muscle spasm and sites of pain. In (A) the ability of the horse to flex laterally to left and right is assessed. In (B) and (C) the ability of the horse to lower (B) and raise its head and neck (C) is assessed.

be unable or unwilling to do this or it may try to turn its body (rather than its neck) around towards the stimulus. It should not be allowed to do this by the handler or it can be placed alongside a stable wall, which will physically stop it moving. If it persists in doing this it may suggest there is a neck problem. Ventroflexion (bending neck down) is tested by placing the food stimulus on the ground just in front of the legs or holding a carrot between them. Dorsiflexion (raising neck up) is much harder to test as even in a small horse it is difficult to hold the food stimulus high enough to test this movement. Feeding the horse off the floor or watching it grazing may demonstrate problems in the caudal neck, with affected animals often straddling the forelimbs to assist in lowering the head.

Orthopaedic Examination

After the neck is examined the horse should be examined for any axial or appendicular orthopaedic abnormality and lameness. This should include: visual inspection and detailed palpation of the limbs, back and pelvis; examination at exercise in hand, on the lunge and ridden/driven (where relevant) at all normal paces; and appropriate flexion tests. If this fails to lead to a definitive diagnosis then localisation of any painful lameness may require regional and/or intrasynovial analgesia techniques. In those neck cases leading to forelimb lameness this will be negative up to, and including, the shoulder region. Bilateral, low grade hindlimb lameness may be easily confused, or even coincidental, with subtle neurological deficits generated by neck pathology as both lead to weakness, gait abnormalities and/or poor impulsion in the hindlimbs. Careful and full clinical examination of the hindlimbs is often necessary to separate the different clinical entities. Some back and pelvic problems, primary or secondary to other lameness (usually hind limb), are also very common in equine clinical practice and can present with similar hindlimb weakness, poor impulsion, toe dragging, gait changes and poor top line muscling, as may be seen in

neck conditions leading to neurological deficits. Poorly muscled, unfit, young and old animals can also confuse the clinical picture further.

Neurological Examination

If during the initial clinical examination of any neck case (abnormal head and/or neck posture or pain), or one with a fore- or hindlimb gait abnormality, there is any suspicion of a neurological deficit, then a full neurological examination should be carried out. Sometimes this rapidly leads to the conclusion that there is not a neurological problem, but in others this is not clear. Further examination at a later time, perhaps with the second opinion of a colleague, can be very helpful in confirming the true nature of the problem. The key elements of a neurological examination are first to identify that there is a neurological problem, second to describe the nature of the neurological deficits and third to localise anatomically the site/s of the lesion/s in the nervous system. Local neurological reflexes and skin sensation in the neck should also be checked, as discussed in Chapter 5.

Diagnostic Imaging

Diagnostic imaging of the neck is discussed in Chapters 7 and 9.

Other Tests

Neuromuscular diseases such as polysaccharide storage myopathies (PSSMs) and equine motor neuron disease (EMND) are differentials of low grade gait abnormalities, weakness and poor impulsion (Chapter 15) and as such may be confused with low level neurological deficits seen in neck pathology. Definitive diagnosis of these diseases relies on the collection and histopathology of muscle biopsies collected from the semimembranosis and dorsosacrocaudalis muscles respectively. Other more advanced neurological tests include the use of electromyelography and transcranial magnetic stimulation, which are outside the scope of this book.

Examination of the Back and Pelvis

Introduction

Back pain is a common presenting complaint from owners and riders in a variety of horses but particularly in performance horses, such as those used in show jumping, eventing and dressage. Often the problems come to the attention of the owner due to a lack of, or poor, performance of the animal or an alteration in gait, rather than actual thoracolumbar pain. The cause of back pain is, however, difficult to pinpoint and differentially diagnose and requires a thorough and systematic approach to examination along with advanced diagnostic aids in specific cases. On many occasions a definitive diagnosis can only be made by eliminating other conditions that may present as possible back pain. There is added confusion in that some animals appear to be 'thin-skinned' or naturally sensitive, and resent palpation of the back. Other horses are 'cold backed', where there is apparent hypersensitivity over the back with transient stiffness and marked dipping of the spine following the rider mounting the horse and sitting in the saddle. These horses often have no other clinical signs and a source of pain is rarely found, although some may have had previous back pain.

Assessment of the degree of pain in a case is complicated by the marked individual variation in the response to pain and this can certainly be affected by the animal's breeding and temperament. Some horses seem to be better able to cope with pain and apparently perform despite its presence.

There are a considerable number of both osseous and soft tissue related primary back problems but in many cases the back pain is caused as a secondary consequence of other problems. Particularly common are lameness conditions of the hind legs, often bilateral, and

on some occasions also associated with fore-limb lameness [1]. Bilateral hindlimb or multiple limb lameness leads to major changes in the gait of the horse with secondary pain in the pelvic and back regions. In addition, many problems related to back pain are due to faulty tack or poor riding. On other occasions inadequately or poorly schooled horses may present with back pain subsequent to their abnormal movement. Finally, and somewhat controversially, there are the apparent or alleged back problems, which are popular with owners, trainers and various 'back people', and which have limited anatomical or pathophysiological evidence for their existence. Such problems include the horse having 'put its back out' or having a 'trapped or pinched nerve'.

Objectives of the Clinical Examination

It is always worthwhile to define the objectives of your clinical examination at the beginning of the process and to separate this into logical progressive stages. This is particularly useful in examining back cases where a haphazard approach will often lead to misdiagnosis and incorrect treatment. First, it is important to define the problem and to confirm that it is indeed a veterinary problem and not a behavioural or schooling issue, or indeed an overestimation of the performance capability of the animal. Behavioural and schooling problems are common, particularly in horses owned/ridden by inexperienced riders and many cases have no evidence of pain-related pathology in the back or elsewhere. Proving this to the owner of the horse can be a major part of the clinical workup of such cases. Horses with axial and appendicular orthopaedic problems can, however, present with behavioural, gait and schooling changes and it is important not to dismiss them casually as an animal that is just being awkward. Some of these changes can be learnt and will in some cases continue even after the original problem has ceased being painful.

Next it is important to define whether back pain is indeed present. The degree of pain within the back of an individual animal can vary enormously depending on: the particular pathology; its duration; its secondary consequences such as muscle spasm and chronic adaptation of posture and conformation; other sources of pain out with the axial skeleton; individual pain tolerance; and the effects of the rider ability and strength.

Whether or not back pain is present, it is also essential that the clinician examines the whole horse for other problems that will affect the horse's performance and, in particular, other orthopaedic problems of the axial skeleton (neck and pelvis) and fore/hindlimbs. Secondary back problems are much more common than primary cases and the majority are due to chronic, often bilateral, hindlimb lameness of the fetlock, hock, proximal suspensory ligament, or stifle. In some cases the addition of pain elsewhere in the axial or appendicular skeleton will trigger off pain in previously present back pathology that has been clinically insignificant. Lower back pain is very common as a secondary consequence of pelvic pathology and the combination of multiple pain sites makes the overall clinical presentation confusing. Neck-related problems can also be confused with back problems or complicate/exacerbate the clinical picture.

The clinical workup should focus on isolating the site/s of pain both in the back, other parts of the axial skeleton and the appendicular skeleton. It is important not to embark on a 'diagnostic imaging fishing trip' where the clinician is looking for a lesion/s within the bony and soft tissue structures without considering whether they are causing pain, and their individual and collective relevance to the animal's overall clinical presentation. Far too often clinicians find a lesion on an image and pin their diagnosis on this without really thinking about it.

Clinical History

Acquiring a good, comprehensive, history is particularly important in those horses presenting with back pain. The clinical signs are varied and multiple, and easily confusable with a number of other clinical problems. After the basic signalment is taken, in the author's opinion, the starting point for the history should be the date of acquisition of the horse, which may be associated with a pre-purchase veterinary examination. Although back problems may have been pre-existing to this point, and it is important to ascertain any prior history, this will have been a comprehensive veterinary examination at a definite point in time from which we can work. It is important to question the owner about the time of onset and the duration of the clinical signs to ascertain whether the problem is acute or chronic. Information on the management of the horse, the particular tack used and the problems regarding performance are all extremely important. The type of work the horse performs and how this has changed, as well as whether the horse shows the signs during free exercise can be helpful. Details regarding the saddle, and whether pads or numnahs are used, and whether these were fitted by a qualified saddle fitter or have changed recently are essential. It is important to assess the rider's size and skill as these will have a direct effect on how the horse is ridden and the forces the horse's back will be subjected to. Detailed information about the horse's performance pre and post the point of any deterioration is useful and there should be particularly close questioning to determine whether the signs may have been occurring earlier than the owner has noticed them. It is vital during the history taking and the examination to assess the temperament, quality of the schooling and equitation of the horse, and the experience of the rider. Many of the problems supposedly related to back pain are in fact due to poor behaviour or schooling of the horse, or poor ability of the rider or handler. If the horse has been ridden by other, perhaps more experienced, riders it is useful to find out how this affected the clinical signs. It is important to note any treatment given, medication, physiotherapy or manipulation, and any response seen.

Further information regarding the clinical history should be focused on previous falls or any acute traumatic incident that may have led to damage to the back. At rest, there may be a history in severe cases of horses having difficulty in straddling to urinate or defaecate, or reluctance to lie down or roll, especially in its stable. The owner may have noted resentment to placement of rugs over the loins or quarters, or during grooming. The farrier may have commented that the horse shows reluctance to having the legs lifted or shod. In some cases there is a history of the horse responding unusually to weight on its back, such as collapsing or roaching, and these horses are sometimes termed 'cold-backed'. This can be learned behaviour, possibly post back pain, and can be a misleading sign that should be viewed with caution. The horse may collapse or roach when backed or ridden, occasionally bucking/rearing on mounting or when ridden, and there may be problems during saddling up or girth tightening. Other points in the history may include resistance to moving backwards or reining back when ridden, and changes in general attitude of the horse both at rest and during exercise.

The history of exercise is extremely important, particularly in helping to differentiate primary from secondary back problems. There may be a history at exercise of unilateral or bilateral hindlimb or multiple leg lameness. On many occasions these are missed by the owner and not picked up until there is a veterinary examination or when the horse is presented to a more experienced owner or trainer. At exercise there may be signs of a lack of enthusiasm for work with a poor and restricted gait, particularly at faster paces. The owner may complain of poorly defined gait changes when ridden, suggesting hindlimb stiffness or decreased impulsion, or, particularly in dressage animals, lack of bend or suppleness in the back. There may be a marked difference between in-hand and ridden gaits. In the jumping horse disinclination to jump, particularly over combination-type fences, may be a feature. When they do jump they may do so with a fixed hollow back, making the horse very flat through the jumps and leading to an increased chance of hitting the jumps. A loss of jumping fluidity, timing and confidence with decreased performance are common complaints. In horses undertaking dressage or other flat work there may be problems in movement, a history of decreasing scores during dressage competitions, a failure to stop or yield to aids, a lack of bend or resistance to collection, a developing sour attitude, and poor impulsion. Finally, back pain can give rise to clinical signs of head shaking and tail swishing and these should always be considered in the differential of this frustratingly difficult syndrome.

Clinical Examination at Rest

The clinical examination at rest needs to be carried out carefully with the examination of the whole horse for other causes of lameness and loss of performance problems. Signs of back pain are often, varied, subtle and inconsistent between individuals and therefore it is important that there is a systematic and logical approach to examination.

Initial Inspection

As with the examination of the neck described above, the author prefers to have the horse stood 'four square' on a flat, hard surface. This is used to carry out a general appraisal of the conformation of its back and fore- and hindlimbs, as well as assessing its general condition and muscling. Specific note is made of whether the horse is long or short in its back with regards to conformation (Figure 6.2) and whether there are any spinal curvatures, such as lumbar kyphosis, thoracic lordosis (Figure 6.3) or scoliosis. The dorsal midline of the back is viewed from behind the horse, if necessary standing on a raised stool or chair, with the horse straight and aligned through its neck, back and quarters. This is a very effective way of assessing the back conformation and muscling. Lateral curvature may also occur due to spastic sclerosis from long-term pain in the back, leading to changes in muscle tension.

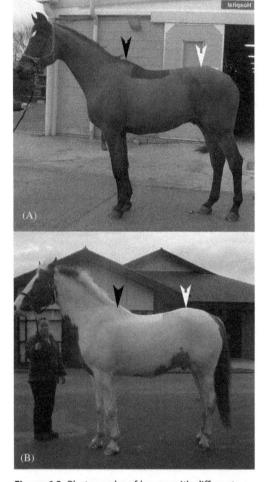

Figure 6.2 Photographs of horses with different conformation. (A) A 'short backed' horse and (B) a 'long backed' horse. This refers to the distance between the withers (black arrowhead) and the *tuber sacrale* (white arrowhead) relative to the other dimensions of the horse.

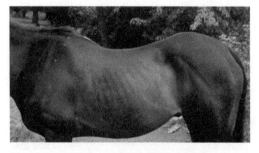

Figure 6.3 A photograph of a horse with age-related lordosis (dipping of the back).

Epiaxial muscle atrophy may also occur due to areas of pain and subsequent reduced movement, or inadequate suitable work [2]. It has recently been shown that both uni- and bilateral back pain will affect both the normal thoracolumbar and pelvic movements in a horse and lead to compensatory changes in motion and muscling [3]. Occasionally, at rest, spasticity and swelling in the epiaxial muscles of the back can be detected visually and confirmed by palpation. At this stage the symmetry of the gluteal and pelvic muscles should also be carefully assessed. Any lumps, scars or saddle marks on the withers or saddle region should be noted and examined further at the palpation stage. They may reflect a poorly fitting saddle or an abnormally positioned or balanced rider. During this visual inspection it is important to start to assess the animal's temperament and general behaviour and whether it is well-schooled and disciplined. Some clinicians believe there is a correlation between nervous or temperamental animals and the incidence of back pain [4], although many horses with a chronic back problem may alter their behaviour or change temperament in response to the pain. In some cases with severe back pain the horse may assume abnormal conformations such as camping the front limbs out in front of it, in a manner rather similar to a laminitic horse, or commonly tucking its limbs and hindquarters underneath it and assuming a rather 'humped' hind limb and lower back posture [5]. In the author's experience this is perhaps more common in horses with persistent pelvic pain, for example in ilial stress fractures in Thoroughbred racehorses.

Symmetry of Pelvis and Hindquarter Muscles

Assessment of the symmetry of the pelvis (bony prominences) and hindquarter muscles is extremely important in differentiating a pelvic or hindlimb lameness problem. It should be carried out as subjectively as possible by standing the horse on a level surface and by using assistant's fingers or tape markers on both prominences of the tuber coxae. The significance of any asymmetry must be considered in the light of other clinical signs and the history. Slight deviations are detectable but may not be significant. It is important to view the pelvis from the left and right sides as well since the angle of the pelvis can change in some conditions (may tilt upwards) and the shape and angle of the tuber sacrale and tuber coxae can vary. It is important at some stage to pull the tail to one side so that it does not interfere with assessment of the tuber ischii and medial thigh muscles. Unilateral muscle wastage over the quarters without any bony asymmetry is common in hindlimb lameness and suggests the most lame limb. Elevation of one tuber sacrale, with or without gluteal muscle wastage, can be seen in problems involving thickening and damage to the dorsal sacroiliac ligament, sacroiliac joint disease and in some racehorses with stress fractures of the wing of the ilium. Lowered tuber sacrale and/or tuber coxae on one side along with muscle wastage may suggest chronic sacroiliac disease although Dyson and Murray [6] noted that only 5% of their confirmed cases of sacroiliac disease had pelvic asymmetry. Lowering of the tuber coxae, without any lowering of the tuber sacrale or tuber ischii, is associated with tuber coxae damage such as old fractures. Lowering or change in shape of the tuber ischii with no alteration to the tuber sacrale or tuber coxae may suggest a fractured tuber ischii.

Palpation of the Thoracolumbar Spine and Pelvis

Palpation of the thoracolumbar spine and pelvis is one of the most important parts of the physical examination and if carried out carefully can be a surprisingly accurate technique for detecting pain [7]. It is important to have the horse standing square on a hard surface, for example in a quiet box with plenty of time allowed for the horse to relax. A start is usually made at the withers and working caudally towards the base of the tail. The fingers are gently, but firmly, run along the

back, first in the midline and then on either side. The process should be repeated a number of times to allow the horse to become accustomed to the examination. There should be symmetry and balance in the horse's reaction to palpation. It is important to assess the feel of the back and the horse's reaction to palpation, and to try to decide whether any reaction is due to pain or behavioural. The horse may guard or splint its back, pelvis or neck when palpated, or even when just approached. There may be muscle fasciculation in the local area or more generally, with prolonged (greater than 2 seconds) time, to the muscles relaxing. The horse may try to move away from the palpation and show abnormal behaviour such as tail swishing, head and ear movement, and even kicking actions. It is important to palpate the tips of the dorsal spinous processes and the interspinous spaces. This is most easily achieved in the lumbar region. Any protrusion or displacement of the summits should be noted and marked on the horse with a small clipped area of hair. Spasm or guarding of the longissimus dorsi muscles can be part of a primary problem or an indicator of deeper pain.

Any skin lesions, white hairs, loss of hair, especially asymmetrically, scars or swellings in the thoracolumbar region should be noted and most often involve the withers or the area immediately under the saddle. They may indicate historical or current problems of saddle fitting or a rider who is riding incorrectly. Swelling and oedema under the saddle may only be transient and should be checked immediately after the saddle is removed.

The saddle should be checked by a master saddle fitter for a proper fit to the individual horse and that there are no abnormalities of the saddle, such as incorrect stuffing and damaged tree. It is important to also check the girth in terms of its type and fit. There should not be any sores or skin lesions where the girth sits around the thorax.

The bony prominences of the pelvis and hip should be palpated firmly to assess their shape, size, position, and pain response.

The left and right tubera sacrale/ischii/coxae of the pelvis and the greater and third trochanter of the femur should be checked and compared. The tips of the sacral spinous processes should also be noted. The dorsal sacral ligament should be assessed for any swelling or pain, as should the tendinous insertions of the longissimus dorsi muscle on to the spinous processes of S2 and S3. The area around the tuber sacrale and working laterally should be carefully palpated for any evidence of pain, fibrosis or thickening. Pain here may be associated with ilial stress fractures in racehorses and also sacroiliac joint disease, and may be represented by marked dropping of the pelvis on that side upon direct pressure. Direct pressure in the caudal lumbar region may reveal secondary pain and muscle guarding in cases with cranial pelvic pathology. The entire area of the pelvis covered by the gluteal muscles plus the upper thigh muscles on the medial and lateral aspects should be palpated for evidence of pain, swelling, spasm, atrophy or change in consistency. The tail and croup region should be assessed for flaccidity, any asymmetry of the tail or tail head muscles and any evidence of cauda equina neuritis.

Manipulation

Careful manipulation can give a considerable amount of information to the examining clinician regarding the source of any back or pelvic pain. Usually the author starts by running a blunt instrument, such as a pen top, from the lateral side of the withers caudally to the tail head. This is repeated on both sides on a number of occasions to note the normal reaction. Alternatively pinching or pressing can be carried out at various points. In the normal horse, pressure on to the caudal thoracic area leads to extension of the spine (dorsal flexion or dip), whereas pressure above the tail head leads to flexion of the spine (ventral flexion or arching), and pressure laterally over the longissimus dorsi muscles causes lateral flexion. It is important to assess the amount and flexibility of movement and whether there are any signs of pain or altered behaviour. In the normal horse these are smooth movements that are easily repeated without any resentment by the horse. Any change in the degree and smoothness of these movements or a response from the horse, such as limb flexion or movement of the tail, kicking, rearing or grunting, may be significant [8]. It is important, however, to make sure that these responses are repeatable. After manipulation the horse may become reluctant to move and assume a rather rigid back conformation. Pain or discomfort may be evident as spasm or guarding of the longissimus dorsi muscle, locally or generally, which can be palpated or sometimes visually noted. The degree of movement on manipulation may reflect the type of horse. Ponies and Cobs, which often have a thicker coat and less reactive behaviour, often show a lesser response than Thoroughbreds or Warmbloods. Specific pelvic manipulation tests have been described in an attempt to confirm pain in the sacroiliac joint or region but the author has found these of limited use beyond what is ascertained from the dorsal, ventral and lateral manipulation tests already described. Rocking the pelvis from side to side by placing direct pressure on the left and right tuber coxae may reveal pain and/or crepitation in some fractures in the ilium.

Examination of Fore- and Hindlimbs

Following assessment of the back and pelvis the conformation and stance of the fore- and hindlimbs should be carefully examined. Any areas of muscle atrophy may suggest long-term chronic lameness or neurological dysfunction. The limbs should be examined individually for swellings, particularly of the joints and other synovial structures. The feet should be examined in detail for shape, symmetry and balance, and hoof testers used carefully to help rule out foot pain. All four limbs should be palpated, in a logical sequence, in both a flexed and standing mode. During this phase the legs and joints should be manipulated, in both flexion and extension.

Rectal Examination

If there is a history of trauma and possible damage to the pelvis or pelvic canal, or one is concerned about the sacroiliac region, sublumbar muscle pain or caudal lumbar vertebral body fractures then a rectal examination may be helpful in detecting sites of pain in these areas. Fractures of the sacrum and pelvic bones may be associated with palpable haematoma whilst gentle rocking of the pelvis may confirm crepitation. Per rectum ultrasonographic examination can also help determine fracture sites and degree of displacement in pelvic and sacral fractures, and extra-articular changes in the lumbosacral and ventral sacroiliac joints. It is useful to carry out a rectal examination pre- and post-exercise to ascertain whether there is any pain following exercise. Palpation and ultrasonographic examination of the aorta and iliac/femoral arteries can also be carried out per rectum to help rule out thrombosis of these structures as a possible differential diagnosis.

Oral Examination

A basic oral examination is useful in all suspected back cases as problems with oral pain will affect the control and movement of the horse. If sedation is required for the use of an oral gag then this part of the overall examination should be carried out after all exercise is finished.

Clinical Examination at Exercise

Initially the horse should be examined in-hand, on a loose rein, on a flat surface and with a competent handler. The horse should be viewed at the walk and trot in a straight line from the back, front and both sides. Careful observation of the gait is important in determining if there is any unilateral or bilateral, fore- or hindlimb lameness. Primary back problems rarely lead to hindlimb or forelimb lameness but occasionally there may be signs of a shifting lameness, unlevelness or evidence of stiffness in the back. Chronic back pain

tends to lead to a restricted hindlimb action with poor hock flexion and, occasionally, unilateral or bilateral dragging of hindlimb toes. If there is more severe pain there may be a wide, straddling, hindlimb gait. Occasionally horses with low grade back pain develop a very close hindlimb gait or 'plaiting', although this may occur for other reasons. Horses with a pelvic-related problem have no specific pathognomic gait pattern and the degree and character of the resulting lameness varies with the specific cause. Fractures of the pelvis give rise to acute and severe lameness if displaced but stress fractures of the ilium may present as a more chronic lameness with intermittent flare-ups. Chronic sacroiliac disease presents very similarly to back pain (which also may coexist) with lack of impulsion in the hindlimb, poor performance and various gait changes at the trot, including plaiting or base wide. Lameness is often worse on a circle and when ridden.

Flexion tests of the fore- and hindlimbs may also be performed. Hindlimb flexion tests are often negative if there is a purely back problem, although they may be positive if there is an underlying hindlimb lameness. Flexion tests of one leg may lead to lameness on the opposite leg in sacroiliac disease as well as resentment during the procedure, and can be a useful initial indicator of a problem in this region.

The horse should be turned tightly in both directions whilst in-hand to assess how well the horse bends and flexes its spine laterally. When the horse has serious back pain there is a loss of suppleness and there may be back spasm leading to difficulty in turning. Horses with hindlimb lameness, cervical pain and neurological deficits may also find this difficult. The horse should also be backed up. In some cases of back pain there may be an initial reluctance to backing with raising of the head and arching of the back followed by back muscle spasm and occasionally dragging of the forelimbs. The horse should also be backed up and down a slope and in some cases of sacroiliac disease there may be evidence of increased resentment to this.

Following the in-hand examination the horse should be lunged for 10–15 minutes on both reins and the horse's gait assessed as previously during this exercise. The author prefers to start this lunging on a grass or all-weather surface to allow the horse to move more naturally initially. If there is a need to accentuate any gait abnormality then the horse can be lunged with due care on a harder surface. The straight line in-hand examination should be repeated after this exercise period. It is important to carefully evaluate the hindlimb action initially at the trot for evidence of a shortened stiff hindlimb gait, poor tracking up, toe-dragging, plaiting, lack of bend in the back with a tendency for the horse to lean out of the circle, head elevation and positioning of the head outside of the circle, and finally for any evidence of spasm in the longissimus dorsi muscle whilst at exercise. Lunging at the canter may show marked signs in horses with back pain but again these are not exclusive. The horse may find it difficult to transfer from one gait to another, particularly from a canter to a trot and a trot to a walk. The horse may have an inability to lead off on the correct leg (disunited gait) and show evidence of poor hindlimb impulsion with a 'bunny hopping' hindlimb gait. The horse may tend to pull its body forward using excessive forelimb action, poor balance within the circle, signs of lack of concentration in the horse's head and tail swishing. These changes may be accentuated by placing a surcingle or saddle on the horse and repeating the exercise.

Ridden Exercise

It is essential to try to observe the horse either ridden or, if it is a driving horse, driven to note what changes during this period of work. The horse should be carefully observed from saddling, when there may be evidence of pain or resentment on girth tightening, through mounting to being ridden. The fit of the saddle, pad or numbnah should be carefully checked, and if necessary a qualified saddle fitter should also be involved. The horse should have ridden/driven exercise carried out with the usual tack and the usual rider/driver. It is important to assess the horse's action, back mobility and attitude at the walk, trot and canter and, if the horse is a jumping horse, also whilst jumping. In a driven horse the horse should be observed whilst the harness is put in place and throughout its normal work programme. It is important to assess the qualifications of the rider/driver for the horse. Gait changes should be assessed further with particular attention paid to any abnormality that occurred on the lunge. In many cases with back pain the changes are exaggerated when ridden/driven, particularly at the canter, the sitting trot or on the turn. It is useful to observe the position of the saddle and rider during exercise and afterwards, because in a horse with back pain the saddle often becomes twisted to one side away from the painful side. Greve and Dyson [9] noted that twisting of the saddle position was most common in horses with hindlimb lameness and that the twisting was towards the side of the lamest limb. The twisting resolved with regional/intrasynovial analgesia techniques. Other causes of saddle twisting included asymmetry of back muscles, poor rider position, incorrect saddle fitting and, rarely, forelimb lameness. All of the latter may occur in synchrony with primary back problems or lead to secondary back pain.

The horse should be allowed to cool down after exercise and then be re-examined in-hand afterwards to assess its action. In some cases there is increased stiffness, which may be related to low grade myopathies or to joint disease elsewhere in the limbs.

During the whole exercise process it is important to talk to the rider/driver to ascertain their feelings and what they are noticing about the horse's action. They will often comment on the lack of hindlimb power, a stiffness to left or right, a 'heavy-handedness' on the forehand with a 'rocking-horse like' action, poor contact on the bit, a lack of rhythm and balance in the stride, and occasionally pain in their own back during or after work on the horse.

Neurological Examination

Horses with suspected back pain should always have a basic neurological examination (Chapter 5) as back pain, altered gait or unusual lameness can all be consistent with a primary neurological problem. Horses with low grade neurological disease may present with low grade hindlimb incoordination, weakness or lameness, which can easily be confused with orthopaedic limb disease, back problems or just plain immaturity of the horse.

Further Management of the Case

At the end of this clinical examination the examining veterinary surgeon should have some indication as to whether she/he is dealing with a primary back problem, a secondary back problem, and whether there is any evidence of fore- or hindlimb lameness or behavioural issues. In some cases there is a clear indication of which direction to pursue, in others there is not.

Re-examination on a separate occasion repeating the methodical examination as before may be helpful in clarifying the position. Using the skills and opinions of other clinicians at the same time can also be very enlightening. In general, the author holds the view that horses may be suffering from back pain if they are changing behaviour, but there are occasions when one has to conclude that it is a behavioural problem and the services of a qualified behavioural consultant are required. On other occasions the services of a fully qualified animal physiotherapist can be most useful in determining whether there are any other sources of pain or stiffness in other areas of the body.

In some cases where there is an issue as to whether pain is present it is possible to use up to 10 days of non-steroidal analgesic administration followed by re-examination to see whether the horse's clinical signs are altered. It is also useful to have the horse's rider/driver to work the horse during this period to assess whether the horse's clinical signs change.

Additional clinical aids to diagnosis include muscle stimulation by a neuroelectrical stimulator, often by an animal physiotherapist, and assessing the subsequent response of the horse. Horses with muscle soreness and guarding may show increased resentment. Full haematology and biological profiles can be useful to eliminate other causes of poor performance, for example myopathies (as discussed in Chapter 15). A standard exercise test can be carried out by assessing the levels of serum aspartate aminotransferase (AST) and creatine kinase (CK), both at rest, immediately postexercise and after 18–24 hours postexercise. The horse is lunged for 10–15 minutes and where there is active muscle damage there may be a rise of 2–5 times resting levels on the postexercise samples.

Other clinical aids include local anaesthetic infiltration. This is usually carried out after identification of specific sites of pain clinically or on evidence of pathology on radiographs, ultrasonograms, or bone scintigraphy. Most commonly this is carried out where there is crowding or over-riding of dorsal spinous processes. The horse's performance signs are recorded before and after injection of a small amount of local anaesthetic into specific sites under radiographic or ultrasonographic guidance. Individual periarticular facet joints of the adjoining thoracolumbar vertebrae have also been injected, under ultrasonographic guidance, with local anaesthetic and/or corticosteroids, and the clinical response of the horse assessed thereafter. The interpretation of this technique is difficult as these injections are effectively intramuscular and may affect the dorsal and ventral rami of the spinal nerves [10]. There is now the widespread use of 'sacroiliac joint local anaesthesia techniques' to assess pain in the sacroiliac joint region and these are described in detail elsewhere. These have been noted to have impressive results on horses with pain in this area [6] but they can lead to serious complications in some horses and may not be as specific to just the sacroiliac joint or region.

On many occasions horses with back pain are treated on the basis of clinical examination only and their response to symptomatic treatment is used to assess how much further to investigate the problem. Some horses respond positively and require no further examinations. On other occasions the horse does not respond to treatment, in the short or long term, and these cases require further clinical examination. Subsequent examination may determine the need for scintigraphic examination, often followed by radiography and ultrasonography of the identified region of interest.

References

1 Landman, M.A., de Blaauw, J.A., van Weeren, P.R. and Hofland, L.J. Field study of the prevalence of lameness in horses with back problems. *Veterinary Records* 2004, August 7; **155**(6):165–168.

2 Stubbs, N.C., Kaiser, L.J., Hauptman, J. and Clayton, H.M. Dynamic mobilisation exercises increase cross sectional area of musculus multifidus. *Equine Veterinary Journal* 2011; **43**(5):522–529.

3 Wennerstrand, J., Gómez Alvarez, C.B., Meulenbelt, R. et al. Spinal kinematics in horses with induced back pain. *Veterinary Comparative Orthopaedics Traumatology* 2009; **22**(6):448–454.

4 Jeffcott, L.B. Back problems. Historical perspective and clinical indications. *Veterinary Clinics of North America: Equine Practice* 1999; (1):1–12.

5 Lesimple, C., Fureix, C., De Margerie, E. et al. Towards a postural indicator of back pain in horses (*Equus caballus*). *PLoS One* 2012; **7**(9).

6 Dyson, S. and Murray, R. Pain associated with the sacroiliac joint region: a clinical study of 74 horses. *Equine Veterinary Journal* 2003; **35**(3):240–245.

7 Ranner, W., Gerhards, H. and Klee, W. Diagnostic validity of palpation in horses with back problems. *Berlin and Munich Tierarztl. Wochenschr.* 2002; **115**(11–12):420–424.

8 Haussler, K.K., Martin, C.E. and Hill, A.E. Efficacy of spinal manipulation and mobilisation on trunk flexibility and stiffness in horses: a randomised clinical trial. *Equine Veterinary Journal* 2010; Suppl., **38**:695–702.

9 Greve, L. and Dyson, S.J. The interrelationship of lameness, saddle slip and back shape in the general sports horse population. *Equine Veterinary Journal* 2014, November; **46**(6):687–694. doi: 10.1111/evj.12222. Epub 2014 Feb 27.

10 Denoix, J.-M. and Dyson, S. The thoracolumbar spine. In: Ross, M.W. and Dyson, S. (eds), *Diagnosis and Management of Lameness in the Horse*, 2nd edn. Saunders, 2001, pp. 592–605.

7

Radiography of the Cervical Spine

Marianna Biggi, Gabriel Manso-Díaz and Renate Weller

Indications for Radiography of the Cervical Spine

As discussed previously in this book, the indications for radiographing the neck include horses showing neurological signs, horses showing signs of musculoskeletal pain and horses that show mechanical impairment of cervical spine mobility:

- The presence of neurological signs, e.g. ataxia that may indicate cervical spinal cord compression.
- Unilateral front limb lameness that cannot be localized to other areas that may indicate a radiculopathy [1].
- History or clinical signs of musculoskeletal pain, including history of a fall and/or the presence of pain on palpation or manipulation of the neck.
- Presence of neck stiffness and restricted range of motion, often noticed by the rider as reluctance to work to one side or other riding problems.
- Neck radiographs are also performed when indicated by other diagnostic techniques. For example, if increased radiopharmaceutical uptake is observed on bone phase scintigraphy (Chapter 9).

In many cases neck problems are associated with unspecific clinical signs, especially loss of performance. Radiographs may help in these cases; however, one has to bear in mind that many radiographic changes in the neck (and elsewhere in the body) can be present without

having any clinical significance and truly pathognomonic changes are rare. This should also be taken into consideration when radiography of the neck is part of a prepurchase exam, a practice that is gaining in popularity.

Radiographic Technique

Plain radiography of the cervical spine can be performed in the standing horse; although myelography has been described in the standing horse [2], it is more commonly performed with the horse under general anaesthesia.

Equipment

Diagnostic quality radiographs of the mid and cranial neck can be obtained with a portable X-ray machine, especially when using digital or computed radiography systems. However, imaging of C6–C7 and C7–T1 usually require high-output X-ray machines to be able to generate the higher exposures necessary for this area.

It is suggested to use large plates (35 cm × 43 cm) so that multiple vertebrae (usually 3) are visible in the same image. This facilitates orientation and is helpful when vertebral alignment is evaluated. The plate is usually positioned with a plate stand or a ceiling suspended holder. If this is not at hand, plates can be taped to the wall or suspended from a sturdy drip stand using a suitably heavy-duty

Equine Neck and Back Pathology: Diagnosis and Treatment, Second Edition. Edited by Frances M.D. Henson.
© 2018 John Wiley & Sons, Ltd. Published 2018 by John Wiley & Sons, Ltd.

plastic bag. For optimal image quality the use of a parallel or focused grid is advisable to reduce scatter radiation, especially in the caudal neck area. Some systems, however, are capable of producing diagnostic images without a grid due to their high sensitivity and excellent noise filters; this not only depends on the equipment but also on the size of the horse.

Patient Preparation and Positioning – The Standing Horse

Intravenous sedation is usually required for examination of the cervical spine in the standing horse. This facilitates positioning, encouraging the horse to lower its head and neck, reduces movement, especially when the plate is positioned close to the head, and allows the horse handler to step away from the primary beam when the images are obtained.

The horse must be positioned square with the weight equally distributed between the four feet. The head is held straight and in a neutral position. It is useful to position the head on a headstand adjusted at the height of the horse's shoulders to obtain a reproducible neck position and reduce movement. If no headstand is available, a bin or bale of shavings can substitute. In some horses obtaining radiographs with the neck in different positions may allow identification of positional lesions, e.g. step formation between adjacent vertebrae may only be obvious in a flexed neck position. Plaits or a thick or dirty mane can create artefacts, making imaging interpretation more challenging, and should therefore be avoided.

For examination of the poll area a rope head collar should be used to avoid metal artefacts. In addition, the pinnae are normally superimposed with the occiput; therefore pulling/taping the ears forward improves interpretation of this region.

In the average size horse four slightly overlapping radiographs are needed to perform a complete examination of the cervical spine. Markers can be placed on the skin to equally divide the neck in four portions. If radiopaque markers (i.e. lead numbers, coins) are used, these are usually positioned ventrally to the cervical spine overlapping the trachea. The postprocessing of many CR and DR systems is influenced by very radiodense markers, resulting in suboptimal image quality. If this is the case less radiodense markers (e.g. plastic wall plugs) might be used.

Radiographic Exposures

Exposure values increase from cranial to caudal and need to be adjusted to the size of the horse, but also the X-ray system used. Exposures need to be increased when using a grid, depending on the type of grid and the focus-film distance. In our hospital we use a 1:16 parallel grid with an FFD of 150 cm.

Examples of exposure settings, using CR and DR systems, in an average size (450 kg) horse are listed in Table 7.1.

Table 7.1 Example of exposure used to radiograph the cervical spine in a 450 kg horse using a high output fixed X-ray machine and both a computed and a direct radiography system with a parallel grid (1:16, FFD 150 cm). Kv: kilovolt, mAs: milliampere-second.

Area to be radiographed	CR		DR	
	Kv	mAs	Kv	mAs
Cranial cervical spine (occiput to C2)	70	20	68	14
Mid cervical spine (C3–C5)	81	40	79	16
Caudal cervical spine (C5–C7)	100	80	93	45
Base of the neck (C6–T1)	100	100	96	71

Image Acquisition

Laterolateral and ventrolateral-dorsolateral oblique sets from both sides should be obtained for a complete investigation of the cervical spine. Ventrodorsal/dorsoventral radiographs of the cranial neck can be reliably obtained in the standing horse. The direction of the beam is determined by the size of the horse and how high/low the X-ray machine can be positioned.

In the average size horse four slightly overlapping laterolateral projections are usually required to image the entire neck. The occipital bone and the first thoracic vertebra should be included in the study. It is crucial to obtain true laterolateral views of the cervical spine to avoid misinterpretation. Occasionally, the X-ray beam must be angled slightly ventrodorsally or dorsoventrally to obtain a diagnostic image, but in the majority of the cases adjusting the position of the horse will be sufficient to correct mild obliquity. In a true laterolateral radiograph the left and right transverse processes should be nicely superimposed.

Ventrolateral-dorsolateral oblique projections from both sides should be part of the standard radiographic protocol since they allow separation of the left from the right articular process joints. In this view the articular process joint closest to the X-ray machine is in outline while enabling the viewer to see through the joint space of the joint closest to the plate. Images are acquired from each side of the neck orienting the X-ray beam ventral to dorsal. The beam is centred about 15 cm ventral to the spine. The plate is positioned perpendicular to the X-ray beam as close as possible to the horse. An angle between 45 and 55 degrees is recommended to image the articular process joints between C4 and C7. A shallower angle (about 35 degrees) is used for the cranial cervical spine [3].

Particular care is needed to correctly centre and orientate the X-ray beam on the plate for oblique views, especially when a grid is used to avoid poor image quality due to grid cut-off. With a ceiling-mounted hospital-based system alignment is often achieved automatically, but manual alignment is more challenging. If automated alignment is not possible, a cheap laser pen taped to the X-ray machine can facilitate proper alignment.

Normal Radiographic Anatomy and Incidental Findings

There are seven cervical vertebrae. Each vertebra, except for the atlas, the axis, C6 and C7, are similar in their anatomy and hence appear similar on radiographs. A detailed description of their anatomy is given in Chapter 2.

The first cervical vertebra (atlas) has no vertebral body or articular processes but two large wings that surround the vertebral canal. In the skeletally immature horse the two halves are separate and a radiolucent line can be seen up to nine months of age. The second cervical vertebra (axis) has a prominent dorsal process. The dens extends from the vertebral body cranially into the fovea dentis of the atlas. The dens originates from a separate centre of ossification, and therefore a radiolucent line is seen cranial to the endplate physis in the skeletally immature horse (up to seven months) (Figure 7.1).

C3, C4 and C5 have a similar anatomy and if three vertebrae in a row have a similar radiographic appearance they can be identified as C3, C4 and C5. C6 can be easily identified since its transverse processes are modified and

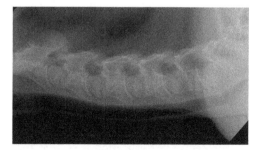

Figure 7.1 Laterolateral radiograph of the cervical spine of a skeletally immature horse (C2 to C7). Note the open cranial and caudal endplate physis.

C7 is usually shorter than the rest of the cervical vertebrae. The vertebral body of C3–C7 is a cylinder that is narrower cranially than caudally. Each vertebral body has a cranial and caudal endplate, the physes of which are visible as radiolucent lines in the immature horse; these fuse at 2 and 4–5 years respectively. The endplates should be smooth and congruent; the cranial endplate is convex and sometimes slightly flattened in the centre. The cranial and caudal endplates of each vertebral body articulate with the adjacent vertebra by means of an intervertebral disc. The disc space is smooth and even in width.

The vertebral arches, together with the dorsal border of the vertebral body delimitate the vertebral canal. The dorsal lamina of each arch should be parallel to the dorsal aspect of the vertebral body so that the vertebral canal is equal in size from cranial to caudal. The vertebral arch provides support for the articular and dorsal processes. Two articular processes are present on the cranial and caudal aspect of each vertebra from C3 to C7 and on the caudal aspect of the axis forming the articular process joints (often called 'facet joints'). The articular process joints are synovial joints with small medial and lateral pouches and a firm joint capsule [4].

The dorsal process is small and rudimental in all vertebrae except for the axis, where it forms a big crest. A variably shaped dorsal process can be identified on the cranial dorsal aspect of C7 in 13% of horses and less commonly on C6 and even C5 [5]. A transverse process is present in all vertebrae other than the axis. C6 has a prominent ventral extension of the transverse processes that allows differentiating C6 from the other vertebrae. This anatomical feature can be absent and/or can be observed in C7 in some horses, which may cause confusion when identifying cervical vertebrae [5]. Visualization of the first thoracic vertebra allows correct vertebral numbering in these cases. Occasionally a small separate centre of ossification is seen at the caudal end of the ventral portion of the transverse process of C6 and this should not be confused with a fracture.

Radiographic Diagnosis of some Conditions Affecting the Cervical Spine

Cervical Stenotic Myelopathy

Compression of the spinal cord is observed in association with cervical stenotic myelopathy and is further discussed in Chapter 12. Dynamic and static forms of compression have been described.

The dynamic form of cervical stenotic myelopathy is more commonly seen in immature horses (<18 months of age). Dorsal subluxation of the vertebral body causes ventral compression of the spinal cord and is responsible for the clinical signs. The degree of compression is usually exacerbated by hyperflexion of the neck. It is thought that subluxation can occur anywhere in the spine, although C3–C4 and C4–C5 are the most commonly affected sites [6].

The static form of cervical stenotic myelopathy is due to narrowing of the vertebral canal or to remodelling of the articular process joints that impinge in the dorsolateral aspect of the spinal cord. Horses affected by static stenosis are usually between 1 and 4 years old; in horses older than 4 years the compression is most commonly related to severe arthropathies of the articular process joints [6].

Subjective Evaluation

Radiographic changes (Figure 7.2) that can be identified in horses with cervical stenotic myelopathy are:

- Malalignment and subluxation between adjacent vertebral bodies resulting in angulation and step formation between vertebrae.
- 'Wedge-shaped' vertebral canal: asymmetric appearance of the vertebral canal, which is narrower at the cranial endplate and wider at the caudal endplate.
- Flaring of the caudal epiphysis of one or multiple vertebrae also known as 'ski jump' formation.

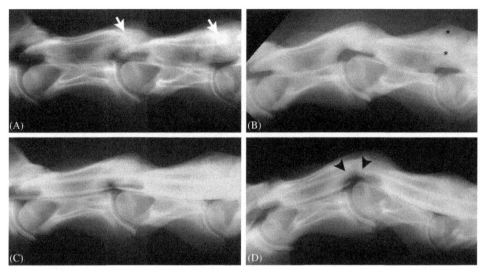

Figure 7.2 Plain laterolateral radiographs (A and B) and myelograms (C and D) centred at the level of C3–C4 of a horse presented for hindlimb ataxia. A and C are obtained with the neck in a neutral position while B and D are hyperflexed. There is caudal extension of the dorsal lamina of C3 and C4 (arrows) and remodelling of the articular process joints of C4–C5 (asterisks). After intrathecal contrast administration (myelogram) there is a normal appearance of the ventral and dorsal column of contrast in the neutral position (C). In the hyperflexed position the cranial physis of C4 is displaced dorsally, causing compression of the spinal cord; there is almost complete loss of the dorsal contrast column (black arrowheads).

- Caudal extension of the dorsal lamina respectively to the cranial endplate of the adjacent vertebra.
- Osteoarthritis of the articular process joints (see below).
- Narrowing of the vertebral canal. Subjective impression of a small vertebral canal height compared to the size of the vertebrae should be verified by a measurement-based evaluation (see below).

Measurement-Based Evaluation: Abnormal Values

Measurements of the width of the vertebral canal are routinely performed in horses where spinal cord compression is suspected. To normalize for size of the horse and magnification of images, the width of the vertebral canal is not used as an absolute measurement but put in relation to a standardized reference measurement. The most commonly used measurements are the intervertebral and intravertebral ratios (Figure 7.3).

The intervertebral ratio is obtained by dividing the minimum sagittal diameter (the distance between the most caudal edge of the dorsal lamina and the most dorsal edge of the endplate of the following vertebral) by the maximum height of the cranial vertebral epiphysis.

The intravertebral ratio is obtained by dividing the minimum sagittal diameter (the minimum width of the vertebral canal at the level of a vertebral body) by the maximum height of the cranial vertebral epiphysis [7].

A recent study comparing intra- and intervertebral ratios between horses with confirmed cervical stenotic myelopathy and horses with other neurological disease showed than the ratio can be used to predict the site of compression. In this study only three horses showed narrowing at the intravertebral site without evidence of narrowing at the intervertebral site, suggesting the importance of obtaining the intervertebral ratio. A cut-off value of 48.5% for the minimum sagittal diameter was suggested as a predictor of ataxia referable to cervical vertebral malformation [8].

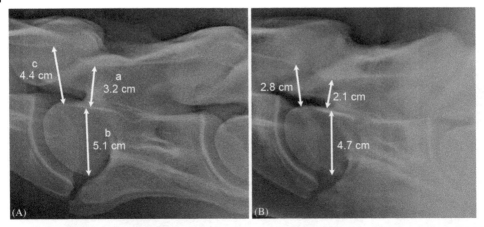

Figure 7.3 Laterolateral radiographic views of C5–C6 showing the positioning of the measurements (double arrowed lines) used to calculate the intravertebral (*a/b*) and intervertebral (*c/b*) ratios. (A) Normal horse. (B) The intravertebral ratio is 44.7%, indicative of stenosis of the vertebral canal; also notice the enlarged articular process joints of C6–C7.

In a recent study the degree of variability in measuring the cervical vertebral ratio has been compared between and within observers. Results showed that measurement error and variability does occur within and among observers and that observer experience in obtaining the measurement does influence the repeatability of measurements [9,10].

Degenerative Joint Disease

Osteoarthritis of the caudal cervical articular process joints has been observed in association with spinal cord compression, neck stiffness and forelimb lameness [1].

Radiographic abnormalities (Figure 7.4) include:

- Enlargement of the articular process joint.
- Periarticular new bone formation.
- Obliteration of the adjacent intervertebral foramen.
- Radiolucent areas associated with the articular process.
- Narrowing/widening of the joint space and irregular joint outline.

There is anecdotal evidence that the caudal cervical articular process joints (C5–C6 and C6–C7) enlarge in mature horses due to the stress placed on these highly mobile joints

and this might not be of clinical significance [11,12]. Conversely, enlargement of the process joint cranial to C5–C6 is very rarely seen in clinically normal horses [13].

Recently a descriptive grading system for enlargement of the caudal cervical articular process joint was developed. Ventral new bone formation was graded based on its relationship with the intervertebral foramen and caudal endplate of the cranial vertebra. Dorsal new bone formation was measured and compared with the height of the vertebral canal. There was no association between the degree of enlargement and breed or discipline of the horse or with the presence of a clinical sign. It was also observed that higher grades were more likely to be observed in older horses [11].

Sometimes asymmetric enlargement of the articular process joints can be seen in a well-positioned lateral–lateral view. In these cases the dorsal border of the two processes is not overlapping and oblique projections should be obtained to confirm which side is more severely affected. Severe enlargement of the articular process joint could potentially extend axially into the vertebral canal, resulting in compression of the spinal cord, or into the intervertebral foramen, compressing the ipsilateral spinal nerve [1]. A static form of spinal compression, leading to hindlimb

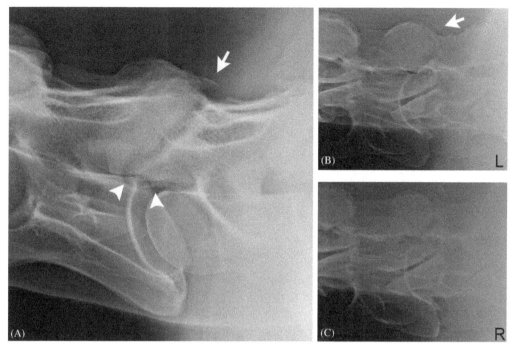

Figure 7.4 Laterolateral (A) and left and right oblique (B and C) radiographic projections of C6–C7 of a horse presented for neck pain. The articular process joints of C6–C7 are asymmetrically enlarged with ventral new bone formation obliterating the intervertebral foramen (arrowheads). There is a large osteophyte formation on the dorsal lateral aspect of the right caudal articular process of C6 (arrows).

ataxia and weakness, has been associated with caudal cervical articular process joints osteoarthritis. Multiple abnormalities are listed as a potential source of compression such as joint effusion, hypertrophy of the joint capsule, periarticular osteophyte formation, hypertrophy of the ligamentum flavum and synovial cyst. Recently the extension of the medial outpouch of the joint within the vertebral canal has been quantified using computed tomography. In this study each process joint was injected to maximal distension and the medial outpouch was measured. It was observed that the joint pouch was extending into the vertebral canal from the dorsolateral direction more than in non-distended joints, but contact between the distended joint pouch and the dura mater was not observed in any of the specimens [4].

The diagnostic value of radiography in the assessment of facet joint osteoarthritis is suboptimal [14]. The combination of both, laterolateral and oblique radiographs increases the diagnostic value (Figure 7.4). Oblique radiographs of the facet joints allow the identification of irregularities on the joint surfaces and osteophyte formation on the articular margin as well as fragments.

Intervertebral disc disease is a barely described entity in horses. A small number of case reports is available in the literature describing protrusion and extrusion of the intervertebral disc. Radiography has a limited diagnostic value for this condition and advanced diagnostic imaging modalities, such as computed tomography and magnetic resonance imaging, would be necessary [15].

Osteochondrosis

Osteochondral fragments can be occasionally identified as well-defined oval bony opacities in close association with the articular margins of the articular process joints. A radiolucent defect in the adjacent articular process can sometimes be identified. Cervical

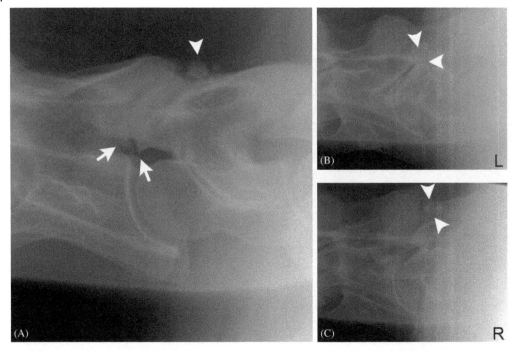

Figure 7.5 Laterolateral (A) and left and right oblique (B and C) radiographic projections of C6–C7. There is remodelling and periarticular osteophyte formation on the ventral and dorsal aspects of the left articular process joint (arrows). There is a single, rounded well-defined osteochondral fragment and a corresponding defect in the caudal dorsal margin of the left caudal articular process of C6 (arrowheads).

osteochondrosis is usually found unilaterally and it is often seen with concurrent radiographic signs of osteoarthritis. The use of oblique views in this particular condition can help in the identification of the affected side and may allow a thorough evaluation of these joints (Figure 7.5).

Cervical Fractures

Fractures of the cervical vertebra usually occur secondary to trauma. The clinical signs are acute in onset but can vary from profound ataxia, inability to lower the neck, abnormal low head carriage or neck stiffness. The severity of neurological signs is an important prognostic indicator. Cervical fractures are usually visible in laterolateral view, but occasionally oblique or ventrodorsal views are required depending on the fracture line location and configuration.

In foals fractures occur more often in the cranial portion of the spine and often involve the dens of the axis, while in adult horses the caudal cervical spine is more likely to be injured [16]. In foals the pathogenesis of an odontoid process fracture is attributed to the poor ability of the open physes to withstand pulling forces when the neck is in flexion, but fractures of the odontoid process have been described in adults secondary to a traumatic event [17]. Fracture of the base of the dens results in dorsal subluxation of the body of the axis, while the dens is kept in position by the odontoid ligaments.

Congenital Malformation

Congenital malformations of the cervical spine in the horse are rare. The most common is occipitoatlantoaxial malformation, which comprises any malformation among the occipital bone, atlas and axis. It can occur in numerous breeds, but is thought to be inherited in the Arabian breed [18]. Common bony abnormalities identified radiographically include fusion of the occiput and atlas (occipitalisation of the atlas) or atlas and axis (atlantalisation of the axis), hypoplastic dens or asymmetric bones [19].

Other congenital abnormalities of the cervical spine are reported infrequently, including butterfly vertebrae, hemivertebrae, block vertebrae, atlantoaxial instability (secondary to ligament laxity) or abnormal transverse process [20].

Ventrodorsal radiographs are recommended to be included as part of the diagnostic workup on foals with suspected cervical malformations [21].

Infectious Diseases

Septic arthritis and osteomyelitis can occasionally occur in the cervical spine. In foals, haematogenous dissemination of bacteria secondary to umbilical infection, pneumonia or enteritis has been described. Septic arthritis of the atlanto-occipital joint has been reported secondary to local spreading from guttural pouch empyema or mycosis. Radiographic findings include single or multiple areas of osteolysis, bone sclerosis and remodelling. The degree of bone destruction varies based on the chronicity of the process; in an early stage of the disease radiographs may appear normal and more sensitive image techniques, such as computed tomography, might be helpful to reach diagnosis. Prognosis for vertebral osteomyelitis is poor to grave, especially if neurological signs are present [22]. Discospondylitis occurs rarely in horses and is more commonly identified in the cervical and cranial thoracic vertebrae. Characteristic radiographic findings include osteolysis of adjacent endplates and vertebral bodies, initial widening and subsequent collapse of the intervertebral disc space, proliferative new bone formation resulting is sclerosis and ventral bridging spondylosis [23].

Neoplasia

Neoplasia of the musculoskeletal system is rare but more commonly described in the axial skeleton. Plasmacellular myeloma, fibrosarcoma, lymphosarcoma, melanoma, undifferentiated sarcoma and haemangiosarcoma have been described in the cervical vertebral spine. The latter might be the most represented based on the literature.

Variable degree of osteolysis and cortical disruption is seen on radiographs. The lesion can be expansile in nature and causing invasion of the vertebral canal and extradural compression of the spinal cord. The degree of compression can be verified using myelography or computed tomography [24].

Soft Tissue Injuries

Soft tissue changes cannot be observed on radiographs; however, enthesiopathies can be visualised. New bone formation on the nuchal crest, involving the origin of the nuchal ligament, is commonly observed and often represents an incidental finding, especially in Warmblood horses. Insertional desmopathy can occur and it is usually associated to trauma to the poll region; it can manifest clinically as reluctance to lower the head, flexing the poll region and headshaking. Occasionally an avulsion fracture from the origin of the nuchal ligament or semispinalis muscles, which originates just lateral to the nuchal ligament, is observed [13]. In rare occasions irregularity of the arch of the atlas can be seen secondary to cranial nuchal bursitis [25] as well as dystrophic mineralization within the adjacent soft tissue [26].

Myelography

Myelography is indicated when compression of the spinal cord is suspected. While it may be possible to identify narrowing of the vertebral canal secondary to bony changes, e.g. vertebral stenosis, vertebral malformations, fractures or subluxation on plain radiographs, identification of spinal cord compression is impossible without the use of positive contrast outlining the spinal cord.

Patient Preparation and Image Acquisition

A radiodense, water-soluble, non-ionic contrast agent (i.e. iohexol) is injected within the subarachnoid space [27]. This technique is usually performed with the patient under general anaesthesia in lateral recumbency, with the head slightly elevated compared to the body. The ears are pulled rostrally and a rectangular area, centred over the foramen magnum, is clipped and aseptically prepared. Cisternal puncture is performed using an 18-gauge 8.3 cm (3.5 inch) spinal needle with the horse's head flexed to an angle of 90 degrees. This can be performed either using a blind technique or using an ultrasound-guided approach [28]. For the blind technique, the wings of the atlas are located; the needle is inserted at the intersection of lines running along the front of the atlas and along the dorsal midline and directed toward the middle of the lower jaw [29]. The needle is then connected to an extension set and a volume of cerebrospinal fluid, approximately 50 ml, is slowly withdrawn; an approximately equal volume of prewarmed contrast medium is slowly injected over 3–4 minutes. Finally, the needle is removed and the head and neck are elevated for 5–10 min, up to 45 degrees from the horizontal to allow the contrast medium to distribute along the cervical spine. Wedge-shaped cushions and a board under the head and neck of the patient facilitate this. Laterolateral radiographs are obtained with the neck in a neutral position, hyperflexed and hyperextended position. To achieve the necessary extreme hyperflexion the horse's head has to be pulled as far as possible between its forelimbs. Tunnel blocks are helpful to facilitate positioning of the plates underneath the neck.

Interpretation

Positive contrast myelography is considered the best antemortem test for diagnosis of extradural compression due to cervical stenotic myelopathy. Multiple criteria have been proposed for the identification of compressed sites. Absolute measurement of the dorsal column of contrast (<2 mm) is considered inadequate to predict cervical vertebral malformation by most authors.

The most commonly used method is a 50% reduction of the minimal height of the contrast column at an intervertebral site compared to the maximal dorsal myelographic column at the level of the vertebral body just cranial to it (Figure 7.2). However, this method was only moderately accurate in detecting horses that did not have extradural compression and it was poor at detecting horses with spinal cord compression [30]. This was also confirmed in a more recent study where it was also noted that sensitivity and specificity of this method varies based on the site and neck position. In the mid cervical spine it was appropriate to use this test only in the neutral position since flexion of the neck will increase false-positive diagnosis. Conversely at the C6–C7 site positioning from flexion to neutral increased the detection of compression sites but also increased false-positive results [31].

Variations in the dural diameter between intravertebral and intervertebral have also been studied and cut-off values also varied between different sites and neck positions [31].

It was concluded that both a reduction of the dorsal column and of the dural diameter are useful techniques for evaluating horses with suspected cervical stenotic myelopathy and that clinicians can vary the degree of reduction and neck positioning to optimizing sensitivity and specificity [31,32].

References

1 Ricardi, G. and Dyson, S.J. Forelimb lameness associated with radiographic abnormalities of the cervical vertebrae. *Equine Veterinary Journal* 1993; **35**:422–426.

2 Rose, P.L., Abutarbush, S.M. and Duckett, W. Standing Myelography in the horse using a nonioninc contrast agent. *Veterinary Radiology and Ultrasound* 2007; **48**:535–538.

3 Withers, J.M., Voute, L.C., Hammond, G. and Lisher, C.J. Radiographic anatomy of the articular process joints of the caudal cervical vertebrae in the horse on lateral and oblique projections. *Equine Veterinary Journal* 2009; **41**:895–902.

4 Claridge, H.A.H., Piercy, R.J., Parry, A. and Weller, R. The 3D anatomy of the cervical articular process joints in the horse and their topographical relationship to the spinal cord. *Equine Veterinary Journal* 2010; **42**:726–731.

5 Santinelli, I., Beccati, F., Arcelli, R. and Pepe, M. Anatomical variation of the spinous and transverse processes in the caudal cervical and the first thoracic vertebrae in horses. *Veterinary Radiology and Ultrasound* 2015; **48**:45–49.

6 Wagner, P.C., Grant, B.D. and Reed, S.M. Cervical vertebral malformation. *Veterinary Clinics of North America: Equine Practice* 1987; **3**:385–396.

7 Moore, B.R., Reed, S.M., Biller, D.S., Kohn, C.W. and Weisbrode, S.E. Assessment of vertebral canal diameter and bony malformation of the cervical part of the spine in horses with cervical stenotic myelopathy. *American Journal of Veterinary Research* 1994; **55**:5–13.

8 Hahn, C.N., Handel, I., Green, S.L., Bronsvoort, M.B. and Mayhew, I.G. Assessment of the utility of using intra- and intervertebral minimum sagittal diameter ratios in the diagnosis of cervical vertebral malformation in horses. *Veterinary Radiology and Ultrasound* 2008; **1**:1–6.

9 Scrivani, P.V., Levine, J.M., Holmes, N.L. et al. Observer agreement study of cervical-vertebral ratios in horses. *Equine Veterinary Journal* 2011; **43**:399–403.

10 Hughes, K.J., Laidlaw, E.H., Reed, S.M. et al. Repeatability and intra-inter-observer agreement of cervical vertebral sagittal diameter ratios in horses with neurological disease. *Journal of Veterinary Internal Medicine* 2014; **28**:1860–1870.

11 Down, S.S. and Henson, F.M.D. Radiographic retrospective study of the caudal cervical articular process joints in the horse. *Equine Veterinary Journal* 2009; **41**:518–524.

12 Butler, J., Colles, C., Dyson, S., Kold, S. and Poulos, P. The spine. In: *Clinical Radiology of the Horse*, 3rd edn. Oxford: Blackwell, 2010, pp. 505–535.

13 Dyson, S.J. Lesions of the equine neck resulting in lameness and poor performances. *Veterinary Clinics of North America: Equine Practice* 2011; **3**:411–610.

14 Tambaschi, M., Dunkel, B., Mullard, J. et al. Latero-oblique radiography as a diagnostic tool for equine cervical osteoarthritis. *Equine Veterinary Journal* 2014; **46**(S47):10–11.

15 Veera, S., Bergmann, W., Wijnberg, I.D., Back, W. and van den Belt, A.J.M. Imaging and pathologic findings in intervertebral disc disease in the equine cervical spine. In: EVDI Annual Meeting Proceedings, Utrecht, 27–30 August 2014, p. 49.

16 DeBowes, R.M. (1990) Management of vertebral fractures. In: White, N.A. and Moore, J.N. (eds), *Current Practice of Equine Surgery*. Philadelphia, PA: J.B. Lippincott, 1990, pp. 187–191.

17 Vos, N.J., Pollock, P.J., Harty, M. et al. Fractures of the cervical vertebral odontoid in four horses and one pony. *Veterinary Record* 2008; **162**:116–119.

18 Mayhew, I.G., Watson, A.G. and Heissan, J.A. Congenital occipitoatlantoaxial malformations in the horse. *Equine Veterinary Journal* 1978; **10**:103–112.

19 Gonda, C., Crisman, M. and Moon, M. Occipitoatlantoaxial malformation in a quarter horse foal. *Equine Veterinary Education*, 2001; **13**:289–291.

20 Rush, B.R. Developmental vertebral anomalies. In: Auer, J.A. and Stick, J.A. (eds), *Equine Surgery*, 4th edn. Philadelphia, PA: W.B. Saunders Co., 2012, pp. 693–699.

21 Griffin, R.L., Bennett, S.D., Brandt, C. and McAnly, J. Value of ventrodorsal radiographic views for diagnosis of transverse atlanto-occipital joint luxation in three American Saddlebred neonates.

Equine Veterinary Education 2007; **19**:452–456.

22 Roberts, B.L., Reimer, J.M., Woodie, J.B. and Reed, S.M. Septic arthritis of the first and second cervical vertebral articulations with vertebral osteomyelitis in a foal caused by *Salmonella*. *Equine Veterinary Education* 2010; **22**:328–333.

23 Sweers, L. and Carstens, A. Imaging features of Discospondylitis in two horses. *Veterinary Radiology and Ultrasound* 2006; **2**:159–164.

24 Raes, E.V., Durie, I., Wegge, B. et al. Imaging findings of a haemangiosarcoma in a cervical vertebra of a horse. *Equine Veterinary Education* 2014; **26**:548–551.

25 Garcia-Lopez, J.M., Janei, T., Chope, K. and Bubeck, K.A. Diagnosis and management of cranial and caudal nuchal bursitis in four horses. *Journal of Veterinary Medical Association* 2010; **237**:823–829.

26 Manso-Diaz, G., Garcia-Lopez, J.M., Maranda, L. and Taeymans, O. The role of computed tomography in equine practice. *Equine Veterinary Education* 2015; **27**:136–145.

27 Burbidget, H.M., Kannegieter, N., Dickson, L.R., Goulden, B.E. and Badcoe, L. Iohexol myelography in the horse. *Veterinary Radiology and Ultrasound* 1989; **21**:347–350.

28 Audigié, F., Tapprest, J., Didierlaurent, D. and Denoix, J.-M. Ultrasound-guided atlanto-occipital puncture for myelography in the horse. *Veterinary Radiology and Ultrasound* 2004; **45**:340–344.

29 Grant, B.D. and Paterson, J. How to perform a myelogram in less than 30 minutes. *Proceedings of the American Association of Equine Practitioners* 2006; **52**:74–77.

30 Mayhew, I.G. and Green, S.L. Accuracy of diagnosis CVM from radiographs. In: Proceedings of the 39th British Equine Veterinary Association Congress, Equine Veterinary Journal, Newmarket, 2000, pp. 74–75.

31 Van Biervliet, J., Scrivani, P.V., Divers, T.J. et al. Evaluation of decision criteria for detection of spinal cord compression based on cervical myelography in horses: 38 cases. *Equine Veterinary Journal* 2004; **36**:14–20.

32 Hudson, N.P.J. and Mayhew, I.G. Radiographic and myelographic assessment of the equine cervical vertebral column and spinal cord. *Equine Veterinary Education* 2005; **17**:34–38.

8

Radiography of the Back

Frances M.D. Henson

Introduction

Radiography is an extremely important diagnostic imaging technique for use in the diagnosis of back pathology in the horse. Radiographic images can be obtained in both the standing animal and under general anaesthesia, although standing radiography is used almost exclusively in clinical practice. This chapter describes the equipment required for radiography of the equine back, the technique for acquiring radiographic images of the back, the normal radiographic anatomy of the equine spine and an introduction to the radiographic appearance of pathology in the equine spine.

Indications for Radiography of the Back and/or Pelvis

The indications for radiography of the back and pelvis include the following:

- The presence of specific areas of suspected pathology. An example of this would be finding heat, pain and swelling in the withers region on a clinical examination, which might indicate a fracture of the dorsal spinous processes (DSPs) of the vertebrae.
- When indicated by another diagnostic imaging technique. An example of this would be where a nuclear scintigraphic examination has identified an area of increased radionuclide uptake in a vertebra.
- As part of a general investigation into back pain.

Technical Difficulties with Radiography of the Equine Back and Pelvis

In the horse, unlike the situation in humans and small animals, radiography is limited to specific areas of the back and pelvis. This limitation is due to the large size of the adult horse and the amount of soft tissue overlaying most of the thoracolumbar spine and pelvis. Both of these factors necessitate the use of extremely high exposures and cause a high amount of scatter, which degrades the radiographic image.

Structures That Can Be Readily Imaged in the Standing Horse

In the standing horse thoracic vertebra T1 is readily imaged on lateromedial projections; however, the scapula overlies the vertebral bodies and DSPs of T2 and T3, and the vertebral bodies of T4–T8. In this region only the DSPs of T4–T8 are imaged. From approximately T9 to L3–L4, the entire vertebral body and DSPs can be seen. From L3 caudally it is extremely difficult to get

Equine Neck and Back Pathology: Diagnosis and Treatment, Second Edition. Edited by Frances M.D. Henson.
© 2018 John Wiley & Sons, Ltd. Published 2018 by John Wiley & Sons, Ltd.

satisfactory pictures of the vertebral body and DSPs; the lumbosacral spine and iliac wings are superimposed and only in foals and small, thin ponies can different structures be visualised. The sacrum cannot be visualised in the standing horse and the pelvis visualised only grossly in comparison to the detail obtained at other sites. In order to obtain images of these areas radiography under general anaesthesia is recommended, although this is expensive and may cause a deterioration in the clinical condition.

Radiographic Technique

Patient Preparation

The horse should be brushed over to check that there is no mud or other substance in the coat that might lead to radiographic artefacts. Before starting the radiographic examination, intravenous sedation is recommended. This has a number of advantages: first it minimises movement of the patient and second it means that the horse needs less close restraint, and the handler can move further away from the horse and hence the X-ray beam. Sedation can, however, cause truncal swaying at high doses. The use of stocks to restrain the horse is a matter of individual veterinarian preference; however, they can be extremely useful where available to minimise movement. Whether or not stocks are available, the horse must be standing straight and must be weight bearing evenly on all four limbs in order to reduce rotational artefacts. Care must be taken to position the head and neck in a neutral position as it has been shown that alterations in head/neck position can alter the distances between the spinous and transverse processes in the thoracic vertebar in horses [1].

To help placement and orientation of radiographs adhesive labels can be used on the coat of the skin to aid the radiographer in spacing out the film series. Alternatively, lead markers can be used to assist in the localisation of specific areas of pathology. This is particularly useful in the presurgical planning

stage when considering surgical removal of clinically significant DSPs.

Equipment

Radiography of the back requires radiographic equipment with an output of up to 150 kV and 250–500 mA. As mentioned above, the large soft tissue mass of the horse and the subsequent scattering of radiation are a limitation to the acquisition of high-quality equine back radiographs. A number of different measures can be taken to help reduce the effect of scatter [2].

First it is recommended that rare-earth film/screen systems are used – this allows the exposure factors to be reduced. A grid (preferably a cross-hatched parallel grid with a ratio of 12:1) is necessary for most radiographs, apart from the summits of the DSPs, to reduce the effect of scattered radiation. In addition, for exposures over 100 kV it is recommended that a lead sheet should be placed behind the cassette to prevent backscatter.

Due to the extensive soft tissue mass of the equine back and the position of the vertebrae and the DSPs, there is a considerable difference in tissue attenuation between the main regions of interest, i.e. the vertebral bodies and the summits of the DSPs. Thus, to image these two different anatomical sites, either two radiographs with different exposures must be taken or a beam filtration device used. With traditional, non-digital radiography it is usually necessary to have a device that permits a higher exposure to be set for the deeper structures of the back while filtering the beam for the summits of the DSPs. There are different ways of achieving this; some clinics have a 'Dodger' beam filter that uses aluminium wedges to achieve beam filtration [3]; other clinics have constructed devices that perform essentially the same function. However, with digital radiography becoming increasingly widespread throughout equine clinics, such filters are not necessarily needed because it is possible to alter the contrast of the radiographs in postacquisitional

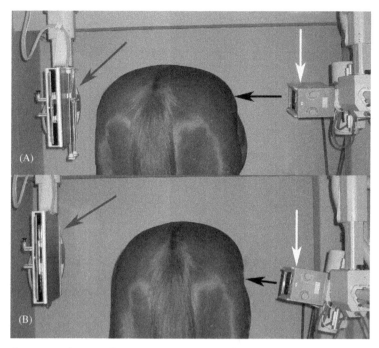

Figure 8.1 Photographs to show the position of the tube head (white arrow), cassette holder (grey arrow) and direction of X-ray beam (black arrow) when acquiring: (A) lateromedial images of the back of the horse and (B) DM20°VL oblique images. (A) The tube head is positioned horizontal to the ground and the beam travels horizontally. (B) The tube head is angled proximally and the beam travels upwards from the tube head. Note, in both photographs, that the cassette holder is aligned with the direction of the tube head angulation and X-ray beam.

processing. Regardless of the method of controlling exposures, close collimation to the region of interest is always recommended in order to enhance image quality if a lesion is detected on survey films.

To obtain standing radiographs of the horse there are a number of ways in which the equipment can be utilised, but ideally the X-ray tube is mounted on an overhead gantry with a linked cassette holder to ensure that the X-ray beam and the film are aligned (Figure 8.1A). The cassette holder can be mounted on the opposite wall or any other suitable upright structure (Figure 8.1A). Large cassettes are required ($35 \times 43\,\mathrm{cm}^2$ recommended) to hold the large radiographic films.

Exposure Values

It is difficult to be prescriptive regarding exposure factors and times for radiography of the equine back because different machines, different technical setups and different sizes of horse mean that what is correct for one situation is under- or overexposed in another. The exposures detailed in Table 8.1 are intended as a rough guide for veterinarians beginning to acquire images of the equine back. They should be altered according to individual situations; use of a detailed record of exposure values used and the outcome is considered good clinical practice.

Positioning and Radiograph Acquisition

Essentially two sets of radiographs are acquired in a 'back series': a set of slightly overlapping *lateromedial radiographs* obtained in order to highlight the DSPs and to allow assessment of the ventral surfaces of the vertebral bodies (usually taken from one side only) and a set

Table 8.1 Radiographic exposures for different areas of the thoracolumbar spine using X-ray machine in an average 500 kg thoroughbred horse.

Radiographic view	Peak (kV)	(mA)	Grid?	Cassette
DSP T3–7 (withers)	75	15	No	Rapid
DSP T8–13 (midthoracic)	80	25	No	Rapid
DSP T13–15 (caudal thoracic)	85	25	No	Rapid
DSP T16–18, L1–4 (thoracolumbar)	90	35	No	Rapid
Thoracic articular facets (oblique)	110	220	Yes	Rapid
Lumbar articular facets (oblique)	110	250	Yes	Rapid
Sacroiliac joint under general anaesthetic	96	500	Yes	Rapid

of slightly overlapping *oblique radiographs* obtained primarily in order to highlight the articular facet articulations (taken from both the left and right of the horse in order to highlight left and right facet joints).

Lateromedial Radiographs

To acquire lateromedial radiographs the beam should be centred 10–15 cm ventral to the dorsal skin surface in order to be centred on the DSP (in an average-sized 500 kg horse, this distance should be adjusted for the size of the horse). The beam is angled horizontally (Figure 8.2A). Three to four radiographs are usually required to image the spine from the withers region to approximately L2–L3; these radiographs should be positioned so that they overlap in order to ensure that no pathology is missed by being marginalised on the edge of a radiograph. The first radiograph is taken of the withers region and subsequent radiographs follow on caudally. In order to image the DSP of T1 a lateromedial radiograph is taken centred over the vertebral body of C6–C7 with the X-ray beam angled horizontally.

Oblique Radiographs

To acquire radiographs of the articular facets the beam is centred 20–25 cm below the dorsum and angled upwards (ventral to dorsal) at an angle of 20–30° (dorsomedial 20° ventrolateral oblique (DM20°VLO); Figure 8.2B). The DM20°VLO view reduces the superimposition of the articulations and, in the lumbar region, reduces superimposition of the transverse processes. Three radiographs on each side (total six) are usually required to image the articular facets (three radiographs to highlight left-hand-side articular facets, and three to highlight right-hand-side ones); again these radiographs should be positioned so that they overlap.

Radiography under General Anaesthesia

Although standing radiography is very useful in most clinical cases, the technique does have its limitations. To obtain optimum lateral views of the caudal lumbar spine, ventrodorsal views of the thoracolumbar spine (in all but the smallest ponies and foals) and ventrodorsal views of the sacroiliac joints, radiography under general anaesthesia is indicated. General anaesthesia is needed because all these views require use of very high exposures; rendering the horse immobile during the acquisition of the images produces diagnostic films because it reduces the movement blur that would otherwise occur.

To obtain radiographs under general anaesthesia the horse should be anaesthetised and positioned with the aid of a hoist. Care must be taken with this positioning and padding/support to ensure that the horse is positioned precisely and that there is no

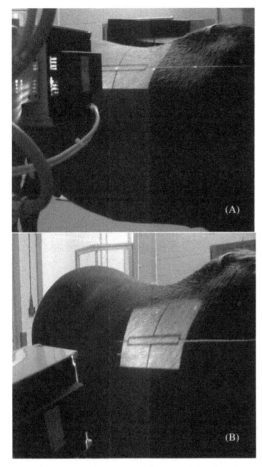

(A)

(B)

Figure 8.2 Photographs to show the centring of the beam and the collimation of the beam used to acquire (A) lateromedial and (B) DM20°VLO radiographs. (A) The beam is centred just above the vertebral bodies of the horse (10–15 cm below the dorsum) and (B) the beam is centred 20 cm distal to this point. The small white markers seen to run from cranial to caudal on the side of the horse are stickers applied to identify where different images have been centred.

rotation of the spine. For lateromedial radiographs, supports under the proximal fore- and hindlimbs are required to ensure that the limbs are parallel with the trunk. To obtain ventrodorsal views the horse should be positioned carefully in dorsal recumbency, again ensuring that there is no rotation of the spine, with the hindlimbs flexed in a neutral ('frog-legged') position.

Of the views that can be obtained under general anaesthesia, radiography of the sacroiliac joint has been well described. To obtain radiographs of the sacroiliac region, the horse is positioned in dorsal recumbency with the legs in a neutral position as described above, with the X-ray beam centred on the midline at the level of the tuber sacrale. This radiographic approach ensures that the X-ray beam strikes the pelvis either perpendicular or slightly caudocranial (no more than 10° angle) to the sacroiliac joint.

Exposures of 96 kV and 500 mA for 5 seconds have been recommended to image the sacroiliac region in warmblood horses of approximately 500 kg [4]. To produce a radiographic image that can be interpreted, Gorgas et al. [4] described a radiographic technique in which active ventilation was performed during the exposure, in order to cause movement and radiographic blurring of superimposed gastrointestinal structures, followed by digital enhancement of the images obtained.

Radiography of the Pelvis – Standing Technique

Standing radiography of the pelvis in the horse is not difficult technically but, due to the large size of the horse, the overlying muscle mass in the pelvic region and the movement that occurs, the resultant images are of poor quality and difficult to interpret. Pelvic radiography is usually performed when a fracture of the ilial shaft is suspected.

A number of different techniques have been described as follows.

Lateromedial Radiography

To obtain lateromedial radiographs, the tube head is positioned lateral to the pelvis and the cassette positioned on the other side of the pelvis, adjacent to the musculature. This approach is rarely performed because it provides little information except in the smallest of ponies, although it has been described as useful in identifying fractures of the tuber sacrale.

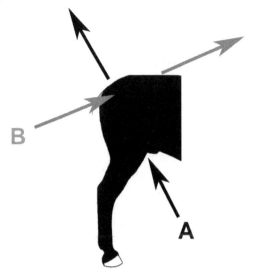

Figure 8.3 A drawing to demonstrate two different radiographic angles for acquiring pelvic radiographs in the standing horse. (A) The direction of the X-ray beam to acquire ventrodorsal radiographs. (B) The direction of the X-ray beam to acquire lateral–oblique radiographs.

Ventrodorsal Radiography

To obtain ventrodorsal radiographs, the tube head is positioned ventrally to the abdomen, just cranial to the hindleg, and the cassette is positioned dorsal to the sacrum (Figure 8.3). The disadvantages of this technique are that centring of the beam and collimation are difficult and imprecise. In addition there is considerable risk to the tube head because it is positioned underneath the horse [5]. However, it is possible to get acceptable quality radiographs using this technique and to identify gross disruptions in the pelvic symmetry or bony displacement.

Lateral–Oblique Radiography (Lateral–Dorsal 30° Lateroventral Obliques)

To obtain lateral-oblique radiographs, the tube head is angled approximately 30° ventrally from the horizontal, centred between the level of the greater trochanter and the base of the tail, approximately two-thirds of the way along the craniocaudal distance between the palpable landmarks of the tuber sacrale

and the tuber ischii (Figure 8.3). The cassette is positioned vertically against the side of the pelvis under examination and the rectum is emptied of faeces in order to provide an air-filled region within the pelvis. It is recommended that a rare-earth screen and stationary parallel grid be used. The radiographic exposure required to image the pelvis depends on the size of the horse and the muscle mass; however, a range of between 90 and 130 kV and between 124 and 400 mA has been described [6].

Normal Radiographic Appearance of the Back

Skeletally Immature Horses

The thoracolumbar spine changes in angulations from birth to about 6 months, with the thoracolumbar spine having a dorsal curvature (kyphosis) that straightens out at 6 months. As discussed in Chapter 1, the cranial and caudal physes of the vertebrae are visible in foals up to approximately 6 months of age (Figure 8.4). From this age they begin to close; the cranial physes begin to close from 6 months onwards and the caudal physes from 24 months onwards. The separate centres of ossification

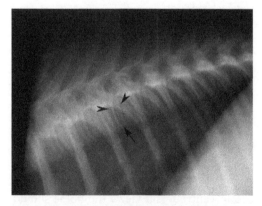

Figure 8.4 A lateromedial radiograph of the vertebral column of a 6-week-old miniature horse. The intervertebral disc space can be seen (arrow) and the open growth plates of the vertebrae are visible (arrowhead).

of the cranial thoracic DSPs (except T1) begin to develop at approximately 12 months of age; the centres of ossification have a very irregular outline and remain separate from the parent bone throughout life.

Skeletally Mature Radiographic Anatomy

The normal structure of the vertebrae is discussed in Chapter 1 and a working knowledge of the normal anatomy should be acquired before radiographic interpretation.

Dorsal Spinous Processes

The DSP of T1 is usually visible on a lateromedial radiograph of the base of the neck; it has a triangular shape and in most horses is approximately the height of the vertebral body. A radiographic study has shown that approximately 75% of horses have the ususal 'long' T1 DSP, with 25% having a shortened, squat DSP [7]. T1 has no separate centre of ossification (Figure 8.5). Advancing caudally,

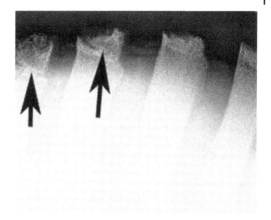

Figure 8.6 A lateromedial radiograph of the dorsal spinous processes obtained in the withers region (thoracic vertebrae T4–T11) to show the radiographic appearance of the summits of these vertebrae. The summits of the more cranial vertebrae show separate centres of ossification (arrow).

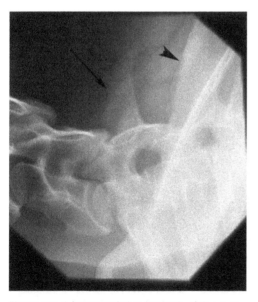

Figure 8.5 A lateromedial radiograph of the vertebral column obtained at the base of the neck to show the radiographic appearance of the first thoracic vertebra (T1; arrow). Note that the dorsal spinous process is markedly enlarged compared with cervical vertebrae (cranial). However, note the cranial edge of the scapular rising up to obscure the dorsal spinal process of T2 (arrowhead).

the DSP of T2 is not usually visible radiographically, but the DSPs of T3–T8 are readily visible on radiography. Each of these DSPs has a clearly visible separate centre of ossification throughout life, which must not be mistaken for a fracture or osteolysis (Figure 8.6). In the withers region T4–T6 have the longest DSPs. The DSPs gradually reduce in length caudally from T6, with the cranial thoracic DSP angled slightly caudal and the caudal thoracic DSP angled slightly cranial. The anticlinal vertebra is usually either T15 or T16 (Figure 8.7). Using the standard standing lateromedial radiographic technique described, the DSPs of vertebrae up to L1–L2 are visible in most horses.

Vertebral Bodies and Discs

The vertebral bodies and related structures of approximately T11 to L1–L2 can be visualised on standing lateromedial radiographs. The cranial and caudal extremities of the vertebral body, articular facets, ventral aspect of the vertebrae, angulation of the vertebrae relative to each other and articulations of the ribs must all be carefully examined.

In mature horses the intervertebral disc spaces are uniform in width from dorsal to ventral, following the curve of the cranial border of the vertebral body (Figure 8.8).

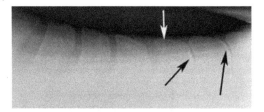

Figure 8.7 A lateromedial radiograph of the dorsal spinous processes obtained in the midthoracic region (thoracic vertebrae T12–T18) to show the direction of angulation of these vertebrae and the radiographic appearance of the summits of these vertebrae. The anticlinal vertebra (T16) is indicated with a white arrow. Cranial to the anticlinal vertebra the dorsal spinous processes (DSPs) point caudally; caudal to the anticlinal vertebra the DSPs point cranially. Cranial to the anticlinal vertebra the DSPs have space between them; caudal to the anticlinal vertebra the DSPs are close together (but not touching). However, there is evidence of remodelling of the adjacent bony surfaces, indicated by sclerosis of the bone (black arrows).

The disc spaces are relatively narrow compared with other species. The cranial and caudal extremities of the vertebrae are smooth, with the caudal extremity appearing sclerotic relative to the cranial extremity. Ventrally the vertebrae are smooth in the normal horse, with

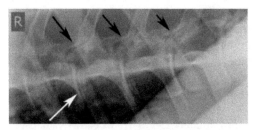

Figure 8.8 A DM20°VLO radiograph of the vertebral bodies obtained in the caudal thoracic region to show the radiographic appearance of the intervertebral discs and the articular facets of the vertebrae. The intervertebral disc spaces are uniform in width from dorsal to ventral (white arrow). The articular facets are seen as radiolucent dog-legged or 'inverted L' shapes at the base of the articular with the rib on this radiograph (black arrows). The two cranial facets indicated are normal articular facet articulations; the most caudal facet has sclerosis associated with the joint edges.

no evidence of new bone formation around the intervertebral disc.

Vertebral Body Articulations

The articular facets of the thoracolumbar vertebrae and the articulations of the ribs are clearly seen on the oblique views. The articular facets are identified as inverted 'L' or dog-legged radiolucent lines dorsal to the vertebral canal (Figure 8.8). The morphology and positioning of the articular facets alter depending on the position of the facet within the spine. The angulation of the facets changes from nearly horizontal in the cranial thoracic spine to almost vertical more caudally and, radiographically, the lumbar articular facets are more radio-opaque and more irregular in structure than in the thoracic region.

The articulations of the ribs are also seen on the oblique projections. The ribs initially course back dorsally and caudally in the cranial thoracic region; more caudally they course ventrally.

Lumbar, Sacral and Coccygeal Vertebrae

It is extremely difficult to obtain diagnostic radiographs of the lumbar and sacral vertebrae in the standing horse, although it can be attempted using a lateromedial technique centred on the region of interest in smaller horses and ponies. The coccygeal vertebrae are more readily imaged and either lateromedial or dorsoventral views can be obtained of this area if required.

Sacroiliac Region

Using the technique described above for radiography of the sacroiliac region, some of the anatomical features of the sacroiliac joints have been described. The cranial sacral borders and the sacral wings are the most readily visible features. Radiographically the cranial sacral borders have been described as having either a 'T' or a 'Y' appearance and the sacral wings as having a butterfly, wing, horn or leaf configuration. However, the significance of these morphological descriptions has not been demonstrated [4].

Pelvis

In the normal pelvis standing radiography reveals the outline of the ilial shaft and the outline of the acetabulum. General anaesthesia is required to visualise the full extent of the pelvis, where the ilial wings, ilial shaft, acetabula, pubis and ischial tuberosities can all be imaged.

An Introduction to Radiographic Abnormalities of the Back and Pelvis

Radiographic abnormalities are commonly seen in the equine back; indeed, it is rare to examine a set of radiographs from a horse and detect no radiographic changes. The challenge to the veterinarian who is investigating the cause of back pain in a horse is first to identify the radiographic changes present and second, and more importantly, to understand the clinical significance of these changes. In this section a brief introduction to the radiographic changes that may be encountered is given. For more specific changes refer to the specific individual chapters referred to in the text.

Congenital Defects

A number of congenital disorders can affect the back of the horse. These can be divided into conditions that are readily detectable clinically (lordosis, scoliosis and kyphosis) and defects that are more usually detected radiographically (hemivertebrae and congenital fusion of the thoracolumbar vertebral bodies or articular processes). Lordosis may be caused by congenital hypoplasia of the articular processes but may also be acquired. Radiographically lordosis is recognised as a ventral convexity of the thoracolumbar spine. Kyphosis, in contrast, is recognised as a dorsal convexity of the thoracolumbar spine. Scoliosis (a twisting of the spine) is best diagnosed on dorsoventral radiographs. In these radiographs scoliosis is recognised radiographically

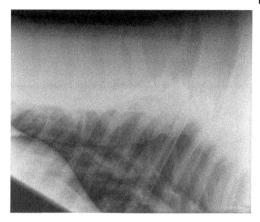

Figure 8.9 A lateromedial radiograph of the thoracic spine of a yearling filly to show marked scoliosis (lateral deviation of the vertebral column). Note the abnormal shape and position of the dorsal spinous process and vertebral bodies. *Source:* Courtesy of Mr R. Pilsworth.

as a deviation of the spine from a normal, straight appearance (Figure 8.9). In addition, wedge-shaped vertebral bodies may be seen. On lateromedial radiographs there is an asymmetry in the positioning of the ribs and an alteration in the length of the vertebral bodies. Radiographically diagnosed congenital defects may be incidental findings on routine radiographic examination or they may be severe, causing back weakness and clinical signs.

Radiographic Abnormalities of the DSP

Radiography of the equine back is most commonly performed in order to identify whether or not the horse is showing evidence of over-riding DSPs (ORDSPs); however, there are many radiographic abnormalities that can be detected in the region of the DSPs in the horse. These include fractured DSPs (Chapter 13). In cases of fractured DSPs the long DSPs are usually noted to be displaced either cranially or caudally. Usually the fractured summit is seen distal to its predicted site on the radiograph. Care must be taken not to confuse separate centres of ossification in the cranial thoracic DSPs (see Figure 8.6) with fractures of the DSPs, as discussed earlier.

The radiographic signs of ORDSPs are basically evidence of two DSPs either being closer together than normal or overlapping/making contact. It must be recognised that many clinically normal horses have DSPs that are in close apposition, particularly in the caudal thoracic and lumbar regions. Indeed, it has been shown that, in one study of normal horses, 34% showed some degree of DSP impingement [3]. *The diagnosis of clinically significant ORDSPs cannot, therefore, be made on radiographic signs alone.* Abnormalities of the DSPs range from DSPs that are close at their summits to overlapped DSPs that have clear radiographic signs of remodelling. The spectrum of changes seen in the DSPs ranges, therefore, from the mildly affected to severely affected. In mildly affected cases the DSPs are close but not in apposition. However, changes at the cranial and caudal cortical borders of the proximal aspect of the DSPs are seen (see Figure 8.7), indicating that contact is occurring, probably when the horse is moving, being ridden or jumping.

This category of ORDSPs can be considered *dynamic ORDSPs*. The changes seen in the DSPs are areas of sclerosis on the cranial and caudal borders of the DSPs, running along their edge (see Figure 8.7) but rarely affecting the central section of the bone. It is of note that it is extremely rare to see sclerosis in the distal portion of the DSPs. More advanced radiographic signs of ORDSPs include marked sclerosis and remodelling of the cranial and caudal borders of the DSPs and the development of cyst-like lucencies within the bones where they are in contact (Figure 8.10). In addition, at the summits of the DSPs, new bone formation can occur (Figure 8.11). In severe cases the DSPs are clearly in apposition or even overlapping (*static ORDSPs*) (Figure 8.12). The radiographic changes seen in ORDSPs have been the subject of a number of grading systems, including those of Pettersson et al. [8], Denoix and Dyson [9] and Desbrosse et al. [10]

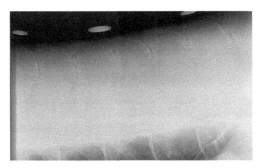

Figure 8.10 A lateromedial radiograph of the dorsal spinous processes (DSPs) obtained in the thoracic region to show the radiographic appearance associated with over-riding DSPs. There is sclerosis associated with the bones that are in contact, remodelling of the DSPs and areas of radiolucency associated with this remodelling. The white, radiodense markers above the bones are markers placed upon the skin to identify the location of individual DSPs before surgical removal of the DSPs. *Source:* Courtesy of Dr J. Kidd.

(Table 8.2). However, there are no published studies correlating the severity of the radiographic changes with clinical pain.

In addition to bony changes caused by ORDSPs, other radiographic abnormalities can be detected. These include enthesiophyte formation on the cranial and caudal borders of the DSPs, presumed to be due to new bone formation within or at the origin/insertion of the interspinous ligament. Similarly, damage to the superspinous ligament (SSL) can lead to periosteal reaction and new bone formation on the summit(s) of the DSPs. In rare cases avulsion of the SSL is diagnosed radiographically by the presence of a detached piece of bone from the summit of the DSPs.

Radiographic Abnormalities of the Vertebral Bodies

New bone formation on the ventral aspect of the vertebrae is an uncommon finding in the horse compared with cats and dogs. This new bone formation is termed 'ventral spondylosis' in the horse (see Chapter 13). The new bone

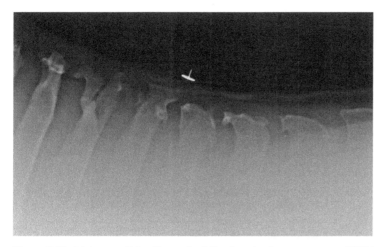

Figure 8.11 A lateromedial radiograph of the dorsal spinous processes (DSPs) obtained in the midthoracic region to show the radiographic appearance associated with marked remodelling of the DSPs. The summits of these DSPs are dramatically remodelled and, in one case, appear to have split. The cause of this remodelling is not known but it may be due to direct trauma to this site. The white, radiodense marker above the bones is placed to identify the location of individual DSPs. *Source:* Courtesy of Dr J. Kidd.

formation that is observed on the ventral aspect of the vertebrae forms a spectrum of changes (Figure 8.13). In some cases small osteophytes are noted on the ventral surface of the vertebral bodies close to the intervertebral disc. In more advanced cases, the new bone formation is sizeable and can fuse beneath the disc space. The clinical

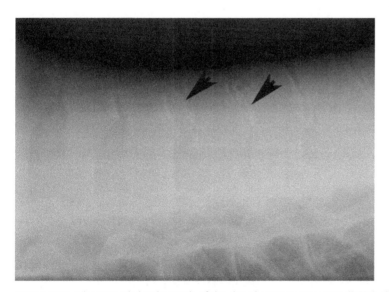

Figure 8.12 A lateromedial radiograph of the dorsal spinous processes (DSPs) obtained in the caudal thoracic region to show the radiographic appearance associated with overlapping DSPs. In this horse the DSPs do not have sufficient room within the back and have overlapped each other (arrows). *Source:* Courtesy of Dr J. Kidd.

Table 8.2 The radiographic grading systems for overriding dorsal spinous processes (DSPs) of Denoix and Dyson [9] and Desbrosse et al. [10]. ISS, interspinous space.

Grade	Radiographic appearance [9]	Radiographic appearance [10]
1	ISS narrowing, mild sclerosis of the cortical margins of the DSPs	Enthesiopathies of the supraspinous ligament
2	Loss of ISS, moderate sclerosis of the cortical margins of the DSPS	Enthesiopathies of the interspinous ligament
3	Severe sclerosis of the caudal margin of the DSPs (can be due to transverse thickening), radiolucencies	Impingement of the DSPs
4	Severe sclerosis of the caudal margin of the DSPs, change in shape of DSPs	Impingement with bone sclerosis and/or osteolysis

Source: Adapted from [9].

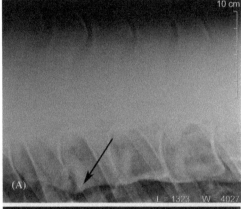
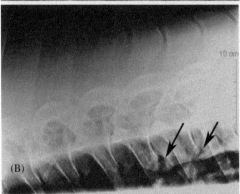

Figure 8.13 (A) A lateromedial radiograph and (B) a DM20°VLO radiograph of the vertebral bodies obtained in the thoracic region to show the radiographic appearance of ventral spondylosis. (A) Ventral spondylosis is seen on the ventral aspect of the vertebra (arrow) (compare with the same normal anatomical site in Figure 8.8). (B) The obliquity of the radiograph demonstrates the extent of the ventral new bone formation and the spondylosis on the vertebra caudal to the one originally identified (arrows).

significance of ventral spondylitis in the horse is not known, but it is recognised that it can be seen occasionally as an incidental finding in some horses.

Radiography is important in the diagnosis of osteomyelitis or neoplasia of the vertebrae, both of which are relatively rare conditions in the horse (Chapter 13). Osteomyelitis leads to new bone formation around the vertebral body, areas of radiolucency in the vertebrae and, in advanced cases, pathological fractures. A distinct disease entity is that of 'fistulous withers' – osteomyelitis of the withers region (T4–T7) – which can occur secondary to the primary soft tissue infection (often a *Brucella* species). On lateromedial radiographs remodelling and new bone formation are seen on the affected DSPs.

Radiography is also used in extreme cases to detect fractures of the vertebral bodies. The most common sites for fractures are the cranial thoracic region (T1–T3), the mid-thoracic region (T9–T16) and the lumbar vertebrae [1]. Radiographic signs of a fractured vertebra include ventral displacement of the vertebrae, apparent shortening or tilting of a DSP and alterations in the angulation of the vertebral bodies. Other radiographic abnormalities that have been reported include poor definition of the articular facets due to callus formation [1]. However, it should be noted that radiography can prove disappointing in the identification of vertebrae fractures and is, of course, limited to T1 and T9 to L1–T2 in its extent. Other imaging modalities, e.g. nuclear scintigraphy, should be considered to confirm the diagnosis or, if radiography does not identify a lesion in a horse with clinical signs, to indicate the presence of a fracture (see Chapter 13).

Radiographic Abnormalities of the Articular Facets

In contrast to radiography of DSPs, radiographs of the articular facets of the mid-thoracic to cranial lumbar spine are difficult to obtain and, in the normal horse, it is not usual to detect radiographic abnormalities. When abnormalities are detected then, at the current time, they are considered to be likely to be clinically significant (see Chapter 13), especially if there is evidence of active bone remodelling demonstrated by nuclear scintigraphy. Evidence of degenerative joint disease of the articular facets of the thoracolumbar spine can be detected on the DM20°VLO view. Articular facet osteoarthritis is recognised on radiography by new bone formation around the facets, loss of joint space (ankylosis) and sclerosis around the joint margins (Figure 8.14). The appearance of affected facets can be compared with the appearance of the facets cranial and caudal to the suspected lesion and to the DM20°VLO of the other side of the horse.

When radiographic changes consistent with a diagnosis of articular facet osteoarthritis are seen, a nuclear scintigraphic examination is recommended (Chapter 9) to provide more detail about active remodelling at this site.

Radiographic Abnormalities of the Pelvis

The only conditions of the pelvis that may be investigated reasonably with radiography are pelvic fractures or sacroiliac pathology. Pelvic fractures can be detected either in the standing horse or under general anaesthesia, as described above, and are seen as marked incongruencies in the ilial shaft or wing. Radiography of the sacroiliac region is technically possible, but due to a number of factors the radiographs obtained can be difficult to interpret. These factors include the large soft tissue mass overlying the area, the presence of ingesta in the pelvis and the orientation of the sacroiliac joints relative to the direction of the X-ray beam. Radiographic changes described in sacroiliac disease include smooth new bone on the caudal aspect of the joint or widening of the sacroiliac joint [11].

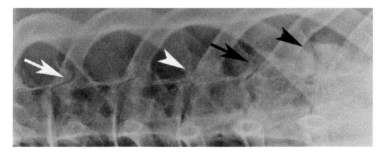

Figure 8.14 A DM20°VLO radiograph of the vertebral bodies obtained in the caudal thoracic region to show the radiographic appearance of osteoarthritis of the articular facets of the vertebrae. A normal articular facet is present cranially in this radiograph (white arrow). A facet that has lost the joint space (ankylosis) is present (white arrowhead). More caudally a moderate amount of new bone formation is seen at one facet (black arrow) and a marked amount of new bone formation is seen in the next facet (black arrowhead). *Source:* Courtesy of Dr J. Kidd.

References

1 Berner, D., Winter, K., Brehm, W. and Gerlach, K. Influence of head and neck position on radiographic measurement of intervertebral distances between thoracic dorsal spinous processes in clinically sound horses. *Equine Veterinary Journal Supplement* 2012.

2 Weaver, M.P., Jeffcott, L.B. and Novak, M. Radiology and scintigraphy. In: Haussler, K.K. (ed.), *Veterinary Clinics of North America Equine Practice: Back Problems*. Philadelphia, PA: W.B. Saunders Co., 1999, pp. 113–130.

3 Jeffcott, L.B. Radiographic examination of the equine vertebral column. *Veterinary Radiology* 1979; **20**:135–139.

4 Gorgas, D., Kircher, P., Doherr, M.G., Ueltschi, G. and Lang, J. Radiographic technique and anatomy of the equine sacro-iliac region. *Veterinary Radiology and Ultrasound* 2007; **48**:6501–6506.

5 May, S.A., Patterson, L.J., Peacock, P.J. and Edwards, G.B. Radiographic technique for the pelvis in the standing horse. *Equine Veterinary Journal* 1991; **23**:312–314.

6 Barrett, E.L., Talbot, A.M., Driver, A.J., Barr, F.J. and Barr, A.R.S. A technique for pelvic radiography in the standing horse. *Equine Veterinary Journal* 2006; **38**:266–270.

7 Santinelli, I., Becati, F., Arcelli, R. and Pepe, M. Anatomical variation of the spinous and transverse processes in the caudal cervical vertebrae and the first thoracic vertebra in horse. *Equine Veterinary Journal* 2016; **48**:45–49.

8 Pettersson, H., Stromberg, B. and Myrin, I. Das thorkolumbe, interspinale Syndrom (TLI) des Reitpferdes – Retriospektiver Vergleich konservativ und chirurgisch behandelter Falle. *Pferdeheilkunde* 1987; **3**:313–319.

9 Denoix, J.-M. and Dyson, S.J., Thoracolumbar spine. In: Ross, M.W. and Dyson, S.J. (eds), *Diagnosis and Management of Lameness in the Horse*, Philadelphia, PA: Saunders, 2003, pp. 509–521.

10 Desbrosse, F.G., Perrin, R., Launois, T., Vanderweerd, J.-M.E. and Clegg, P.D. Endoscopic resection of dorsal spinous processes and interspinous ligaments in ten horses. *Veterinary Surgery* 2007; **36**:149–155.

11 Jeffcott, L.B. Radiographic appearance of equine lumbosacral and pelvic abnormalities by linear tomography. *Veterinary Radiology* 1983; **24**:204–213.

9

Nuclear Scintigraphy and Computed Tomography of the Neck, Back and Pelvis

Sarah Powell

This chapter is an evolution of the original chapter on nuclear scintigraphy of the back and pelvis written for the First Edition of this book by the late Alastair Nelson. The chapter has been updated and the content has been expanded to include computed tomography (CT).

Introduction

The limitations of radiography and ultrasonography of the equine vertebral column and pelvis are well recognised and offer restricted evaluation of these complex areas. The introduction of equine nuclear scintigraphy almost 4 decades ago [1] proved a significant step forward and 'bone scanning' was rapidly established as the gold standard for imaging the equine vertebral column and pelvis (Figure 9.1) [2]. In contrast to radiography, nuclear scintigraphy permits visualisation of the whole back and pelvis and allows identification of physiologic and pathologic alterations in bone metabolism, rather than relying on changes in bone morphology. In comparison to nuclear scintigraphy, CT is a relatively recent introduction to equine imaging, which has become more widely available over the last decade. CT has logistical limitations for imaging the equine axial skeleton due the size of the patient relative to the gantry bore size or 'aperture' and necessity for general anaesthesia. Table and gantry adaptations of standard CT systems designed to accommodate equine patients more easily have increased the number of horses undergoing CT examination of the head and cranial neck, in many cases under standing sedation. However, at the time of writing, CT of the equine back and pelvis is relatively rarely carried out in clinical cases.

Nuclear Scintigraphy

Indications for nuclear scintigraphy of the neck, back and pelvis include but are not restricted to the following:

- High index of suspicion for bone pathology, such as radiographically silent fracture or infection.
- To assess the relevance of radiographic findings, such as impinging dorsal spinous process or caudal cervical facet modelling.
- To image the axial skeleton, which is difficult to image comprehensively with other techniques, such as the pelvis and thoracolumbar spine.
- As part of a general investigation into poor performance or multilimb lameness.
- Where horses are not amenable to diagnostic local anaesthesia.
- Vascular phase studies can be used to detect pelvic conditions, such as thrombosis of the iliac arteries.

Equine Neck and Back Pathology: Diagnosis and Treatment, Second Edition. Edited by Frances M.D. Henson.
© 2018 John Wiley & Sons, Ltd. Published 2018 by John Wiley & Sons, Ltd.

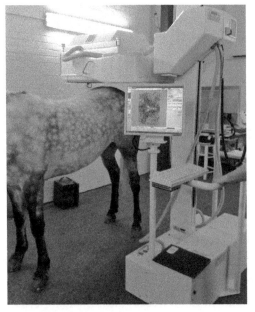

Figure 9.1 Scintigraphy of the pelvis carried out on the MiE Scintron HR Equine Scanner, which has a large, rectangular field of view. (*For a colour version of this figure, see the colour plate section.*)

Mechanism of Action

Nuclear scintigraphy produces images based on the physiologic function of the tissue rather than representing tissue anatomy. Scintigraphic images do not resolve structures for direct visualisation; rather interpretation relies on the recognition of patterns of abnormal increased radionuclide uptake (IRU), which can predict certain pathologic conditions [3,4] (Figures 9.2 and 9.3). The radiolabelled agent (radiopharmaceutical) is bound within the organ of interest and the location of the agent is then detected, historically using a

point probe that has been superseded in most facilities by imaging the location of the agent using a gamma 'camera' more correctly called a gamma detector.

Tracer agents are chosen depending on the target tissue. The standard agent used for bone phase imaging in horses is technetium-99m (^{99m}Tc)-labelled methylene diphosphonate (MDP) or hydroxymethylene diphosphonate (HDP). The disintegration of the ^{99m}Tc results in the emission of gamma rays with a peak energy of 140 keV.

The radioisotope is injected intravenously and is distributed via the bloodstream to the skeleton over the following 2–3 hours. The agent then attaches to exposed hydroxyapatite within osseous tissues. The uptake is therefore related to the metabolic activity of the bone, the osteoblastic activity and/or the blood supply to the tissues [3]. The agent is therefore taken up to a greater extent by the metabolically active parts of the skeleton, which can be seen as areas of increased radionuclide uptake ('*hot spots*'), which may be normal (such as the joints and open growth plates) or abnormal (such as areas of pathologically increased bone turnover). In rare cases, an area of photopenia (abnormally reduced uptake of the radionuclide) is detected (e.g. septic osteomyelitis or sequestrum [5]).

Procedure for Scintigraphy of the Neck, Back and Pelvis

The procedure for imaging the neck, spine and pelvis is similar to that for other areas. In contrast to imaging of the distal limbs, it is less important for the horse to be exercised

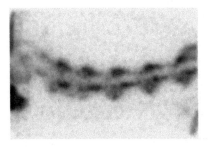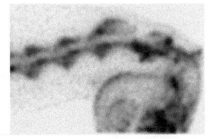

Figure 9.2 Normal scintigraphic appearance of the equine cervical spine.

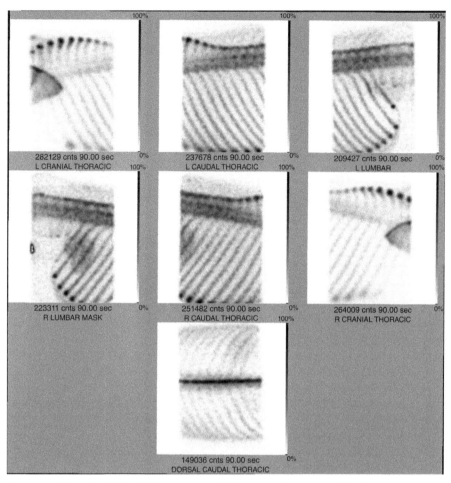

Figure 9.3 Normal scintigraphic appearance of the equine thoracic and lumbar spine.

directly prior to injection of the radiopharmaceutical, as blood flow to the axial skeleton is unlikely to be rate limiting. Intravenous administration is usually via an indwelling catheter abiding by the specific radiation safety guidelines of the facility. The use of a catheter is particularly important if the cervical vertebrae are of interest to avoid perivascular deposition of the radiopharmaceutical in non-cooperative patients, which will reduce the dose available to the remainder of the skeleton and cause superimposition over the cervical spine on resultant images. Following injection, the horse remains in the stable for 120–180 minutes prior to the acquisition of bone (delayed) phase images (Table 9.1). Bone phase imaging

is the most commonly performed method for examination of the equine neck, spine and pelvis. The time delay of between 2 and 3 hours allows clearance of the radioactivity from the soft tissues. If venous (vascular) phase images are required administration of the radiopharmaceutical must take place within the scintigraphy suite, as images must be acquired immediately. If soft tissue (pool) phase images are required image acquisition should ideally take place within 3–15 minutes. A diuretic should be administered 30–60 minutes prior to image acquisition in all cases undergoing delayed phase imaging, not just those in which the pelvis is included in the study. This reliably results in evacuation of the bladder prior to the horse entering the

Table 9.1 The three phases of scintigraphic examination of the spine and pelvis.

Phase	Time postinjection (min)	Anatomic structures	Pathologic example
Vascular	0–3	Blood vessels	Iliac thrombosis
Pool	3–15	Soft tissues	Muscle tears
Delayed	120–180	Bone	Fractures

scintigraphy room, therefore reducing the radiation dose to handlers and reducing superimposition of the bladder on the bony structures of the pelvis.

Image Acquisition of the Cervical, Thoracic and Lumbar Spine

The horse should be imaged with the gamma detector positioned from both left and right sides. The horse should be adequately sedated with the head positioned on a headrest to minimise motion. Images of the cervical spine and withers should be acquired with the gamma detector perpendicular to the spine (lateromedial to the skeleton) (Figure 9.2). Images of the thoracic and lumbar spines should be acquired with the gamma detector positioned dorsolateral 45° ventromedial oblique (DL45°VMO). This oblique positioning reduces the distance of the gamma detector from the skin surface, reduces scatter and offsets the facet joint and the rib articulations, which can therefore be assessed independently. Dorsoventral views of the thoracic and lumbar spine and ventrodorsal views of the cervical spine may be advantageous. For clinics using the newer, larger, rectangular field of view systems (90 cm) the spine can be imaged in 5 lateral views (2 cervical, 3 thoracic/lumbar) taken from both sides, with a DV view included where necessary (Figure 9.3). More images are necessary for those using older systems with smaller (60 cm), circular gamma detectors. Reducing the number of projections taken for any reason is ill advised as subtle abnormalities may be missed and comparison between left and right sides is essential.

Image Acquisition of the Pelvis

Routine examination of the pelvis includes a dorsoventral image (which may need to be split into cranial and caudal areas depending upon the field of view of the gamma detector). Both iliac wings including the *tubera coxae* should be included in this image. Where two images are necessary one should be centred over the *tubera sacrale* and the second more caudal images should centre over the coxofemoral joints. A DL45°VMO of each iliac wing and lateromedial views centred on the coxofemoral joints are also routine and also to include the *tuber ishii*, the pubis and the caudal part of the iliac shaft. Additional oblique images of the coxofemoral and tail head can also be acquired (Figure 9.4).

Technicalities of Image Acquisition

An image matrix of 128×128 is routinely used. Despite the increased resolution of a higher matrix size, counts are usually not sufficient to support the use of a 256×256 matrix commonly used for distal limb imaging. A total of 2–3 K counts per image are required to produce a diagnostic quality image.

Dynamic, rather than static, acquisitions are standard. This involves the acquisition of between 25 and 90 short 'frames' of between 1 and 3 seconds. The information from these frames is summed together and corrected for motion to produce the final image.

Motion correction software is necessary when imaging the neck, back and pelvis of horses under standing sedation and the technology varies between software providers. The real-time 'Paralyzer' motion correction

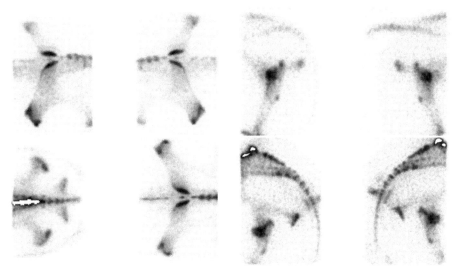

Figure 9.4 Standard views showing a normal scintigraphic appearance of the equine pelvis.

software available with the recently introduced MiE Scintron system has significantly improved the quality of the scintigraphic image of the equine spine and pelvis (Figure 9.5).

Postprocessing of the image can be done either 'horse side' or later at DICOM-viewing work stations, which are now commonplace in veterinary hospitals. Image contrast and grey scale alterations, image masking, regions of interest and profiling are all available to

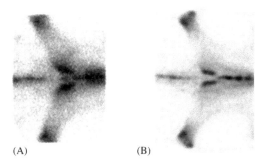

(A) (B)

Figure 9.5 Dorsoventral scintigraphic images of the equine pelvis from two systems. (A) This system has a smaller field of view and poorer quality motions correction software. (B) Image acquired by MiE Scintron HR system with a 90 cm rectangular field of view and 'Paralyser' software to give superior image quality.

the user but are outside the scope of this chapter and can be found in more specialised texts [6].

Image Interpretation

The resultant image depends not only on the amount of radioactivity detected by the gamma detector (in turn related to distribution of the radiopharmaceutical and distance of the tissues from the detector) but also the degree of attenuation by overlying tissues (bone and soft tissue). For example, the scapula attenuates radionuclide detection of the cranial thoracic spine and radionuclide detection of the pelvis is attenuated by the gluteal musculature. Soft tissue thickness may vary greatly between individuals and it is important for the radiologist to have an appreciation of the body type of the animal from which the images have been acquired. For example, very subtle, diffuse IRU in the region of a lumbar facet joint of a draught breed may represent the relevant pathologic process as focal, intense IRU in the region of a lumbar facet joint of a Thoroughbred. Muscle wastage can also alter the attenuation between the left and right sides of the same individual and should be taken into account. Horses of advanced age and those with reduced exercise intensity level (especially box rest) leading up to the scan can also reduce the activity of the skeleton. Conversely, immature horses will have more active skeletons, particularly in the region of the growth plates and should not be confused with pathological remodelling. Finally, an increase in radionuclide uptake does not necessarily equate to a pathologic process or indeed pain! Increased bone remodelling may be physiologic or pathologic and other diagnostic and clinical techniques may be necessary to determine if the process is pathologic and if there is associated pain.

The Normal Scintigraphic Appearance of the Spine and Pelvis of the Horse

Over the decades, substantial data has been acquired regarding the 'normal' pattern of radionuclide uptake in the horse [6] (Table 9.2). In addition, patterns common to horses used for various disciplines are recognised to the experienced user and may represent a spectrum of 'normal variation' in these horses.

Scintigraphic Abnormalities of the Spine

Caudal Cervical Facet Joint Osteoarthrosis
Radiographic evidence of caudal facet joint enlargement and modelling is not uncommon, particularly in older horses (Chapters 7 and 12).

Table 9.2 Table to describe the scintigraphic appearance of the back and pelvis in the routinely obtained scintigraphic views in a normal horse modified from the original version by Alastair Nelson in the first edition. These descriptions should be read in conjunction with Figure 9.3. DLVMO view = dorsolateral–ventromedial oblique, DV view = dorso–ventral view, DSP = dorsal spinous processes.

Region	View	Scintigraphic description
Cranial thoraco-lumbar spine	Lateromedial	The DSPs of T3–T8 seen dorsally and caudally. There are marked areas of increased uptake on the caudal border of the scapula (S) and associated with the summits of the dorsal spinous processes of T3–T8. These are normal 'hot spots'. It has been suggested that the increased radionuclide in these summits is because these areas retain separate centres of ossification (SCO) and thus remodelling continues to occur throughout life. In addition, higher counts will be seen in the tips of the DSP in the withers region due to the lack of soft tissue coverage.
Mid thoraco-lumbar spine	Lateromedial	In this view the vertebral bodies (V) are visible and show uniform uptake of radionuclide in a dorsal and ventral plane. There is a mild increase in uptake in the last 4 or 5 thoracic vertebrae. The ribs (R) are also clearly visible, running ventrocaudally from the vertebral column. The ribs have an even distribution of radionuclide uptake throughout their length. The summits of the DSP T9 and caudally do not show significant increases in radionuclide uptake in the normal horse and can be difficult to distinguish from the soft tissue background.
Mid thoraco-lumbar spine	DLVMO	This view is used in order to obtain information about the articular facets (AF) of the spine. Camera angulation means that the facets are no longer superimposed as they are in the lateromedial view above. The articular facets of the vertebral column are seen to form a parallel line of radionuclide uptake above the vertebral bodies (VB). This uptake is continuous with no focal areas of increased uptake visible.
Mid thoraco-lumbar spine		A straight vertebral column with uniform radionuclide uptake throughout the vertebral bodies.

Table 9.2 (*Continued*)

Region	View	Scintigraphic description
Caudal thoraco-lumbar spine	Lateromedial	The scintigraphic uptake is similar to that seen in the mid-thoracic region with the vertebral column dominating in the cranial aspect of the image. There is uniform radionuclide uptake in the vertebral bodies, ribs and dorsal spinous processes as seen more cranially. Caudally in the image, however, the kidney (K) will be revealed as a large area of increased radionuclide uptake just distal to the vertebral column overlying ribs 16–18.
Caudal thoraco-lumbar spine	DLVMO	As in the mid thoracolumbar spine view, this view separates the articular facets. However, in this region care must be taken to identify both kidneys on the oblique views of the cranial lumbar region as they may be superimposed over the vertebrae and give a false impression of increased uptake in the bone.
Caudal thoraco-lumbar spine	DV	This view reveals a straight vertebral column with uniform radionuclide uptake throughout the vertebral bodies. The kidneys are seen as areas of increased radionuclide uptake either side of the midline.
Cranial pelvis	DV	In this view the *tuber sacrale* (TS) are always seen as areas of increased radionuclide uptake. In the normal horse they appear as paired comma-shaped 'hot spots' just either side of the midline. The bladder shadow is often seen as a large area of increased radionuclide uptake just behind the *tuber sacrale*, usually in the midline, although the bladder shadow can be very asymmetric and to mimic pelvic pathology. In some cases, where there is a significant amount of radionuclide retained in the bladder, it is not possible to ascertain whether or not there is any pathology in the pelvis and it is recommended that a repeat scintigraphic examination be made 6 hours later/following urination. Alternatively, angulation of the camera head in a craniocaudal direction can help distinguish between uptake within the bladder and genuine uptake within the pelvis itself.
Cranial pelvis	DLVMO	This view highlights the iliac wings. Dorsally the *tuber sacrale* (TS) are seen as 'hot spots', whilst ventrally the *tuber coxae* (TC) are marked areas of increased uptake. Uptake in the iliac (IW) wing is relatively low and should be evenly distributed.
Cranial pelvis	Lateromedial	The *tuber sacrale* are seen as a focal area of increased radionuclide uptake in the dorsocranial aspect of the view and the hip joint is seen in the middle of the view. The hip joint is an area of relatively poorly defined increase in uptake. In this view some detail of the proximal femur can be seen, for instance the greater trochanter.
Caudal pelvis	DV	In this view the paired tuber sacrale are still present and the sacrum is seen in the midline. To either side of the sacrum the hip joint is seen as a focal area of increased uptake.
Caudal pelvis	Lateromedial	In this view the hip joint is seen as an area of a relatively poorly defined increase in uptake. Again, in this view some detail of the proximal femur can be seen, for instance the greater trochanter (GT). The *tuber ischii* (TI) can be seen as an area of increased uptake caudal to the hip.
Caudal pelvis	Caudal view	This view is obtained by positioning the camera behind the horse. The coccygeal vertebrae are seen in the midline of the image and the paired *tuber ischii* are seen either side of the midline.

Scintigraphic evaluation can enable the clinician to assess the relevance of radiographic findings. C5/C6 and C6/C7 are most commonly affected. As with IRU in the thoracic and lumbar facet joints, mild IRU in the caudal cervical facet joints is not always associated with pain. Clinical significance in subtle cases can be assumed if reduced cervical mobility, poor performance or, in some cases, forelimb lameness is also a feature. Uptake in the region of the facet joint should be equal to that in the vertebral laminar processes of the same vertebrae.

Thoracic and Lumbar Facet Joint Osteoarthrosis

IRU in the facet joints of the thoracic and lumbar region may be seen in cases of facet joint arthrosis, which can be a cause of poor performance, apparent back pain or even lameness in certain individuals. The pattern of IRU can range from focal abnormal IRU in a single facet joint to more diffuse IRU with a number of joints affected. The obliquity of the gamma detector during acquisition is essential to offset the facet joints from the rib articulations and lumbar transverse processes to enable detection of subtle IRU (Figure 9.6). DV views allow comparison with the contralateral side within the same image. Ultrasonography and radiography can be further used to evaluate and monitor injury.

Conditions of the Dorsal Spinous Processes

Subtle focal IRU associated with the summit of the thoracic dorsal spinous processes (DSP) can be seen in normal horses in the absence of pathology or pain [7,8] and a combination of radiographic and scintigraphic findings is not necessarily an indication of pain [9]. A ratio of radionuclide uptake in the DSP compared to that in the 15th or 16th rib has been described [8], but not in clinical cases. Assessing the relevance of IRU in the DSPs depends on the pattern of uptake and the results of diagnostic local analgesia, where possible in horses with presenting signs of back pain (Chapter 13) [10]. Relatively subtle IRU in a small number of DSPs in the saddle region can prove to be clinically significant (Figure 9.7).

IRU within the dorsal spinous processes (DSPs) can be associated with a number of conditions, including traumatic injury (most commonly in the cranial thoracic region or 'withers'), impinging or over riding dorsal spines (most commonly in the midthoracic and lumbar regions or may be due to

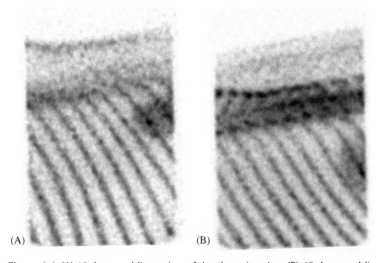

(A)   (B)

Figure 9.6 (A) 10 degree oblique view of the thoracic spine. (B) 45 degree oblique view of the thoracic spine further offsets the dorsal spines, facet joints and rib articulations to allow clearer differentiation of these structures.

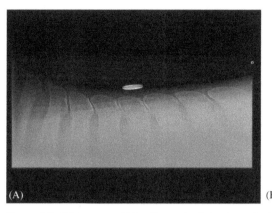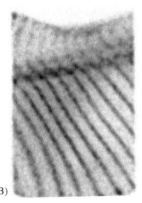

Figure 9.7 (A) Lateromedial radiograph of the thoracic dorsal spines showing several areas of impingement in a horse with severe bucking behaviour. (B) The corresponding scintigraphic image of the same horse. Local anaesthesia confirmed the presence of pain associated with the back and surgical resection of several dorsal spines was curative.

remodelling of the DSP at the insertion of the supraspinous and/or interspinous ligaments.

Vertebral Body Fractures

Vertebral body fractures may result from trauma at any level of the spine (seen most commonly in foals) or as a form of stress injury in the thoracic and lumbar spine of horses used for racing [11]. Traumatic injuries may present as focal IRU, which may be sufficiently intense to 'steal counts' from the surrounding skeleton despite the soft tissue attenuation. Image quality may be poor in horses presenting with ataxia. Vertebral body stress injuries may show only very mild IRU and may be missed due to attenuation of gamma rays from overlying soft tissue or if patient motion reduces image quality. Depending on location, vertebral body fractures may be visible radiographically and may be assessed in more detail on computed tomographic imaging.

Ankylosing Spondylosis/Discospondylosis/ Discospondylitis

IRU in the region of the vertebral bodies may be due to discospondylosis or discospondylitis, the former most commonly seen in the thoracic or lumbar spine, while the latter may be seen at any site including the sacrum (Figure 9.8). One or more vertebral bodies may show focal IRU of variable intensity depending of the stage of disease. The pattern of uptake is similar irrespective of whether infection is a feature, but a septic process may show more intense IRU. Further investigations will be necessary to differentiate infectious from non-infections conditions. Careful analysis of the image and the minimal motion artefact should enable the site of the IRU to be differentiated from the rib articulation or facet joints. Depending on location and equipment available, radiographic evaluation may be possible.

Sacroiliac Disease/Dysfunction

Nuclear scintigraphy of the normal [12] and abnormal [13,14] equine sacroiliac region has been reported and is widely used to evaluate sacroiliac dysfunction (SID) in clinical cases (Chapter 14). Due to the location within the pelvis and relative position of the iliac wings, scintigraphy may be considered the gold standard for imaging this region. The sacroiliac region is assessed on the oblique and dorsal views described above. Uptake may be diffuse or more linear positioned adjacent and abaxial to the *tubera sacrale* (Figure 9.9). Most experienced clinicians familiar with the technique would be comfortable assessing the images visually; however, images may also be subject to

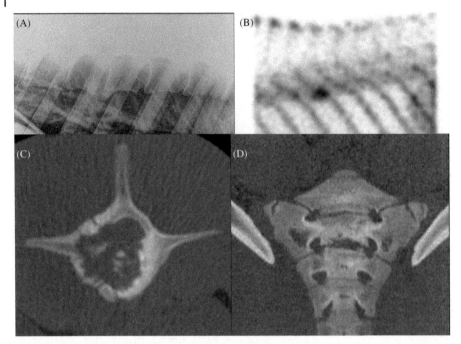

Figure 9.8 (A) Lateromedial radiograph of the thoracic vertebral bodies showing discospondylosis which correlates with an area of increased radionuclide uptake on the scintigraphy image of the same horse (B). (C) Discospondylitis causing severe destruction of the lumbar vertebrae in a foal. (D) Sacral vertebral discospondylosis in a weanling.

profile analysis [12] and region of interest analysis [13,14] for subjective assessment. Care should be taken to account for asymmetry in the gluteal musculature when comparing uptake in the left and right sacroiliac joints. IRU in one or more sacroiliac regions is not uncommon in horses with concurrent lameness due to pain more distally within the same or contralateral limb, without apparent pain originating from the region of the sacroiliac joint. IRU in the sacroiliac region may occur due to local inflammation following recent diagnostic local analgesia to the region.

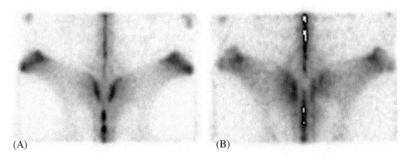

Figure 9.9 (A) Dorsoventral view of the pelvis showing normal scintigraphic uptake through the sacroiliac region. (B) Dorsoventral view of the pelvis showing mild diffuse IRU in the left sacroiliac region and mild, focal uptake in the right sacroiliac region.

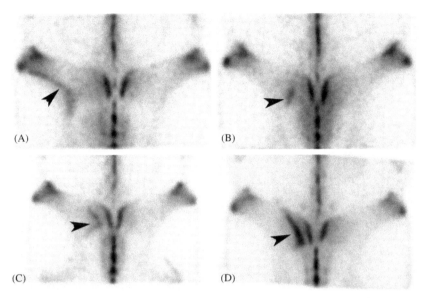

Figure 9.10 Dorsoventral views of the pelvis showing IRU in the left ilium at four different locations, all consistent with stress injury of the left wing of the ilium (arrowheads).

Pelvic Fractures

One of the most useful and potentially life-saving applications of equine scintigraphy, recognised soon after its clinical development, was the ability to detect stress fractures within the pelvis of the Thoroughbred race-horse [11,15]. Stress fracture screening remains one of the most clinically relevant uses of this technique today. Superimposition of the activity from the urinary bladder has been mentioned earlier in this chapter and is particularly important if early stress remod-elling of the iliac wing and shaft are to be detected. Stress fractures of the iliac wing may present as IRU at several locations (Figure 9.10) and, with varied intensity, ultraso-nographic imaging can be useful to detect callus formation and monitor healing. Specific injuries (such as iliac wing stress fractures, pelvic trauma and coxofemoral joint pathol-ogy) are recognised and covered in some detail elsewhere in this text (Chapter 13).

Rib Fractures

Focal IRU in one or more ribs is a not an uncommon finding in horses undergoing scintigraphic examination due to poor performance and 'resistive' behaviour, and occasionally in horses presenting with fore-limb lameness (Figure 9.11). Interpretation is usually straightforward. Depending on the field of view of the detector, more ventral injuries may not be detected on standard views and additional images may be war-ranted in horses presenting with these signs. The diagnosis can usually be confirmed and heeling monitored ultrasonographically. Diagnostic local analgesia may assist in con-firming an association between the scinti-graphic finding and the presenting complaint.

Miscellaneous IRU in the Back and Pelvis

Linear IRU is in the paravertebral and gluteal musculature but can be seen at any site (Figure 9.12). This finding is not uncommon in the racing Thoroughbred and can be dra-matic, involving multiple muscle bellies, or be more subtle, and may mimic pelvic stress fractures. Despite the common assumption that this indicates a previous episode of exer-tional rhabdomyolysis this is not always reported in the clinical history or confirmed on blood profiles and may be seen as an incidental finding.

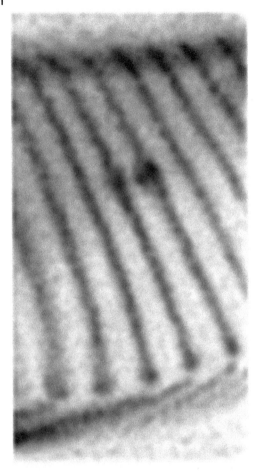

Figure 9.11 Lateral view of the left thoracic region showing two areas of IRU in the ribs. Rib fractures were confirmed ultrasonographically.

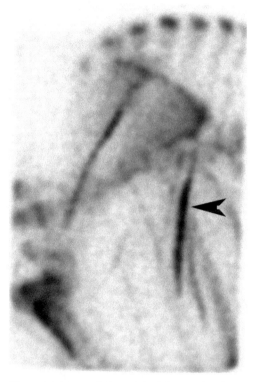

Figure 9.12 Lateral view of the left scapular showing linear IRU in the long head of the triceps.

Limitations of Scintigraphy of the Spine and Pelvis

As with all equine imaging techniques, successful application depends upon a rigorous knowledge of normal, normal variants, imaging artefacts and prevalence of subclinical disease. Following the expenditure and time implications of carrying out a scintigraphic examination, revealing the sometimes elusive 'hot spot' can tempt the clinician to assume relevance where none exists, particularly in an anatomic area where definitive confirmation of pathology and/or pain is frustratingly difficult. This may be the main limitation to achieving the correct diagnosis and improving case management and outcomes in a proportion of cases. In human imaging, basic scintigraphy is being superseded by positron emission tomography (PET) scanning, and magnetic resonance imaging (MRI) and computed tomography (CT) allow greater evaluation of disease processes and clinical relevance. PET and MRI scanning are, at the time of writing, not feasible to image the vertebral column and pelvis in the overwhelming majority of equine patients. Due to technical considerations horses may be more amenable to CT imaging and data are starting to emerge that may forward our knowledge significantly in coming decades.

Computed Tomography

Indications for CT of the Neck, Back and Pelvis

A body of knowledge regarding CT diagnosis of conditions of the head and limbs has grown in recent years [16]. The literature is yet to contain detailed information regarding the normal and pathologic CT appearance of the equine spine due to logistical problems of imaging these areas with the current technology, though a number of case reports appear in the literature [17]. The neck is the most accessible region of the spine to image and CT has proven useful primarily where traditional imaging techniques (radiography/ scintigraphy) have localised the site of injury but concerns remain about the specific disease process and/or the structures involved. CT offers greater detail in this complex anatomic area and the unique ability to directly visualise the spinal cord [17,18]. The back and pelvis of most horses are simply too large to be imaged in this way in the live animal. Postmortem imaging, with prior 'de-bulking' of the overlying musculature necessary in some specimens, gives us a tantalising insight as to how our diagnostic capabilities could be expanded in the future [19]. Imaging the back and pelvis in smaller breed adult horses, foals and weanlings is possible [20] but requires general anaesthesia and may be contraindicated where neurologic deficits are a feature or fracture pathology is suspected. However, on rare occasions when CT holds the possibility of a diagnosis and subsequent treatment where traditional techniques have failed, these potential risks are legitimately overcome. However, selecting cases in this way results in practices collecting a small number of examples of often rare conditions. Routine scanning of poor performance cases for sports injury detection is yet to become reality.

Mechanism of Action

CT uses X-ray technology to generate cross-sectional images and relies on the principle that X-ray beams can be used to measure the density of the tissue through which they pass by calculating the attenuation coefficient of the tissue.

The CT tube emits X-rays (typically with energy levels between 20 and 150 keV) whilst rotating around the patient. The CT detector, placed at the opposite side of the gantry,

measures the transmission of the X-ray beam through a full scan of the body and generates a large number of attenuation coefficient data for the tissue. The computer software then applies complex mathematical algorithms to convert this raw data into a reconstructed image that consists of a pixel matrix, each of which represents a voxel (volume element) of the tissue of the patient. The value of the attenuated coefficient for each voxel corresponding to each pixel needs to be calculated. Each CT image is typically composed of a square matric of $512 \times 512 = 262\,144$ pixels (one for each voxel).

Procedure for CT of the Neck, Back and Pelvis

The head and cranial/midneck can be scanned under standing sedation using CT systems modified to do this (Figure 9.13). The remainder of the spine and pelvis currently

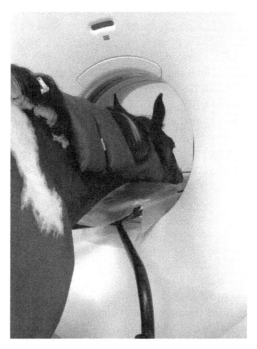

Figure 9.13 A horse positioned with the head extended into the gantry of a CT machine adapted to scan horses under standing sedation. Sandbags placed over the neck can assist in keeping the head stable.

requires general anaesthesia. For standing horses most establishments have the horse standing on a platform with the head extended into the gantry. The platform moves with zero inertia (typically an air skates systems) by a direct connection to the adapted CT system table, which pushes or pulls the horse through the gantry. Sedation protocols vary between sites; however, relatively profound sedation is necessary compared to that used for radiographic procedures. Nervous or head-shy horses may prove poor candidates for this procedure. The specific local rules for each facility will dictate the number of people allowed to be present in the room during the exposure (if any) and the required distance from the gantry during acquisition. The table speed used for horses under standing sedation may be necessarily slower that that used for horses under general anaesthesia to prevent horses becoming alarmed by the table motion. In the author's experience a maximum table speed of 2 cm per second is recommended. Earplugs and blindfolds may help disassociate the horse from its environment, but these are no substitute to adequate sedation and experienced handlers. Motion artefact may be more of an issue in standing horses and studies should be scrutinised carefully for patient motion, which can mimic pathology.

Horses scanned under general anaesthesia are placed in dorsal recumbency in most cases for examinations of the neck, back and pelvis. Dorsal recumbency has the advantage that alignment of the spine perpendicular to the X-ray beam is optimised. When imaged in lateral recumbency, extension of the spine is hard to achieve and flexion or rotation of the vertebral bodies and associated joints can affect image interpretation. Neonates may be imaged under relatively light sedation in sternal or lateral recumbency (though they generally resent dorsal recumbency) if general anaesthesia is contraindicated. Topograms or 'scout' scans are utilized to allow the extent of the area of interest to be defined. Axial images are acquired in an acquisition width typically between 1 and 2 mm, voltage (kVp) 120, current (mAs) 200 and tube rotation time

0.5 s. Image reconstruction width is typically between 0.625 and 1.25 mm in bone and soft tissue kernels respectively for optimal visualisation of skeletal and soft tissue/neural structures.

CT Anatomy and Normal Variation

Aspects of the anatomy additionally or more comprehensively visualised on CT include the axial aspect of the facet joints, vertebral canal, spinal cord and nerve roots [18], intervertebral discs and the ligaments that extend along substantial portions of the spine and pelvis (including the nuchal, supraspinous and sacral ligaments) and detail of their bony attachments. Detailed CT descriptions of the normal equine spine and pelvic anatomy are lacking in the literature. As is the case with the introduction of any new imaging technique assigning clinical significance to findings, particularly in areas not amenable to diagnostic local analgesia, presents a serious challenge. For example, incidental bone proliferation at the occipital attachment of the nuchal ligament and semispinalis capitis insertions is not uncommon in clinically normal horses, although it is also seen in cases of nuchal ligament injury. It is likely that a wide spectrum of normal variation (particularly with respect to bone remodelling at the site of ligamentous attachments and joints in the lumbosacral region, for example) will be seen in clinically normal horses.

Computed Tomographic Abnormalities of the Equine Spine and Pelvis

Poll Injuries and Conditions of the Nuchal Ligament

The poll and nuchal ligament region is amenable to CT imaging under standing sedation in most horses and this technique is therefore now more widely used for assessment of such conditions. Nuchal ligament injury has been reported previously [21]. Diagnosis of traumatic injury to the nuchal ligament, occipital bone and semispinalis capitis tendons can be associated with thickening and hypoattenuation of the nuchal ligament and tendons, loss of tissue margins and occipital bone fragmentation (Figure 9.14). Nuchal ligament enthesiopathies have been postulated as a cause of poor performance and non-specific neck pain, but the clinical relevance of bone remodelling at the nuchal ligament attachment on the occipital bone is complicated by the presence of proliferative bone in some normal horses.

Vertebral Fractures

Spinal fractures are usually associated with traumatic incidents in the paddock or high-speed incidents during racing/competition

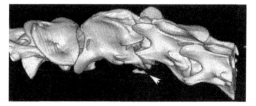

Figure 9.15 Three-dimensional reconstruction of the cranial cervical region of a horse with multiple traumatic fractures of the third cervical vertebra following an incident in the starting stalls; cranial is to the left. A fracture fragment from the transverse process of Ce3 can be seen ventrally (white arrow). The left cervical facet joint between Ce2 and Ce3 is luxated, the caudal articular process of Ce2 is displaced ventral to the cranial articular process of Ce3.

(Figure 9.15). Fracture detection and comminution is more easily assessed on CT images as compared with radiography [22]. However, horses with suspected fracture pathology may be poor candidates for general anaesthesia. Foals are particularly susceptible to epiphyseal fractures and luxations. Vascular channels, particularly those made more prominent by increased bone mineral density of the surrounding bone should not be confused with fissures or fractures.

Cervicovertebral Malformations

Cervicovertebral malformations are a common cause of 'wobbler syndrome' in horses, resulting from malformation and/or malarticulation and facet joint degeneration causing compression of the spinal cord. CT features may include spinal cord compression and in chronic cases osteoarthrosis (Figure 9.16) and osteochondrosis of the articular processes. CT myelography can be carried out to assess any relevant spinal cord compression (Figure 9.17) [23,24].

Scoliosis

Equine congenital scoliosis ('sway back') is not uncommon. Subtle forms may be difficult to detect clinically and may partially resolve or correct with increasing maturity and cause no ill effects in the long term. More severe cases are assumed to be performance limiting for

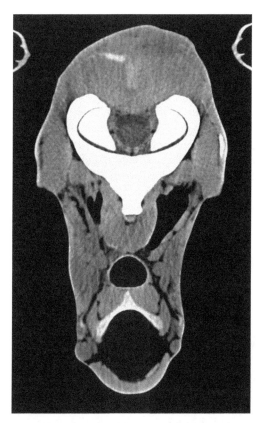

Figure 9.14 Computed CT image of the cranial neck at the level of the atlantooccipital junction acquired under standing sedation. There is moderate swelling of the soft tissues. This horse had ruptured the right SSC tendon after rearing over backwards when tied up in the stable.

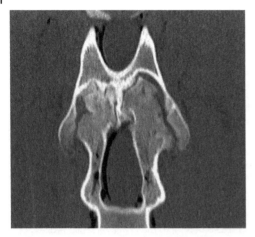

Figure 9.16 Multiplanar reformatted CT image in the dorsal plane through the facet joints of the cervical vertebrae in a hose with a congenital cervical vertebral malformation. Cranial is at the top of the image. There is extensive degeneration of the facet joint articulations between the 4th and 5th cervical vertebrae.

athletic horses or pose other problems such as saddle fit in the future. CT assessment of congenital scoliosis has been reported in the literature [25] and has been used by the author for objective assessment of the severity of and subsequent correction of a small number of cases (Figure 9.18). Hypoplasia of the facet joints and rib articulation causing axial rotation in combination with lateral deviation may be a feature in more severe cases.

Discospondylitis and Spinal Abscesses

Spinal abscesses are rare in horses. Radiography (predominantly) and scintigraphy are typically used in adult horses to assist diagnosis. Foals may be amenable to CT imaging [26]. Most spinal abscesses originate from preexisting osteomyelitis/discospondylitis due to bacteraemia and haematogenous spread of the pathogen. Severe irregular destruction of the vertebral endplates and adjacent bone is seen often in combination with bone deposition primarily on the ventral aspect of the affected area. Pathologic fracture of the bone and fragmentation may be a feature (Figure 9.19).

Spinal Masses Causing Spinal Cord Compression

Masses (neoplasms and cyst-like lesions) within the equine vertebral canal and pelvis are rare and infrequently reported in the literature, though melanoma, haemangiosarcoma, squamous cell carcinoma and lymphoma are reported. The CT appearance has yet to be described and will depend on the nature of the tumour, but is likely to include osteolysis, extradural soft tissue causing spinal cord compression and pathologic fracture. Involvement of the paravertebral musculature may be a feature in locally invasive neoplasms. Synovial cysts may be a feature of vertebral malformations and osteochondrosis and one case of a

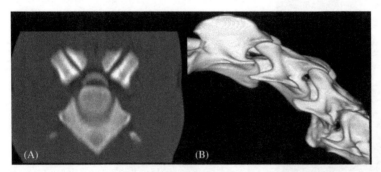

(A) (B)

Figure 9.17 (A) Axial CT myelogram image of the same horse as in Figure 9.16. This slice is taken at the level of the facet joints between the 3rd and 4th cervical vertebrae at the level of the dorsal displacement of the cranial aspect of the 4th cervical vertebra. Contrast delineates the space surrounding the dorsal aspect of the spinal cord, which is not continuous around the ventral aspect of the spinal cord. (B) CT of the vertebral column.

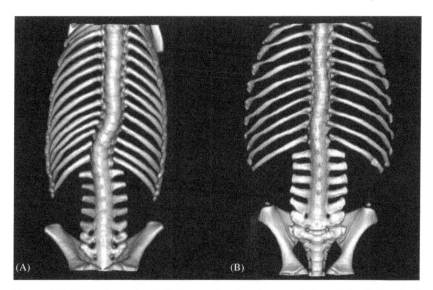

Figure 9.18 Three-dimensional CT images showing the ventral view of the thoracolumbar spine of a Thoroughbred foal with scoliosis at: (A) 1 week of age, (B) 8 weeks of age (right). The degree of scoliosis has improved considerably. This horse went on to train and race successfully.

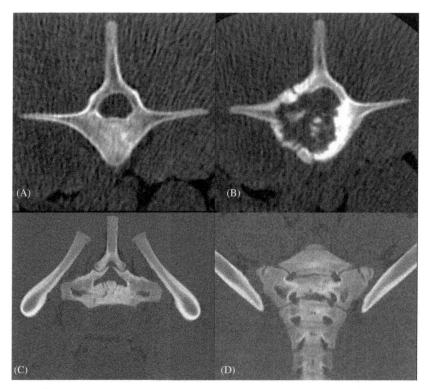

Figure 9.19 (A) Normal CT appearance of the lumbar vertebrae of a 4-week-old foal. (B) Severe bone destruction in a 4-week-old foal with a spinal abscess. (C and D) Images of discospondylitis in a weanling Thoroughbred between the 1st and 2nd sacral vertebrae.

spinal hydatid cyst has been seen by the author (Figure 9.20).

Sacroiliac Joint and Lumbosacral Dysfunction

As discussed above, sacroiliac dysfunction is usually diagnosed using scintigraphy and/or diagnostic local analgesia. Ultrasonography permits evaluation of the ventral aspect of the sacroiliac joints and can be useful in detecting modelling changes. The majority of horses are too large to be accommodated by the CT gantry and the owner may be reluctant to anaesthetise horses for diagnostic imaging procedures. CT imaging of clinical cases has usually therefore been carried out postmortem in horses euthanized for multisite orthopaedic disease. As with the majority of conditions of the spine and pelvis, CT findings have not yet been reported but are likely to include alterations in bone density

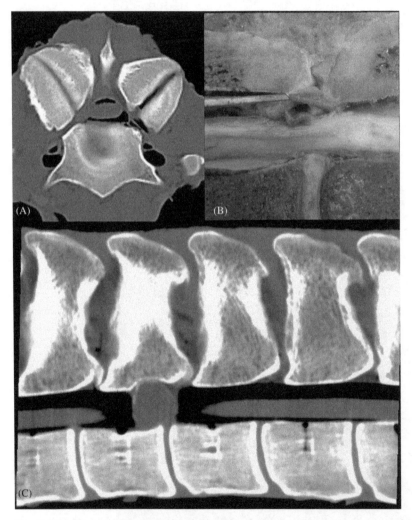

Figure 9.20 (A) Axial CT image (left is to the left) of a horse presenting with signs of ataxia. Soft tissue swelling axial to the cervical facet joint between the 3rd and 4th cervical vertebrae was detected with enlargement of the facet joint consistent with arthrosis. A subsequent postmortem examination (B) revealed a synovial cyst was present at this location. (C) A multiplanar reformatted image of a Warmblood gelding presenting with ataxia. A well-circumscribed soft tissue mass is visible within the spinal canal, displacing the spinal cord in the midthoracic regions, which proved to be a hydatid cyst at postmortem.

and compact bone thickness, varying degrees of bone modelling at the articulation, osteophytosis, etc. (Figure 9.21). The limited number of horses who have been imaged suggest a spectrum of physiologic and pathology remodelling. Osteophytes surrounding the intertransverse joint have been observed in close proximity to the S1 nerve roots and are postulated as a cause for hindlimb lameness and gait abnormalities (Figure 9.21).

Limitations of CT of the Equine Neck, Back and Pelvis

Despite the wealth of information, computed tomographic evaluation of spinal and pelvic pathology affords the clinician technical and logistical problems due to the size of the horse remain. Technological advancements take time and, in some respects, are bound by the fundamental physics of medical imaging. The need for general anaesthesia is likely to always have an impact on the number of horses having the benefit of a CT scan, even if the newer large-bore scanners can accommodate more areas of interest. Routine CT scanning of the back and pelvis of poorly performing athletic horses is unlikely to become a reality in the near future. The ability of clinicians to interpret the huge volume of diagnostic data would be a challenge of perhaps equal magnitude.

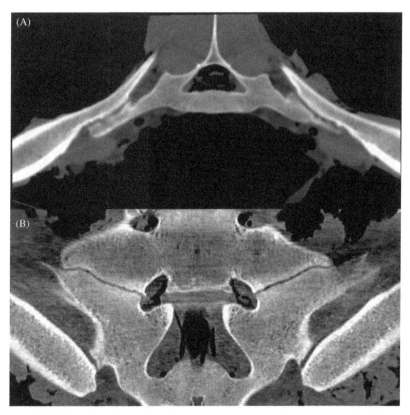

Figure 9.21 (A) Multiplanar reformatted CT images of the sacroiliac region of a 12-year-old pony gelding. Modelling changes of the sacroiliac region are present. (B) Multiplanar reformatted CT images of the intertransverse joints between the 1st sacral and 6th lumbar vertebrae of an 8-year-old warm blood gelding showjumper. Modelling of the intertransverse joints was visible ultrasonographically. The CT image reveals a large osteophyte on the axial aspect of the joint close to the S1 root.

References

1 Ueltschi, G. Bone and joint imaging with ^{99m}Technetium-labelled phosphates as a new diagnostic aid in veterinary orthopaedics. *Journal of the American Radiological Associations* 1977; **18**:80–84.

2 Archer, D.C., Boswell, J.C., Voute, L.C. and Clegg, P.D. Skeletal scintigraphy in the horse: current indications and validity as a diagnostic test. *Veterinary Journal* 2007; **173**:31–44.

3 Twardock, A.R. Equine bone scintigraphyic uptake patterns related to age, breed and occupation. *Veterinary Clinics of North America Equine Practice* 2001; **17**(1):75–94.

4 Levine, D.G., Ross, B.M., Ross, M.W., Richardson, D.W. and Martin, B.B. Decreased radiopharmaceutical uptake (photopenia) in delayed phase scintigraphy images in three horses. *Veterinary Radiology and Ultrasound* 2007; **48**:467–470.

5 Dyson, S.J., Pilsworth, R.C., Twardock, A.R. and Martinelli, M.J. Equine Scintigraphy. Part II; Chapter 1–5. In: *Atlas of Normal and Abnormal Patterns of Uptake*, 2003, pp. 117–238. ISBN 0-9545689-0-7.

6 Dyson, S.J., Pilsworth, R.C., Twardock, A.R. and Martinelli, M.J. Equine Scintigraphy. Part I; Chapter 5, Image acquisition, post processing, display and storage. In: *Atlas of Normal and Abnormal Patterns of Uptake*, 2003, pp. 53–68. ISBN 0-9545689-0-7

7 Ehrlich, P.J., Seeherman, H.J., O'Callaghan, M.W., Dohoo, I.R. and Brimacombe, M. Results of bone scintigraphy in horses used for show jumping, hunting, or eventing: 141 cases (1988–1994). *Journal of American Veterinary Medical Association* 1998, November 15; **213**(10):1460–1467.

8 Erichsen, C., Eksell, P., Widström, C. et al. Scintigraphy of the sacroiliac joint region in asymptomatic riding horses: scintigraphic appearance and evaluation of method. *Veterinary Radiology Ultrasound* 2003, November–December; **44**(6): 699–706.

9 Erichsen, C., Eksell, P., Holm, K.R., Lord, P. and Johnston, C. Relationship between scintigraphic and radiographic evaluations of spinous processes in the thoracolumbar spine in riding horses without clinical signs of back problems. *Equine Veterinary Journal* 2004, September; **36**(6):458–465.

10 Walmsley, J.P., Pettersson, H., Winberg, F. and McEvoy, F. Impingement of the dorsal spinous processes in 215 horses: case selection, surgical technique and results. *Equine Veterinary Journal* 2002; **34**:23–28.

11 Haussler, K.K. and Stover, S.M. Stress fractures of the vertebral lamina and pelvis in Thoroughbred racehorses. *Equine Veterinary Journal* 1998; **30**:374–381.

12 Dyson, S., Murray, R., Branch, M. et al. The sacroiliac joints: evaluation using nuclear scintigraphy. Part 1: The normal horse. *Equine Veterinary Journal* 2003, May; **35**(3):226–232.

13 Dyson, S., Murray, R., Branch, M. and Harding, E. The sacroiliac joints: evaluation using nuclear scintigraphy. Part 2: Lame horses. *Equine Veterinary Journal* 2003, May; **35**(3):233–259.

14 Tucker, R.L., Schneider, R.K., Sondhof, A.H., Ragle, C.A. and Tyler, J.W. Bone scintigraphy in the diagnosis of sacroiliac injury in twelve horses. *Equine Veterinary Journal* 1998 September; **30**(5):390–395.

15 Pilsworth, R.C., Shepherd, M.C., Herinckx, B. and Holmes, M.A. Fracture of the wing of the ilium, adjacent to the sacroiliac joint, in Thoroughbred racehorses. *Equine Veterinary Journal* 1994; **26**:94–99.

16 Tucker, R.L. and Sande, R.D. Computed tomography and magnetic resonance imaging of the equine musculoskeletal conditions. *Veterinary Clinics of North America: Equine Practices* 2001, April; **17**(1):145–157, vii, Review.

17 Sleutjens, J., Cooley, A.J., Sampson S.N. et al. The equine cervical spine: comparing MRI and contrast-enhanced CT images with anatomic slices in the sagittal, dorsal,

and transverse plane. *Veterinary Quarterly* 2014; **34**(2):74–84.

18 Claridge, H.A., Piercy, R.J., Parry, A. and Weller, R. The 3D anatomy of the cervical articular process joints in the horse and their topographical relationship to the spinal cord. *Equine Veterinary Journal* 2010, November; **42**(8):726–731.

19 Collar, E.M., Zavodovskaya, R., Spriet, M. et al. Caudal lumbar vertebral fractures in California Quarter Horse and Thoroughbred racehorses. *Equine Veterinary Journal* 2015, September; **47**(5):573–579.

20 Schliewert, E.C., Lascola, K.M., O'Brien, R.T. et al. Comparison of radiographic and computed tomographic images of the lungs in healthy neonatal foals. *American Journal of Veterinary Research* 2015, January; **76**(1):42–52.

21 Saunders, J. and Bergman, H.J. Chapter 42. In: Swartz, T. and Saunders, J. (eds), *Veterinary Computed Tomography*. Wiley-Blackwell, pp. 451–456. ISBN: 978-0-8138-1747-7.

22 Trump, M., Kircher, P.R. and Fürst, A. The use of computed tomography in the diagnosis of pelvic fractures involving the acetabulum in two fillies. *Veterinary Comparative Orthopaedics and Traumatology* 2011; **24**(1):68–71.

23 Janes, J.G., Garrett, K.S., McQuerry, K.J. et al. Cervical vertebral lesions in equine stenotic myelopathy. *Veterinary Pathology* 2015, September; **52**(5): 919–927.

24 Janes, J.G., Garrett, K.S., McQuerry, K.J. et al. Comparison of magnetic resonance imaging with standing cervical radiographs for evaluation of vertebral canal stenosis in equine cervical stenotic myelopathy. *Equine Veterinary Journal* 2014, November; **46**(6):681–686.

25 Wong, D.L., Miles, K. and Sponseller, B. Congenital scoliosis in a quarter horse filly. *Veterinary Radiology and Ultrasound* 2006, May–June; **47**(3):279–282.

26 Garcia, E.B., Biller, D.S., Beard, L. et al. Computed tomographic myelography of a foal with discospondylitis and extradural spinal cord compression due to a vertebral abscess. *Goravanahally Equine Veterinary Education* 2015; **27**(2):75–80.

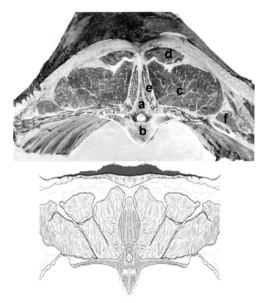

Figure 2.11 The cross-sectional anatomy of thoracic vertebra 1. A postmortem section B line diagram: A = dorsal spinous process, b = vertebral body, c = *longissimus dorsi*, d = *longissimus dorsi (spinalis)*, e = *multifidus*, f = *ilio costarum*.

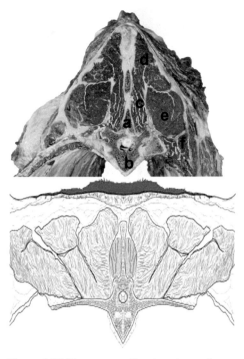

Figure 2.12 The cross-sectional anatomy of thoracic vertebra 7. A postmortem section B line diagram: a = dorsal spinous process, b = vertebral body, c = *multifidus*, d = *longissimus dorsi (spinalis)*, e = *longissimus dorsi*, f = *ilio costalis*.

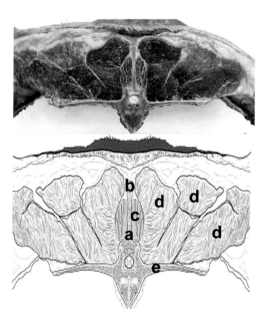

Figure 2.13 The cross-sectional anatomy of lumbar vertebra 2. A postmortem section B line diagram: a = dorsal spinous process, b = supraspinous ligament, c = *multifidus*, d = *longissimus dorsi*, e = transverse process.

Equine Neck and Back Pathology: Diagnosis and Treatment, Second Edition. Edited by Frances M.D. Henson.
© 2018 John Wiley & Sons, Ltd. Published 2018 by John Wiley & Sons, Ltd.

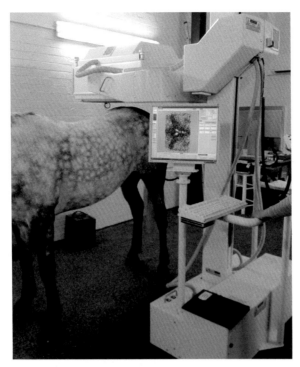

Figure 9.1 Scintigraphy of the pelvis carried out on the MiE Scintron HR Equine Scanner, which has a large, rectangular field of view.

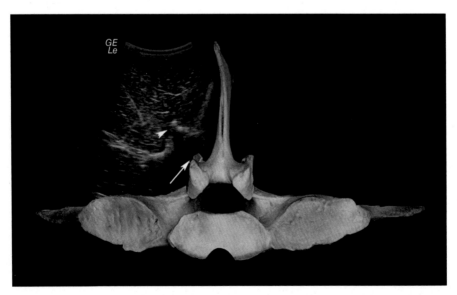

Figure 10.4 A postmortem specimen of a vertebra and a transverse ultrasonogram of the same region to demonstrate the ultrasonographic view of articular facets. The articular facet is seen at the base of the dorsal spinous process in the postmortem specimen (arrow points to the angle of the joint). In the ultrasonogram the facet is seen to form a sharp angled structure at the base of the dorsal spinous process (arrowhead points to the angle of the joint).

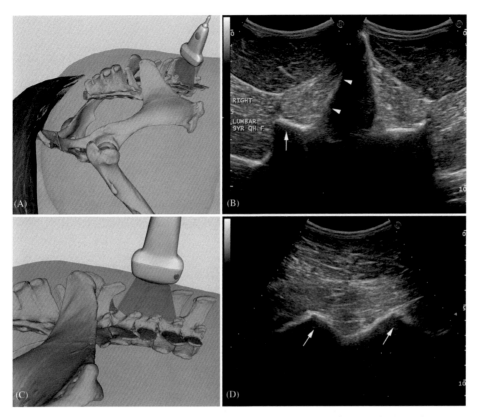

Figure 10.7 The ultrasonographic appearance of the articular facets of the lumbar vertebra. (A) Transducer position to obtain a transverse view of the lumbar vertebra. (B) Normal transverse ultrasonogram of the right (arrow) and left articular facets and dorsal spinous process (arrowheads). (C) Transducer position to obtain a longitudinal image of the lumbar articular facet joints. (D) Normal longitudinal ultrasonogram showing the undulating appearance of the articular facet joints (arrows) of the lumbar spine. Images obtained with 3.5 MHz curvilinear transducer, scanning depth = 12–15 cm.

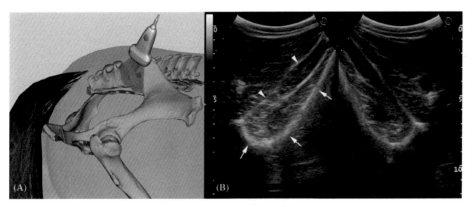

Figure 10.13 The ultrasonographic appearance of the sacrum. (A) Transducer position to obtain a transverse image of the lateral aspect of the sacrum. This view is obtained by sliding the transducer caudally from a longitudinal image of the ilial wing. Each side is evaluated independently by scanning to the left and right of the dorsal sacral processes. (B) A composite transverse ultrasonogram to show the ultrasonographic image of the sacrum (arrows) obtained using the technique shown in (A). The long (or lateral) portion of the right and left dorsal sacroiliac ligaments (arrowheads) are also visible and have an echogenic linear appearance that parallels the lateral aspect of the sacrum.

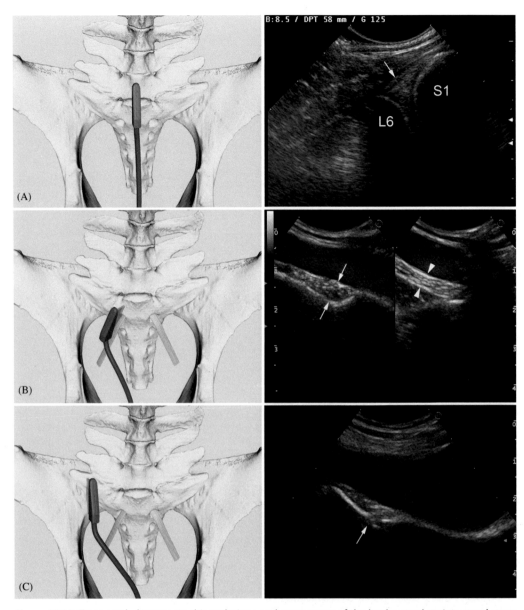

Figure 10.14 Transrectal ultrasonographic technique and appearance of the lumbosacral region, sacral nerve roots and sacroiliac joints. (A) Transducer position to obtain a transrectal ultrasonogram (top right image) of the ventral aspect of the lumbosacral junction. The vertebral bodies of L6 and S1 have smooth bony surfaces. The intervertebral disc (arrow) has a somewhat triangular shape and a homogeneously hypoechoic appearance. (B) Transducer position to obtain a transrectal ultrasonogram of the sacral nerve roots of S1 (middle right image). The nerve is round to oval in shape on transverse views (arrows) and shows linear fibers on longitudinal views (arrowheads). (C) Transducer position to obtain a transrectal ultrasonogram of the sacroiliac joint (arrow, bottom right image). Images obtained with 8.5 MHz microconvex transducer, scanning depth = 5–6 cm.

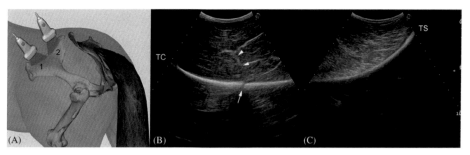

Figure 10.15 The ultrasonographic appearance of the ilial wing as it extends from the tuber sacrale (TS) to the tuber coxae (TC). (A) Transducer placements to obtain longitudinal views of the ilial wing. (B) Longitudinal ultrasound image corresponding to the location of transducer 1 in A. (C) Longitudinal ultrasound image corresponding to the location of transducer 2 in (A). The normal ilial wing has a smooth convex bony surface with the exception of an artifactual defect (arrow) in its bony surface, created by refraction of sound waves by the overlying fascial planes (arrowheads). Images obtained with 4.0 MHz curvilinear transducer, scanning depth = 14 cm.

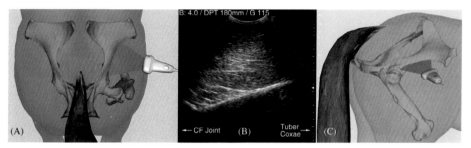

Figure 10.16 The ultrasonographic examination of the ilial body (shaft). (A) Dorsal view showing the transducer orientation to obtain longitudinal views of the ilial body. (B) A longitudinal ultrasonogram of the normal ilial body as it extends from the *tuber coxae* to the coxofemoral joint region. (C) Lateral view showing the transducer orientation to obtain a longitudinal view of the ilial body. Image obtained with 4.0 MHz curvilinear transducer, scanning depth = 18 cm.

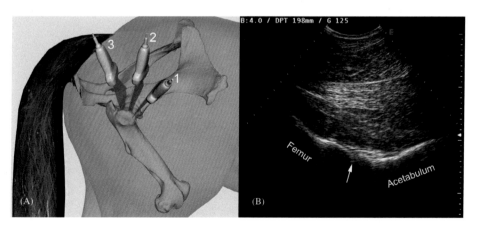

Figure 10.17 The ultrasonographic examination of the coxofemoral joint. (A) Transducer positioning to obtain transverse views of the cranial (1), craniodorsal (2) and dorsal (3) surfaces of the coxofemoral joint. (B) Transverse ultrasonogram to show the normal appearance of the cranial aspect of the coxofemoral joint (arrow). This image was obtained with transducer orientation 1 shown in (A). The tight articulation between the acetabulum and femoral head is visible in most horses. All bony surfaces should be smooth. Image obtained with 4.0 MHz curvilinear transducer, scanning depth = 20 cm.

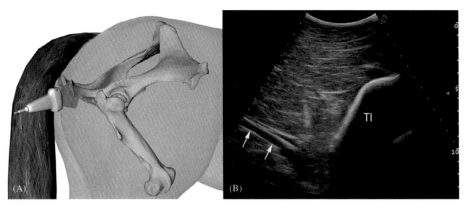

Figure 10.19 The ultrasonographic examination of the *tuber ischii (TI)*. (A) Transducer placement to obtain a longitudinal view of the *tuber ischii* and its ventral muscle attachments. (B) A normal ultrasonogram to show the appearance of the *tuber ischii*. The *tuber ischii* is seen to have a sloping bony contour and normal ventral muscle attachments. Multiple blood vessels (arrows) are often visible during evaluation of the *tuber ischii*. These are at risk for laceration and hemorrhage in horses with TI fractures. Image obtained with 3.5 MHz curvilinear transducer, scanning depth = 13 cm.

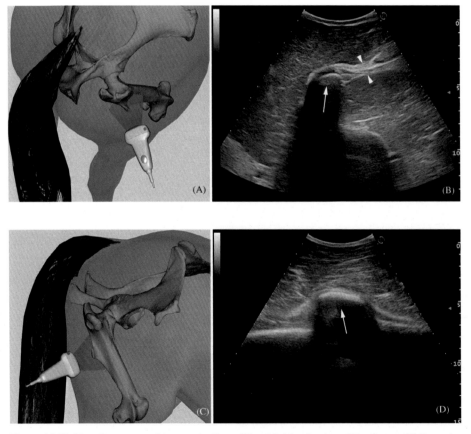

Figure 10.20 The ultrasonographic examination of the third trochanter of the femur. (A) Transducer placement to obtain a transverse ultrasonogram of the third trochanter. (B) A normal transverse ultrasonogram of the third trochanter (arrow) showing its superficial location relative to the body of the femur. The tendinous attachment of the superficial gluteal muscle is also visible (arrowheads). (C) Transducer placement to obtain a longitudinal view of the third trochanter of the femur. (D) A normal longitudinal ultrasonogram of the third trochanter (arrow) showing its slightly convex surface.

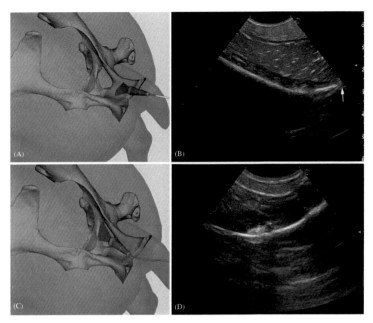

Figure 10.21 The transrectal ultrasonographic examination of the ischium and pubis. (A) Transducer placement to evaluate the ischium using a microconvex transducer. (B) A transrectal ultrasonogram showing the smooth bony surface of the left ischium (lateral is to the left). The gap created by the pubic symphysis should not be mistaken for fracture (arrow). (C) Transducer placement to obtain a longitudinal view of the pubis using a microconvex transducer. (D) A transrectal ultrasonogram to show the smooth sloping bony surface of the right pubis (lateral is to the right). Ultrasonographic images obtained with 8.5 MHz microconvex transducer, scanning depth = 5–6 cm.

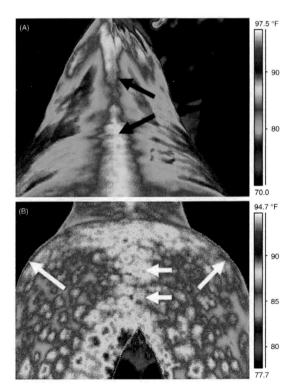

Figure 11.1 Two thermograms to show the normal pattern of distribution of body surface temperature. (A) Thermogram of the thoracolumbar region of the back of a normal horse; the midline is the warmest area (yellow stripe) (black arrows). (B) Thermogram of the lumbosacral and gluteal region of the back of a normal horse; the warmest area (yellow) is along the midline and from tuber coxae to tuber coxae (white arrows).

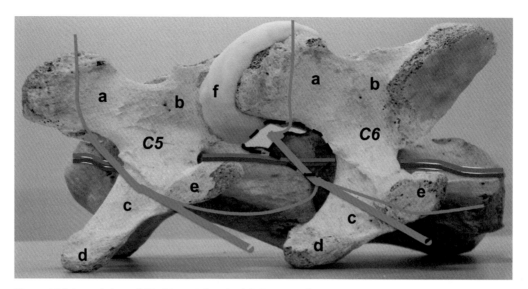

Figure 12.1 Lateral view of C5–C6, cranial to the left (a = cranial articular process, b = caudal articular process, c = transverse process, d = cranial tubercle, e = caudal tubercle, f = articular process joint in yellow. Green = segmental spinal nerves, red = paravertebral blood vessels, purple = paravertebral sympathetic nerve, black dotted line defines intervertebral foramen).

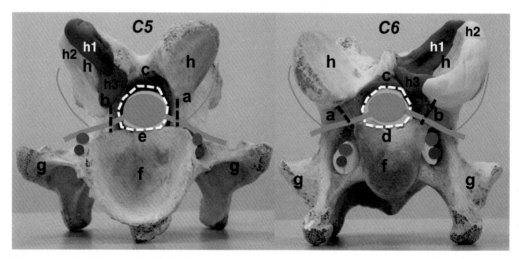

Figure 12.2 Cranial view of C5 (left) and caudal view of C6 (right) (a = right articular process, b = left articular process, c = vertebral arch, d = cranial epiphysis, e = caudal epiphysis, f = margins of intercentral joint, g = transverse process, h = articular surface of articular process joint, with blue/yellow/red/white denoting the joint outpouches, green = segmental spinal nerves, grey = spinal cord, white dotted line = vertebral canal, black dotted line = intervertebral foramen, red = paravertebral blood vessels, purple = paravertebral sympathetic nerve).

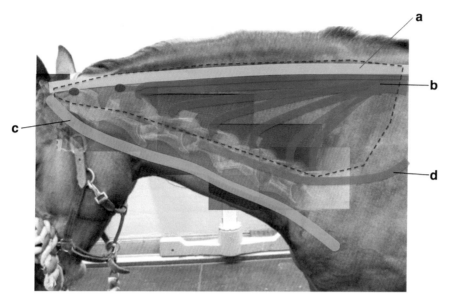

Figure 12.4 Relevant structures within the cervical region, overlayed with laterolateral radiographs of the cervical spine and caudal skull (yellow = nuchal ligament, funicular part, blue = nuchal ligament, lamellar part, purple circles = nuchal bursae, green = brachiocephalicus muscle, orange = spinalis muscle, red area within dotted line = semispinalis and splenius muscles).

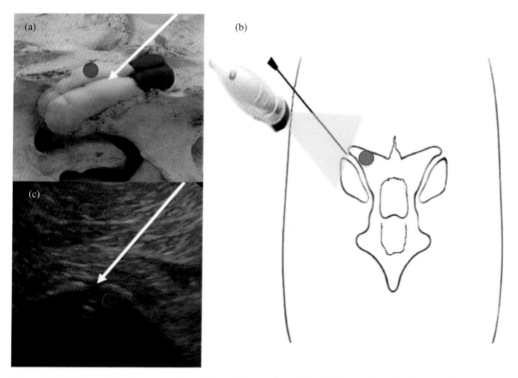

Figure 12.8 (a) Dorsolateral aspect of cervical articular process joint (APJ), cranial to left, showing the APJ pouches (white, yellow, blue). (b) Schematic diagram showing the position of ultrasound probe and spinal needle relative to the skin surface and vertebral cross-section. (c) Ultrasound image of the dorsolateral aspect of an APJ, dorsal to right, with a white arrow representing the needle approach. In all images the red dot signifies the caudal articular process of the cranial vertebral, which is located dorsally to the joint space.

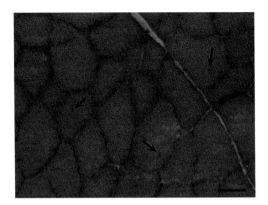

Figure 15.1 *Semimembranosus* muscle biopsy sample. 11-year-old TBx mare with a history of repeated episodes of exertional rhabdomyolysis. Note the internalised nuclei (arrows). Haematoxylin and eosin stain. Bar = 50 μm.

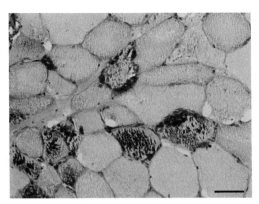

Figure 15.2 *Semimembranosus* muscle biopsy sample stained with periodic acid Schiff (PAS) following diastase digestion. 8-year-old Cob gelding with exertional rhabdomyolysis. Note the abundant pink staining inclusions in multiple fibres, consistent with abnormal polysaccharide and a diagnosis of polysaccharide storage myopathy. Bar = 50 μm.

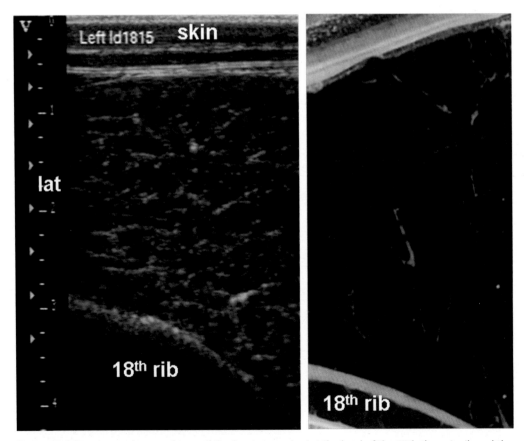

Figure 15.3 Transverse ultrasound scan of the *longissimus dorsi* at the level of the 18th thoracic rib and the corresponding dissection. Muscle tissue appears less echogenic than the connective tissue enveloping the muscle fascicles, resulting in a speckled appearance.

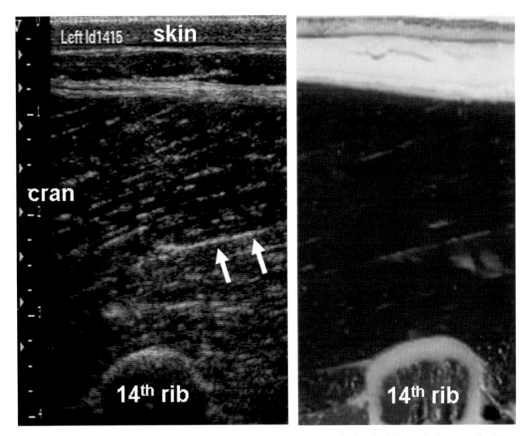

Figure 15.4 Longitudinal ultrasound scan of the *longissimus dorsi* at the level of the 14th thoracic rib, 15 cm ventral to the midline and the corresponding dissection. Muscle is less echogenic compared to the connective tissue, the muscle fascicles appear as multiple, parallel, linear lines and aponeurotic sheets appear as distinct hyperechonic lines within muscles (arrows) and separating muscle bellies.

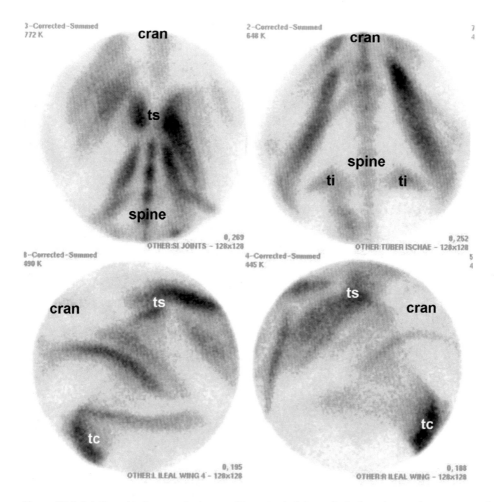

Figure 15.5 Scintigraphic images of a horse with acute rhabdomyolysis three hours after injection of Tc^{99m}-methylendiphosphonate. The top two images show two dorsal views of the pelvis region, the two bottom images show a left lateral oblique and a right lateral oblique image (tc = *tuber coxae*, ts = *tuber sacrale*, ti = *tuber ischii*). Note the striped/linear increase in radiopharmceutical uptake over the musculature typical for this condition.

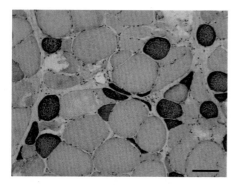

Figure 15.6 *Sacrocaudalis dorsalis medialis* muscle biopsy specimen. 2-year-old filly with marked muscle atrophy and weakness, labelled (immuno-peroxidase) with an antibody to slow myosin heavy chain. Note the angular atrophy of particularly the darker, type I fibres, characteristic of equine motor neurone disease. Bar = 100 μm.

10

Ultrasonography

Mary Beth Whitcomb, Luis P. Lamas and Marcus Head

Introduction

Whilst radiography and nuclear scintigraphy are excellent diagnostic imaging techniques for imaging bony back and pelvis pathology, ultrasonography is the imaging modality of choice for imaging the superficial soft tissues of this region. Ultrasonography can be performed in the thoracic spine, the lumbar spine, the sacroiliac region and the pelvis.

10.1 Ultrasonography of the Thoracic Spine

Luis P. Lamas and Marcus Head

Ultrasonography of the thoracic spine is performed:

- When specifically indicated on the basis of the clinical examination, i.e. a swelling is detected in the region of the supraspinous ligament (SSL, Chapter 2) or there is focal pain on palpation.
- When indicated by other diagnostic imaging techniques, e.g. to further investigate articular facet osteoarthritis identified by radiography and nuclear scintigraphy and the soft tissue at their osseous insertions.
- As part of a general investigation into back pain and/or loss of performance.
- To facilitate the administration of diagnostic analgesia or regional medication.

General Considerations

The horse should be adequately restrained, preferably in stocks and the hair clipped from the dorsal midline. The area to be ultrasound scanned is then cleaned and ultrasound coupling gel applied. Ultrasonography of this region can be done with linear/curvilinear and sector scanners using frequencies between 2.5 and 12 MHz depending on the structure to be viewed.

Ultrasonography of the thoracic spine allows assessment of the following important structures:

- SSL
- Intraspinous ligament (ISL)
- Muscles
- Dorsal spinous processes (DSP) of the vertebrae
- Articular processes (facet) joints of the vertebrae (APJ)

Supraspinous Ligament and Interspinous Ligament Ultrasonography

As outlined above, ultrasonography of the soft tissues of the thoracolumbar region is used to identify anatomical structures and any abnormalities in the SSL, the ISL and the muscles. As discussed in Chapter 2, the SSL is the continuation of the more elastic nuchal

Equine Neck and Back Pathology: Diagnosis and Treatment, Second Edition. Edited by Frances M.D. Henson.
© 2018 John Wiley & Sons, Ltd. Published 2018 by John Wiley & Sons, Ltd.

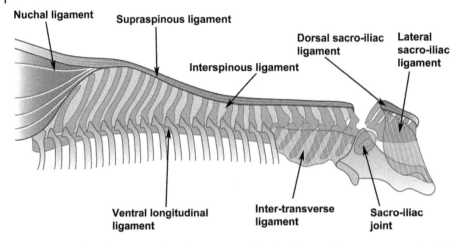

Figure 10.1 A line diagram to show the position of the significant soft tissue structures in the back. *Source:* Courtesy of Professor L.B. Jeffcott.

ligament, which originates at the occipital bone and has its most caudal insertion on to the last lumbar vertebra [1] (Figure 10.1). As the SSL runs caudally it becomes progressively stiffer. It is thicker in the cranial thoracic region and the lumbosacral area [2]. The SSL has multiple attachments to the tendinous portion of the *longissimus dorsi* muscles, which contributes to the stabilizing function of the ligament. The SSL lies directly beneath the skin and a variable amount of subcutaneous adipose tissues with the ventral fibres of the ligament coursing downwards to become continuous with the ISL, which attaches to the cranial and caudal margins of adjacent DSPs.

Ultrasonographic Technique

Ultrasonographic evaluation should be performed using a high-frequency linear ultrasound probe (7.5–12 MHz). A 7.5 MHz probe is most routinely used. The hair should be clipped with a #40 blade in a 3–4 cm wide strip. In most routine cases this clip is begun at the base of the withers as lesions of the SSL are uncommon cranial to this point [3]) and continued caudally to the caudal sacral region. Evaluation requires a systematic and thorough approach. It is important to image the entire thoracolumbar portion of the ligament using both longitudinal (long-axis) and transverse (cross-sectional, short-axis) images.

Longitudinal Section

In longitudinal section the ligament is seen as a horizontal structure with a prominent fibre pattern present on the midline (Figure 10.2A).

Transverse Section

In transverse section the ligament is seen as a small oval hyperechoic structure that is better identified in the spaces between adjacent DSPs (Figure 10.2B). The ligament should be examined for the following characteristics:

Echogenicity. The normal SSL has a heterogeneous echogenicity (Figure 10.2A). The dorsal portion of the SSL is generally more hyperechoic than the ventral fibres and the ISL, which are more hypoechoic. The change in echogenicity occurs because of the difference in SSL fibre orientation between the dorsal and ventral parts of SSL. As the SSL fibres become deeper, their angle increases, resulting in a decrease in echogenicity due to the loss of the perpendicular orientation of the US beam. Immediately adjacent to the dorsal margin of

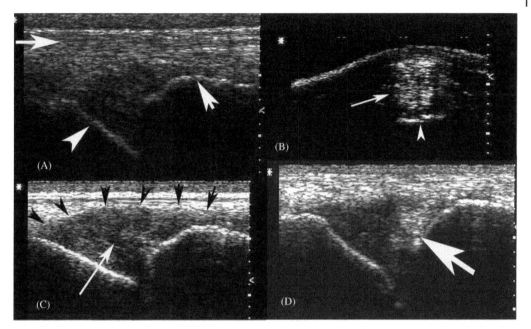

Figure 10.2 Ultrasonograms to show the ultrasonographic appearance of the supraspinous ligament (SSL). (A) Longitudinal section showing the normal appearance of the ligament. The ligament runs over the summits of the dorsal spinous processes (arrowheads) and is seen to be a horizontal structure. The fiber pattern is visible (arrow). (B) Transverse section through the SSL (arrow) as it runs over the summit of a dorsal spinous process (arrowhead). (C) A hypoechoic lesion (blacker) within the supraspinous ligament (arrow). This hypoechoic lesion extends dorsally into the body of the supraspinous ligament (black arrowheads). (D) A hyperechoic lesion (whiter) within the supraspinous ligament (arrow) adjacent to a dorsal spinous process.

the DSPs there is a hypoechoic cap (1 mm approximately), formed by the fibrocartilaginous pad over each DSP.

The normal echogenicity of the SSL can be altered in a number of ways. Both hyperechoic and hypoechoic regions may be detected on an ultrasound scan (Figure 10.2C and D). The clinical relevance of these findings is discussed in Chapter 13.

Fibre pattern. A linear fibre pattern should be present in the dorsal portion of the ligament. Fibre pattern scoring systems used in other structures [4] could theoretically be used for the SSL, although this is not currently in common use. Adjacent to the DSP and in the interspinous region, the fibre pattern is difficult to assess because of the change in fibre direction, as discussed previously (Figure 10.2A).

Objective measurements. A normal range of measurements of the SSL has not been determined. However, some generalisations about the size of the ligament can be made.

Longitudinal section measurements. In the longitudinal section the ligament thickness should be measured in the dorsoventral plane at the level of the middle of the DSP summit. Care must be taken to avoid misinterpretations caused by possible differences in the contour of adjacent DSPs. Comparing the dimensions of adjacent sections of the ligament is an acceptable and recommended method of size evaluation.

Transverse section measurements. In transverse section the SSL is continuous with the thick echogenic thoracolumbar fascia on either side [2] and so accurate measurements are hard to make. Comparing the dimensions of adjacent sections of the ligament is an acceptable method of size evaluation.

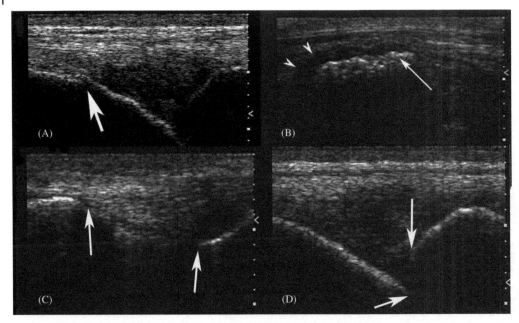

Figure 10.3 Ultrasonograms to show the ultrasonography of bone in the thoracic region. (A) Enthesiopathy. The supraspinous ligament has been torn away from the summit of the dorsal spinous process and a small piece of bone has become detached (arrow). (B) The normal appearance of the summit of the dorsal spinous process (DSP) of the 6th thoracic vertebra on a transverse (cross-section) scan. Note the roughened appearance of the secondary centre of ossification in the summit of this bone (arrow). Note also the cartilage cap overlying the summit, seen as a hypoechogeneic region (arrowheads delineate the lateral margin), between the bone and the overlying supraspinous ligament. (C and D) Ultrasonograms to identify the proximity of two DSPs in the longitudinal plane. (B) DSPs are clearly separate in this horse in the caudal thoracic region (the white arrows show the caudal edge of one DSP and the cranial edge of the next DSP). (C) DSPs are very close together (the white arrows show the caudal edge of one DSP and the cranial edge of the next DSP).

Entheseopathy. Insertional desmopathy of SSL can be readily identified using ultrasonography. Insertional desmopathy occurs when the fibres of the SSL become pulled from the dorsal surface of the DSP and this is reflected in an alteration in the appearance of the DSP. On ultrasonography, the main characteristic of enthesiopathy is the irregular shape of the dorsal surface of the DSP (Figure 10.3A), although an increase in echogenicity of the SSL may also be seen. The presence of small hyperechoic detached fragments of bone from the dorsal margins of the DSPs is associated with more severe cases (avulsion fractures). When an avulsion fracture is suspected, low exposure radiographs of the area may be taken for further evaluation. In the more cranial DSPs the incomplete centres of ossification should not be confused with avulsion fractures, as noted in Chapter 8.

Ultrasound of the Muscles of the Thoracic Spine

Muscular ultrasonography is discussed in detail in Chapter 15.

Ultrasonography of the Bone

Although the deeper structures of the vertebral column are not accessible, ultrasonography of some of the more superficial ones is possible. Ultrasonography of the summits of the DSPs and the articular facets of the thoracolumbar spine has been described. In addition it is possible to use ultrasonography of these regions to facilitate ultrasonographic guided injections, for example to medicate the articular facets in cases of osteoarthritis (Chapter 13).

Ultrasonography of the Dorsal Spinous Processes

Ultrasonography can provide very useful information about the summits of the DSP and their relationship to one another. In the normal horse the dorsal surfaces of the summits of the DSPs of T7–T18 are smooth and are seen as a hyperechoic line horizontal to the skin. In contrast the summits of T3–6, with their separate centres of ossification, have roughened summits (Figure 10.3B).

Ultrasonography can provide information on the interspinous spaces between the DSPs – the space can be seen in normal regions of the spine (Figure 10.3C), but in cases where there is contact between the DSPs this space is lost (Figure 10.3D) (Chapter 13). Desmitis of the SSL following impingement of the DSPs has not been recognised as a clinical entity although an ultrasonographic appearance consistent with entheseopathies is often present with overriding DSP due to the bone modelling that as occurred.

Ultrasonography of the DSP can also be used to identify fractures of the DSP, although these can usually be clearly seen on radiography (Chapter 13) and other, far less common, conditions, such as congenital malformations and developmental variations in the interspinous spaces [5].

Ultrasonography of the Articular Processes (Facets)

Ultrasonography of the thoracolumbar articular process joints (APJ) (facet joints) is performed fairly routinely. The AJP complex is formed by the caudal articular process of the cranial vertebra, the synovial intervertebral articulation and the cranial articular process of the adjacent vertebra [6] (Chapter 2). As discussed in Chapter 13, pathology at the APJ of the thoracolumbar spine is considered, at the current time, likely to be a significant cause of back pain in the horse [7]. In most cases radiographic examination and/or nuclear scintigraphic examination will have alerted the clinician to the possibility of lesions at a specific site. Ultrasonographic examination of the affected area of the thoracolumbar area and particularly the lumbar articular APJ is a very useful procedure, and with practice and good equipment is a very sensitive way of detecting enlargement of the APJ that are commonly affected by osteoarthritis and stress fractures. In addition, this ultrasonography technique will also enable ultrasound-guided injection of the joints to be performed.

Technique

The APJ are best imaged using a convex low-frequency (2.5 to 5 MHz) transducer. As described above, the hair is clipped from the region to be imaged, extending 6–12 cm from the midline depending on the size of the horse, the skin is cleaned and ultrasound coupling is applied.

The APJ are most usefully imaged in transverse views (perpendicular to the midline). In order to obtain images of the articular facets, place the probe 2–4 centimetres to the side of the midline of the back and tilt the probe head back and forth (towards the head and then the tail) until the joint is visible. The DSP can be used as a convenient reference point within the ultrasound scans. By starting cranially and moving slowly towards the tail each joint will appear sequentially. The APJ are located differently with respect to the DSP at different levels of the spine [6]. Denoix describes that in the midthoracic region the APJ are located in the middle of the apex of the cranial vertebra, by approximately T16 the APJ are located at the level of the interspinous spaces and that in the caudal thoracic and lumbar area the APJ are located in the middle of the apex of the caudal vertebra.

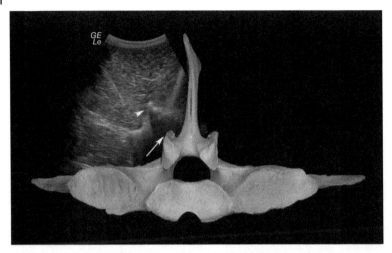

Figure 10.4 A postmortem specimen of a vertebra and a transverse ultrasonogram of the same region to demonstrate the ultrasonographic view of articular facets. The articular facet is seen at the base of the dorsal spinous process in the postmortem specimen (arrow points to the angle of the joint). In the ultrasonogram the facet is seen to form a sharp angled structure at the base of the dorsal spinous process (arrowhead points to the angle of the joint). (*For a colour version of this figure, see the colour plate section.*)

The APJ can be imaged either on transverse scans or on longitudional scans. On transverse sections the joints appear as the corner of a square at the junction of the dorsal and transverse processes (Figure 10.4). With a good quality scanner, it is possible to differentiate the cranial and caudal articular processes of each vertebra. It is useful to compare each joint with the ones immediately cranial and caudal to it and to the contralateral joint. In a normal horse the right and left APJ are symmetrical. Longitudinal scans also allow identification of the facets. On a longitudinal scan the bone surfaces are regular and, again, the right and left articular facets are symmetrical. The advantage of the longitudinal scan is that it permits a comparison of adjacent joints simultaneously.

A number of abnormalities of the APJ has been described. These abnormalities have been classified into 8 types [6]. In most cases, however, it is not possible to see sufficient detail of the APJ to be able to classify the lesion. This may be due to a number of factors, including the large size of the patient, the capabilities of the ultrasound machine and the operator's experience. It is usually possible to assess and identify any asymmetries of the APJ, loss of the facet joint space (indicative of articular facet osteoarthritis) and the presence of proliferative new bone formation. New bone formation is the most commonly identified ultrasonographic abnormality detected at this site and is identified by the production of an enlarged, irregular outline associated with the facet.

Ultrasound Guided Injection in the Thoracic Spine

As mentioned above, the technique of APJ ultrasonography is extremely useful in that it permits ultrasound guided injections of diseased facet joints, as described by Denoix [8]. Ultrasonography of the APJ of the cervical spine is discussed in Chapter 12, while this chapter describes the injection of thoracolumbar APJ.

In order to medicate the region surrounding the APJ the skin should be clipped and prepared asceptically. Ultrasonography is used to identify the APJ in the transverse plane, as previously discussed. A spinal needle is then introduced through the skin and aimed towards the facet. The needle should be angled at 45° to the skin surface and the site of entry is between 2 and 6 cm from the midline, depending on the size of the horse. The ultrasound image will allow the needle to be traced in real time as it passes through the soft tissues towards the joint. In the majority of cases an intra-articular injection is not possible, either due to the angle of the facet, poor image quality on the ultrasound, new bone formation or joint ankylosis. In these cases the medication is injected periarticularly in the region of the *multifidus*. In addition. an ultrasound guided technique of injection of the nerves proposed to innervate the articular facets has been described [9]. The APJ are innervated by the medial branch of the dorsal ramus (the spinal nerve splits into dorsal and ventral rami once it exits the intervertebral canal, Chapter 5). This nerve branch runs in a groove on the base of the articular process of the caudal vertebra in direct contact with the cranial aspect of the transverse process of that vertebra. In order to desensitise this nerve the ultrasound probe is placed 3 cm lateral to the median plane transversally and the APJ identified. Once the characteristic APJ has been identified the scanner is repositioned 5 cm caudally and a needle is introduced obliquely at an angle of 45° until it hits bone. Local anaesthetic solution can then be injected.

10.2   Ultrasonography of the Pelvis, Lumbar Spine and Sacrolliac Region

Mary Beth Whitcomb

Introduction

Although nuclear scintigraphy and radiography are useful in the evaluation of horses with back or pelvic abnormalities, ultrasound is frequently used as the primary imaging modality for soft tissue and osseous abnormalities in the ambulatory and hospital setting. While hospitals are more likely to be equipped with the transducers necessary to perform a complete exam, a standard tendon or rectal format transducer owned by many ambulatory practitioners can be used to evaluate many of the structures presented here. It is recognized that examination and interpretation of some of the structures discussed in this chapter can be technically challenging to the novice and intermediate ultrasonographer. Armed with a solid understanding of osseous and soft tissue anatomy, experience will provide the dedicated veterinarian with an adequate skill level to evaluate many horses.

The clinical presentation of horses undergoing lumbar/sacroiliac ultrasound is typically quite different from that of horses presenting for pelvic ultrasound. Therefore, the ultrasonographic techniques to evaluate the lumbar and sacroiliac regions will be presented separately from the pelvis in this chapter.

Lumbar Spine and Sacroiliac Region

Many horses that present for examination of the lumbosacral region have a history or clinical finding of pain on palpation. Less frequently, horses present for diffuse or focal lumbar swelling or tuber sacrale asymmetry. Other indications include increased radiopharmaceutical uptake on nuclear scintigraphy, lameness not abated by diagnostic anesthesia of the hind limbs, a positive response to sacroiliac joint anesthesia, behavioral changes perceived by the owner as related to back pain and known trauma to the region. Differentiation between lumbar and sacroiliac pain is difficult in most horses and ultrasonographic investigation of both regions is recommended using both transcutaneous and transrectal approaches.

Multiple transducers are required to perform a complete exam. A high-frequency (8–18 MHz) linear transducer should be used for evaluation of the dorsal spinous processes and supraspinous ligament of the lumbar spine as well as the short dorsal sacroiliac ligaments. A midrange frequency (4–8 MHz) microconvex transducer may be useful to visualize the sacroiliac ligaments in large horses or those with significant subcutaneous fat accumulation. This transducer is also useful for transrectal examination of the caudal lumbar and lumbosacral disc spaces, right and left sacroiliac joints, ventral aspect of the sacrum and sacral nerve roots, although a standard rectal transducer set at its highest frequency can also be used. A low-frequency (2–5 MHz) curvilinear transducer is often necessary for evaluation of the lumbar articular facets and transverse processes, especially in large horses. Although a microconvex transducer can penetrate to the depths required to visualize these structures, diagnostic images are often only obtainable in young or thin horses with this transducer. A program suitable for musculoskeletal use (tendon, small parts, etc.) should be selected, although an abdominal program may be helpful when using the low-frequency curvilinear transducer.

Alcohol saturation is often adequate in young or thin horses, but clipping the hair with #40 blades is necessary to obtain diagnostic images in many horses. Significant dorsal fat accumulation in well-fed or overweight horses can significantly impede image quality. In such cases, clipping the hair will provide the examiner with the best opportunity to obtain diagnostic images. Furthermore, the skin of the back can be quite thick, especially in ponies, and may require razor shaving in order to obtain images of the lumbar or sacroiliac region.

Transcutaneous Evaluation

Lumbar Spine

Evaluation of the lumbar spine should begin with the DSPs and SSL. In the lumbar region they are evaluated using transverse and longitudinal techniques at a depth setting of 4–6 cm. The use of a standoff pad may help to maintain skin contact in thin horses with prominent DSP. Each DSP should demonstrate a relatively smooth, flat to convex shape, although occasional small surface defects can be seen in horses without a history of back problems. The DSP are more superficially located in the cranial lumbar spine and become deeper relative to the skin surface as the exam progresses caudally. DSP should be regularly spaced and aligned along the dorsal midline.

The SSL is located between the skin surface and the dorsal spinous processes along the length of the lumbar spine. Its size and shape varies as it extends caudally from the DSP of L1 to L6. At L1 and L2, it has a small, slightly crescent shape on transverse views, becomes progressively larger from L3 through L5 (Figure 10.5) and may show an undulating or 'S'-shaped appearance at L6 (Figure 10.6). Echogenicity is somewhat variable, especially in the mid to caudal lumbar regions and between the DSP due to the varying orientation of fibers as they insert on to the cranial aspect of each DSP. On longitudinal views, fiber pattern should appear relatively linear, overlying each DSP, but will appear to be somewhat irregular between DSPs.

The right and left APJ of the lumbar spine are best visualized by placing the transducer (low-frequency curvilinear) perpendicular to the long axis of the spine, slightly to the right and left of the midline respectively. The APJ are located 8–10 cm from the skin surface and therefore scanning depth should be set at 10–15 cm. Normal articular facets will show a step-like appearance on transverse views (Figure 10.7A and B). Mild cortical irregularity may be present in horses without clinical signs. Longitudinal views are obtained by placing the transducer parasagittally approximately 4–5 cm to the right and left of the midline. APJ should be regularly spaced, should not be contiguous with adjacent facets and should show an undulating appearance (Figure 10.7C and D).

The transverse processes of the lumbar spine extend to the right and left of the vertebral bodies in a nearly horizontal plane. They can be evaluated using transverse and longitudinal views by following their bony

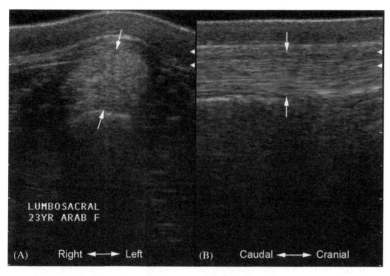

Figure 10.5 The ultrasonographic appearance of the normal supraspinous ligament in the midlumbar region at the dorsal spinous process of L4. (A) Transverse and (B) longitudinal images. The ligament has a round to oval shape at this level with a slightly mottled echogenicity. Image obtained with 10.0 MHz linear transducer, scanning depth = 4 cm.

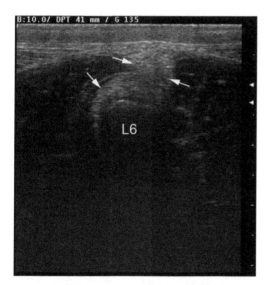

Figure 10.6 The ultrasonographic appearance of the supraspinous ligament in the caudal lumbar region at the dorsal spinous process of L6. A transverse ultrasonogram shows an undulating appearance of the ligament at this level that may change with head position or as the horse shifts weight between hind limbs. Image obtained with 10.0 MHz linear transducer, scanning depth = 4 cm.

surfaces from the midline to their abaxial extents using the same transducer and machine settings as for the articular facets. All bony surfaces should be smooth. Although clinically significant abnormalities of the transverse processes are infrequent, evaluation should not be neglected. Interpretation is relatively straightforward and the exam can be performed in a timely fashion.

Sacroiliac Ligaments

Ultrasound of the sacroiliac area is very helpful for the diagnosis of pathology in this site [10]. The short dorsal sacroiliac ligaments (DSIL) are paired structures that originate on the right and left *tuber sacrale* and course caudally alongside the dorsal sacral processes to their insertions on the caudal sacral process. These ligaments are located relatively close to the skin surface and a shallow depth setting of 4–7 cm should be used. Large horses may require an increased depth setting and a decreased frequency setting to obtain adequate penetration and visualization. Each ligament should be evaluated individually by locating the *tuber sacrale* to the left and right of the midline and then following each

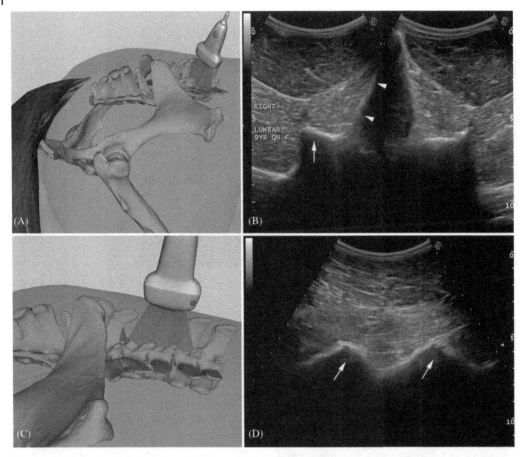

Figure 10.7 The ultrasonographic appearance of the articular facets of the lumbar vertebra. (A) Transducer position to obtain a transverse view of the lumbar vertebra. (B) Normal transverse ultrasonogram of the right (arrow) and left articular facets and dorsal spinous process (arrowheads). (C) Transducer position to obtain a longitudinal image of the lumbar articular facet joints. (D) Normal longitudinal ultrasonogram showing the undulating appearance of the articular facet joints (arrows) of the lumbar spine. Images obtained with 3.5 MHz curvilinear transducer, scanning depth = 12–15 cm. (*For a colour version of this figure, see the colour plate section.*)

ligament caudally to its insertion. At the origin, the ligament has a thin crescent shape on transverse views (Figure 10.8), becomes somewhat round to oval shaped in the midligament region (Figure 10.9) and is semicircular at its insertion on to the sacrum (Figure 10.10). Echogenicity is fairly homogeneous and fiber pattern is linear in most horses; however, some variability in both parameters will be seen in normal horses. Such variability can complicate detection of many mild and even moderate injuries. There is also considerable anatomic variation between horses due to caudal continuation of the thoracolumbar

fascia (TLF) that joins the short DSIL caudal to the *tuber sacrale*. The TLF inserts along the medial border of each short DSIL in most horses. Less commonly, the TLF is located dorsal to the short DSIL prior to their confluence, creating a nearly bipartite appearance (Figure 10.11). Such an appearance will be bilaterally symmetrical and should not be confused with injury.

Although clinical abnormalities of the *tuber sacrale* are uncommon, they should be evaluated in conjunction with the short DSIL. Each *tuber sacrale* should demonstrate smooth bony contours in adult horses; however, minor

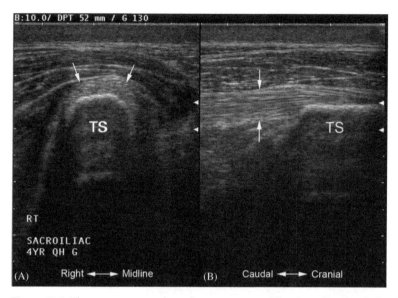

Figure 10.8 Ultrasonograms to show the appearance of the short dorsal sacroiliac ligament (DSIL) at its origin on the right tuber sacrale (TS). (A) Transverse and (B) longitudinal ultrasonographic images of the right short dorsal sacroiliac ligament (arrows). Note the smooth bony surface of the TS in this adult horse. Image obtained with 10 MHz linear transducer, scanning depth = 5 cm.

surface irregularities have been reported. Care should be taken with interpretation of distance measurements from the skin to the bony surfaces of each *tuber sacrale*. Measurements can vary significantly depending on the limb position as well as transducer placement/pressure on the skin surface. Care should also be taken when evaluating foals and juvenile horses, due

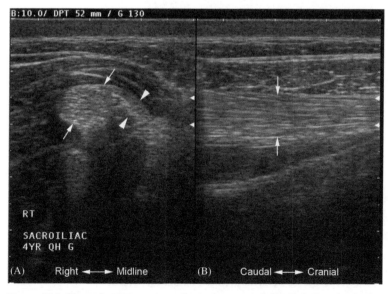

Figure 10.9 Ultrasonogram to show the appearance of the short dorsal sacroiliac ligament (DSIL) at the midligament region. (A) Transverse and (B) longitudinal ultrasonographic images of the right DSIL. The caudal extension of the thoracolumbar fascia (arrowheads) is visible medial to the right short DSIL (arrows). Image obtained with 10 MHz linear transducer, scanning depth = 5 cm.

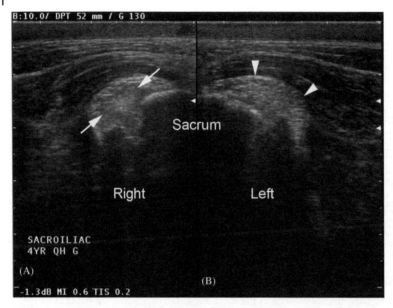

Figure 10.10 Transverse ultrasonogram to show the insertion of the (A) right and (B) left short dorsal sacroiliac ligaments (DSIL) on to the sacrum. (B) The left insertion is normal (arrowheads); however, a central hyperechoic core lesion (arrows) is present within the right DSIL (A). Image obtained with 10 MHz linear transducer, scanning depth = 5 cm.

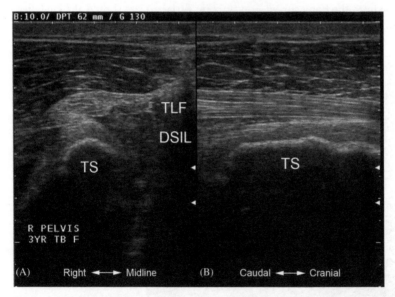

Figure 10.11 Ultrasonogram to show an alternative relationship between the thoracolumbar fascia (TLF) and short dorsal sacroiliac ligament (DSIL) at the level of the tuber sacrale (TS). (A) Transverse ultrasonogram and (B) longitudinal ultrasonogram. The TLF is located dorsal to the short DSIL at the level of the TS. This anatomic variation is considered within normal limits, but is less commonly seen than a medial insertion of the TLF on to the short DSIL, shown in Figure 11.5. Image obtained with 10 MHz linear transducer, scanning depth = 6.2 cm.

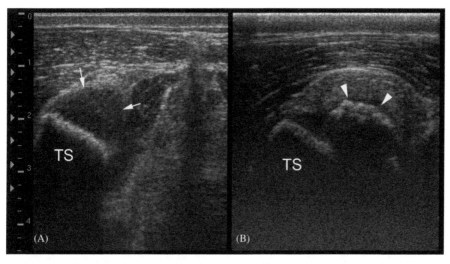

Figure 10.12 Ultrasonograms to show the transverse ultrasonographic images of the tuber sacrale (TS) in a 2-month-old foal (A) and a 2-year-old colt (B). Note the hypoechoic cartilage cap (arrows) overlying the ossified portion of the TS in the foal (A) and the irregularly shaped, hyperechoic area of ossification (arrowheads) within the TS cartilage of the juvenile horse (B). Varying degrees of ossification will be present in horses up to 4 years of age and are within normal limits. Image obtained with 10 MHz transducer, scanning depth = 4.5 cm.

to the fact that a large portion of each *tuber sacrale* is cartilaginous due to incomplete ossification. Normal cartilage is hypoechoic with a slightly speckled appearance. The underlying subchondral bone of the *tuber sacrale* will therefore have an altered shape compared to adults (Figure 10.12A). Varying degrees of ossification of the cartilage caps will be present in juveniles up to even 3–4 years of age (Figure 10.12B). Such findings are typically bilaterally symmetrical, and comparison can be helpful to differentiate bony pathology such as fractures or osteomyelitis from normal ossification.

Transcutaneous evaluation of the lateral surfaces of the sacrum should be attempted in all horses suspicious for sacral fracture. The transducer is positioned perpendicular to the long axis of the spine, slightly to the right and left of the midline, caudal to the tuber sacrale and ilial wings (Figure 10.13A). Bony surfaces should be smooth and slightly concave (Figure 10.13B). Transcutaneous visibility of the sacrum is highly variable, even with a low-frequency curvilinear transducer. Diagnostic images may not be possible in many horses,

and close transrectal inspection is recommended in horses suspicious for fracture. The long component of the DSIL can also be imaged during transcutaneous ultrasound of the sacrum. The long DSIL has a thin linear appearance that extends obliquely to the right and left of the sacrum (Figure 10.13B).

Transrectal Ultrasound

Transrectal ultrasonography is an important aspect of the lumbosacral exam and includes evaluation of the lumbosacral junction, sacral nerve roots, sacroiliac joints and ventral aspect of the sacrum [11]. All structures are located in close proximity to the rectal mucosa and therefore a musculoskeletal or small parts program should be selected with a shallow depth setting of 3–4 cm. The transducer (rectal or microconvex) is directed dorsally along the midline to first locate the disc space of L6–S1 at approximately midforearm to elbow's length (Figure 10.14A). The bony surfaces of the vertebral body of L6 and sacrum should be smooth. The disc space will

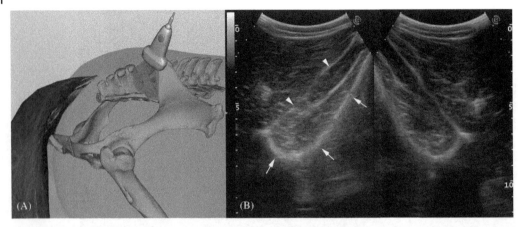

Figure 10.13 The ultrasonographic appearance of the sacrum. (A) Transducer position to obtain a transverse image of the lateral aspect of the sacrum. This view is obtained by sliding the transducer caudally from a longitudinal image of the ilial wing. Each side is evaluated independently by scanning to the left and right of the dorsal sacral processes. (B) A composite transverse ultrasonogram to show the ultrasonographic image of the sacrum (arrows) obtained using the technique shown in (A). The long (or lateral) portion of the right and left dorsal sacroiliac ligaments (arrowheads) are also visible and have an echogenic linear appearance that parallels the lateral aspect of the sacrum. (*For a colour version of this figure, see the colour plate section.*)

appear somewhat triangular with a homogeneously hypoechoic appearance. Hyperechoic foci within the disc are frequent findings in horses without lumbosacral pain. To visualize the disc spaces of L5–L6 and L4–L5, the transducer is advanced further cranially along the midline. These disc spaces will appear smaller than the lumbosacral junction. The transducer is then moved caudally from the lumbosacral junction and slightly to the right or left of the midline, until the concave surface of the right or left first sacral foramina, respectively, is seen. Depending on transducer orientation, this will produce a transverse or longitudinal image of the sacral nerve roots of S1 (Figure 10.14B). The nerve roots of S1 and S2 are large enough to be evaluated in most horses and show a round to oval, heterogeneous appearance on transverse views and a linear fiber pattern on longitudinal views. The right and left sacroiliac joints are identified by sliding the transducer laterally from an image of the right or left first sacral foramina respectively. The normal joint should appear tightly articulated with relatively smooth bony surfaces (Figure 10.14C). Evaluation of the ventral aspect of the sacrum can also be performed to assist in the diagnosis of sacral

fracture. Visible step defects and bony fragmentation are consistent with fracture; however, care should be taken not to misinterpret neural foramina as fractures.

Ultrasonographic Examination of the Pelvis

The primary indication for ultrasonographic evaluation of the equine pelvis is to rule out fracture [12,13]; however, ultrasound can also assist in the diagnosis of other *coxofemoral* joint disorders such as effusion/synovitis, osteoarthritis and luxation/subluxation [14]. In contrast to small animal patients, fractures are usually unilateral in horses and comparison to the contralateral hemipelvis can therefore be useful when findings are questionable. Ultrasound has many advantages compared to nuclear scintigraphy and radiography for the diagnosis of pelvic fractures [15]. Ultrasound is relatively inexpensive and can be performed in the ambulatory setting without the risks and costs associated with transportation to a referral hospital. There are no exposure risks to personnel and general anesthesia is not necessary. Although ultrasound frequently provides a rapid diagnosis in horses

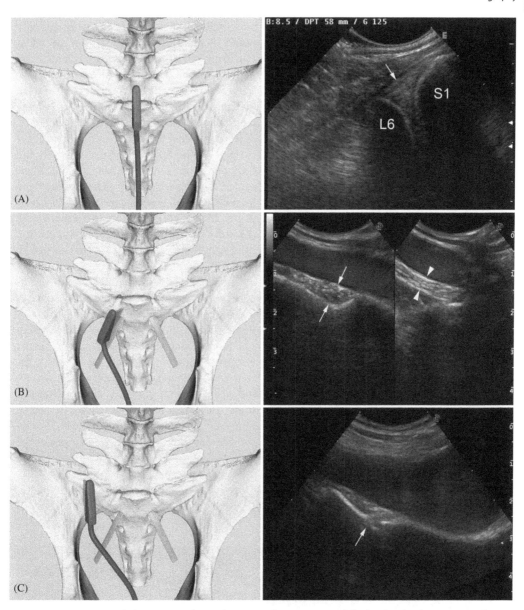

Figure 10.14 Transrectal ultrasonographic technique and appearance of the lumbosacral region, sacral nerve roots and sacroiliac joints. (A) Transducer position to obtain a transrectal ultrasonogram (top right image) of the ventral aspect of the lumbosacral junction. The vertebral bodies of L6 and S1 have smooth bony surfaces. The intervertebral disc (arrow) has a somewhat triangular shape and a homogeneously hypoechoic appearance. (B) Transducer position to obtain a transrectal ultrasonogram of the sacral nerve roots of S1 (middle right image). The nerve is round to oval in shape on transverse views (arrows) and shows linear fibers on longitudinal views (arrowheads). (C) Transducer position to obtain a transrectal ultrasonogram of the sacroiliac joint (arrow, bottom right image). Images obtained with 8.5 MHz microconvex transducer, scanning depth = 5–6 cm. (*For a colour version of this figure, see the colour plate section.*)

with pelvic fractures, nuclear scintigraphy and/or radiography should be considered in highly suspect cases when ultrasonographic examination is negative.

Many horses can be evaluated using alcohol saturation of the hair coat. Improved image quality is possible by clipping the hair with #40 clipper blades, washing with soap and water and application of ultrasound gel. Clipping is often necessary in large, overweight or thick-coated horses. Evaluation of the *tuber sacrale, tuber coxae* and *tuber ischii* is performed with a high or midrange frequency transducer, as these structures are relatively superficially located [16,17]. Evaluation of the bony surfaces of the ilial wing, ilial body and *coxofemoral* joint must be performed with a low-frequency (2–5 MHz) curvilinear transducer. Transrectal ultrasound should be performed in all amenable cases, regardless of rectal palpation findings. It is not uncommon to identify a fracture using transrectal ultrasound in horses that were negative on rectal palpation [18]. Furthermore, fractures of the ischium and pubis are rarely visible on transcutaneous examination.

Deep Structures of the Pelvis

The ilial wing is most easily evaluated on longitudinal views by following a line drawn between the ipsilateral *tuber sacrale* and *tuber coxae*. The scanning depth should be set at 10–15 cm. Multiple slices through the ilial wing should be performed with special attention paid to the caudal border of the ilial wing in Thoroughbred racehorses due to their propensity for stress fractures in this location. The normal ilial wing has a smooth concave surface (Figure 10.15). The examiner should be careful not to misinterpret 'edge' artefacts caused by refraction of sound waves from fascial planes of overlying muscle bellies (Figure 10.15B). This creates an artifactual gap in the bony surface at the mid to lateral portion of the ilial wing that may be confused with fracture.

The ilial body is evaluated by following its cortical surface from the *tuber coxae* towards the coxofemoral joint region. The ilial body demonstrates a smooth sloping bony surface on longitudinal views that becomes deeper relative to the skin surface as it nears the coxofemoral joint (Figure 10.16). An increased scanning depth of 15–20 cm is therefore required to visualize the entire bony surface. Similar to the ilial wing, longitudinal views are most useful to visualize step defects created by fractures, but transverse views may also be used in some cases.

Evaluation of the coxofemoral joint is performed by sliding the transducer slightly

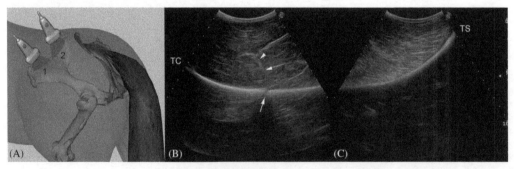

Figure 10.15 The ultrasonographic appearance of the ilial wing as it extends from the tuber sacrale (TS) to the tuber coxae (TC). (A) Transducer placements to obtain longitudinal views of the ilial wing. (B) Longitudinal ultrasound image corresponding to the location of transducer 1 in A. (C) Longitudinal ultrasound image corresponding to the location of transducer 2 in (A). The normal ilial wing has a smooth convex bony surface with the exception of an artifactual defect (arrow) in its bony surface, created by refraction of sound waves by the overlying fascial planes (arrowheads). Images obtained with 4.0 MHz curvilinear transducer, scanning depth = 14 cm. (*For a colour version of this figure, see the colour plate section.*)

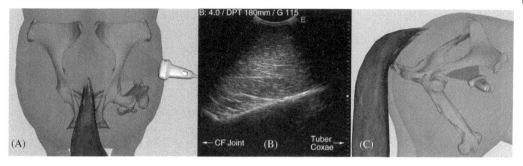

Figure 10.16 The ultrasonographic examination of the ilial body (shaft). (A) Dorsal view showing the transducer orientation to obtain longitudinal views of the ilial body. (B) A longitudinal ultrasonogram of the normal ilial body as it extends from the *tuber coxae* to the coxofemoral joint region. (C) Lateral view showing the transducer orientation to obtain a longitudinal view of the ilial body. Image obtained with 4.0 MHz curvilinear transducer, scanning depth = 18 cm. (*For a colour version of this figure, see the colour plate section.*)

caudally from a longitudinal image of the ilial body (Figure 10.17A) [19]. This produces a transverse image of the acetacular rim and femoral head at the cranial aspect of the coxofemoral joint (Figure 10.17B). Scanning depth is similar to that used for the ilial body (15–20 cm). The joint should appear tightly articulated, and all bony surfaces should be smooth and free of step defects. Visible joint effusion is an unusual finding in normal horses [20]. Examination of the craniodorsal and dorsal aspects of the coxofemoral joint

is performed by sliding the transducer slightly dorsal and caudal from the cranial view and then rotating the transducer 70–90 degrees in a clockwise direction when evaluating the left hemipelvis or in a counterclockwise direction when evaluating the right hemipelvis (Figure 10.17A). The transducer should be directed somewhat ventrally to avoid obstruction by the greater trochanter of the femur. The caudal and ventral aspects of the joint are not visible ultrasonographically.

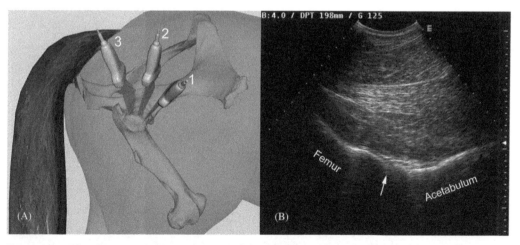

Figure 10.17 The ultrasonographic examination of the coxofemoral joint. (A) Transducer positioning to obtain transverse views of the cranial (1), craniodorsal (2) and dorsal (3) surfaces of the coxofemoral joint. (B) Transverse ultrasonogram to show the normal appearance of the cranial aspect of the coxofemoral joint (arrow). This image was obtained with transducer orientation 1 shown in (A). The tight articulation between the acetabulum and femoral head is visible in most horses. All bony surfaces should be smooth. Image obtained with 4.0 MHz curvilinear transducer, scanning depth = 20 cm. (*For a colour version of this figure, see the colour plate section.*)

Superficial Structures of the Pelvis

The appearance of the *tuber sacrale* was described earlier in the chapter in conjunction with evaluation of the short DSIL. Evaluation of the *tuber coxae* is performed by following the ilial wing from medial to lateral until the transducer is located directly over the tuber coxae or by placing the transducer directly on the point of the hip. The *tuber coxae* is located close to the skin surface and requires a shallow scanning depth of 4–6 cm. The normal *tuber coxae* has a relatively smooth cortical surface, although some surface irregularities are within normal limits (Figure 10.18). Comparison to the contralateral side can be used in horses that are suspicious for fracture. Evaluation of the musculature ventral to the *tuber coxae* is important, as fracture fragments are typically displaced ventrally due to distraction by muscle attachments. Lastly, evaluation of the *tuber ischii* is performed by placing the transducer in the region of its palpable bony prominence approximately 20–30 cm ventral to the base of the tail. Compared to the *tuber sacrale* and *tuber coxae*, the *tuber ischii* requires an increased scanning depth of 6–12 cm. The normal *tuber ischii* has a smooth sloping appearance (Figure 10.19). Multiple large vessels are located in this region and are often visualized while scanning the *tuber ischii*. Similar to *tuber coxae* fractures, *tuber ischii* fractures are often readily apparent due to ventral distraction of fracture fragments by the *semimembranosus* and *semitendinosis* muscles. Similar to the *tuber sacrale* described earlier in this chapter, care should be taken when evaluating pelvic tuberosities in foals and juvenile horses due to their cartilaginous centers of ossification. As ossification progresses, hyperechoic areas of ossification will become visible within the cartilage and these should not be mistaken for fracture. Contralateral comparison can be useful in suspect cases.

Although not part of the pelvis, evaluation of the third trochanter of the femur should also be performed [21]. Horses with third trochanter fractures often have a similar history and clinical findings as horses with pelvic injury [22]. The third trochanter is located on the caudolateral aspect of the proximal third of the femur and can be evaluated with both transverse and longitudinal views. Transducer orientation and its normal ultrasonographic appearance are shown in Figure 10.20. Evaluation is straightforward and fractures are easily recognizable in many cases. The third trochanter is the primary attachment site for the superficial gluteal muscle, which often

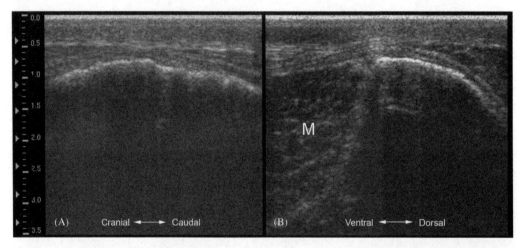

Figure 10.18 Ultrasonograms of the *tuber coxae*. (A) A normal transverse ultrasonogram and (B) a normal longitudinal ultrasonogram. The *tuber coxae* shows a smooth to variably irregular bony surface and ventral muscle attachments (M). Note the close proximity of the tuber coxae to the skin surface (within 1–2 cm). Image obtained with 10 MHz linear transducer, scanning depth = 3.5 cm.

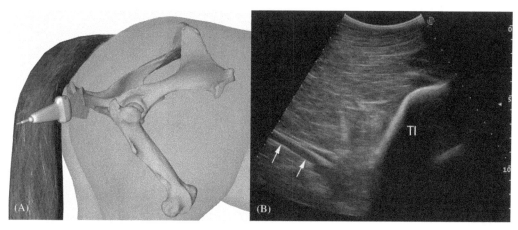

Figure 10.19 The ultrasonographic examination of the *tuber ischii* (*TI*). (A) Transducer placement to obtain a longitudinal view of the *tuber ischii* and its ventral muscle attachments. (B) A normal ultrasonogram to show the appearance of the *tuber ischii*. The *tuber ischii* is seen to have a sloping bony contour and normal ventral muscle attachments. Multiple blood vessels (arrows) are often visible during evaluation of the *tuber ischii*. These are at risk for laceration and hemorrhage in horses with TI fractures. Image obtained with 3.5 MHz curvilinear transducer, scanning depth = 13 cm. (*For a colour version of this figure, see the colour plate section.*)

causes cranial displacement of fracture fragments.

Transrectal Examination

Either a standard rectal transducer or a mid-range frequency microconvex transducer can be used. All pelvic bony surfaces are located in close proximity to the rectal mucosa. A shallow scanning depth of 4–8 cm and a musculoskeletal or small parts program should be used. The bony surface of the ischium is readily evaluated by directing the transducer ventrally upon entry into the rectum and then sweeping from left to right. The ischium should be smooth, although mild roughening and occasionally a slight gap will be seen along its midline symphysis (Figure 10.21A and B).

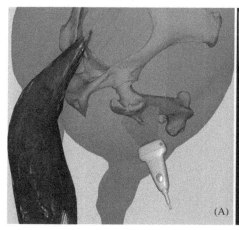
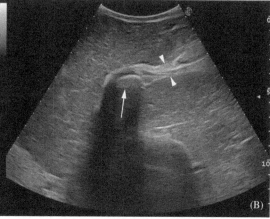

Figure 10.20 The ultrasonographic examination of the third trochanter of the femur. (A) Transducer placement to obtain a transverse ultrasonogram of the third trochanter. (B) A normal transverse ultrasonogram of the third trochanter (arrow) showing its superficial location relative to the body of the femur. The tendinous attachment of the superficial gluteal muscle is also visible (arrowheads). (C) Transducer placement to obtain a longitudinal view of the third trochanter of the femur. (D) A normal longitudinal ultrasonogram of the third trochanter (arrow) showing its slightly convex surface. (*For a colour version of this figure, see the colour plate section.*)

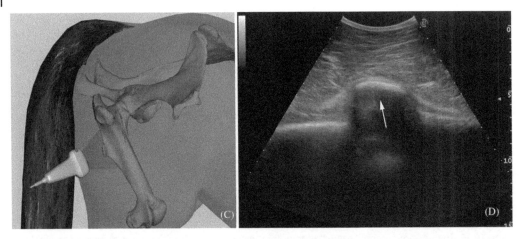

Figure 10.20 (*Continued*)

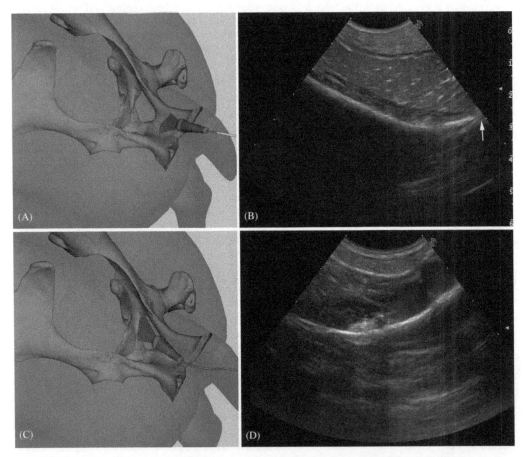

Figure 10.21 The transrectal ultrasonographic examination of the ischium and pubis. (A) Transducer placement to evaluate the ischium using a microconvex transducer. (B) A transrectal ultrasonogram showing the smooth bony surface of the left ischium (lateral is to the left). The gap created by the pubic symphysis should not be mistaken for fracture (arrow). (C) Transducer placement to obtain a longitudinal view of the pubis using a microconvex transducer. (D) A transrectal ultrasonogram to show the smooth sloping bony surface of the right pubis (lateral is to the right). Ultrasonographic images obtained with 8.5 MHz microconvex transducer, scanning depth = 5–6 cm. (*For a colour version of this figure, see the colour plate section.*)

To visualize the pubis, the transducer is moved further into the rectum, past the obturator foramen until the concave bony surface of the pubis is seen (Figure 10.21C and D). The transducer should again be swept from left to right to visualize the entire extent of the pubis, although in many horses each side must be evaluated independently by retracting the transducer until the ipsilateral ischium is found before again moving cranially over the ipsilateral obturator foramen to the ipsilateral pubis. The axial surfaces of the acetabulum and ilial body can also be seen with transrectal ultrasound and should demonstrate a smooth bony surface. Evaluation of these regions is most easily accomplished with a rectal transducer.

References

1 Getty, R. *Sisson and Grossman's The Anatomy of Domestic Animals*, 5th edn. Philadelphia, PA: W.B. Saunders, 1975.

2 Denoix, J.M. Ligament injuries of the axial skeleton in the horse: Supraspinal and sacroiliac desmopathies. In: Rantanen, N.W. (ed.), *Dubai International Equine Symposium*, 1996, pp. 273–286.

3 Henson, F.M., Lamas, L., Knezevic, S. and Jeffcott, L.B. Ultrasonographic evaluation of the supraspinous ligament in a series of ridden and unridden horses and horses with unrelated back pathology. *BMC Veterinary Research*, 2006.

4 Genovese, R.L., Rantanen, N.W., Simpson, B.S. and Simpson, D.M. Clinical experience with quantitative analysis of superficial digital flexor tendon injuries in Thoroughbred and Standardbred racehorses. *Veterinary Clinics of North America: Equine Practice* 1990; **6**:129–145.

5 Haussler, K.K., Stover, S.M. and Willits, N.H. Developmental variation in lumbosacropelvic anatomy of Thoroughbred racehorses. *American Journal of Veterinary Research* 1997; **58**:1083–1087.

6 Denoix, J.M. Lesions of the vertebral column in poor performance horses. In: *World Equine Veterinary Association Symposium*, Paris, 1999.

7 Denoix, J.M. Ultrasonographic evaluation of back lesions. In: Haussler, K.K. (ed.), *Veterinary Clinics of North America: Equine Practice*. Philadelphia, PA: Saunders, 1999, pp. 131–139.

8 Denoix, J.M. Apport des injections echoguidees pour les treatment locaux et intra-articulaires. In: *French Equine Veterinary Association*, Angers, 1995.

9 Vandeweerd, J.M. et al. Innervation and nerve injections of the lumbar spine of the horse: A cadaveric study. *Equine Veterinary Journal* 2007; **39**:59–63.

10 Tomlinson, J.E., Sage, A.M. and Turner, T.A. Ultrasonographic abnormalities detected in the sacroiliac area in twenty cases of upper hindlimb lameness. *Equine Veterinary Journal* 2003; **35**:48–54.

11 Nagy, A., Dyson, S. and Barr, A. Ultrasonographic findings in the lumbosacral joint of 43 horses with no clinical signs of back pain or hindlimb lameness. *Veterinary Radiology and Ultrasound* 2010; **51**(5):533–539.

12 Almanza, A. and Whitcomb, M.B. Ultrasonographic diagnosis of pelvic fractures in 28 horses. In: Proceedings of the American Association of Equine Practitioners, 2003.

13 Shepherd, M.C. and Pilsworth, R.C. The use of ultrasound in the diagnosis of pelvic fractures. *Equine Veterinary Education* 1994; **6**:23–27.

14 Brenner, S. and Whitcomb, M.B. Ultrasonographic diagnosis of coxofemoral subluxation in horses. *Veterinary Radiology and Ultrasound* 2009; **50**(4):423–428.

15 Geburek, F., Rötting, A.K. and Stadler, P.M. Comparison of the diagnostic value of ultrasonography and standing radiography

for pelvic-femoral disorders in horses. *Veterinary Surgery* 2009; **38**(3):310–307.

16 Tomlinson, J.E., Sage, A.M. and Turner, T.A. Ultrasonographic examination of the normal and diseased equine pelvis. In: Annual Convention of American Association of Equine Practitioners, 2000.

17 Tomlinson, J.E., Sage, A.M., Turner, T.A. and Feeney, D.A. Detailed ultrasonographic mapping of the pelvis in clinically normal horses and ponies. *American Journal of Veterinary Research* 2001; **62**,1768–1775.

18 Goodrich, L.R., Werpy, N.M. and Armentrout, A. How to ultrasound the normal pelvis for aiding diagnosis of pelvic fractures using rectal and transcutaneous ultrasound examination. In: Annual Convention of the American Association of Equine Practitioners, 2006.

19 Whitcomb, M.B. and Vaughan, B. Ultrasonographic evaluation of the coxofemoral joint. In: Proceedings of the American Association of Equine Practitioners 2015; 61:346–354.

20 Rottensteiner, U., Palm, F. and Kofler, J. Ultrasonographic evaluation of the coxofemoral joint region in young foals. *Veterinary Journal* 2012; **191**(2): 193–198.

21 Shields, G.E., Whitcomb, M.B., Vaughan, B. and Wisner, E.R. Abnormal imaging findings of the femoral third trochanter in 20 horses. *Veterinary Radiology and Ultrasound* 2015; **56**:466–473.

22 Bertoni, L., Seignour, M., de Mira, M.C. et al. Fractures of the third trochanter in horses: 8 cases (2000–2012). *Journal of the American Veterinary Medical Association* 2013; **243**:261–266.

11

Thermography

Tracy Turner

Introduction

Back problems are considered a major cause of altered gait or performance in horses. Unfortunately the characterization, localization and identification of the painful area can be problematic. The incidence of back problems in general practice has been reported as 0.9% [1] and has been estimated as 2.2% of lameness cases [2]. The equine back covers a large area, it includes the axial skeleton from the withers to the sacroiliac joint and sacrum and it is covered with thick muscles and fascial tissues and the numerous ligaments. It is the complex nature of this large structure that makes diagnosis so difficult. Clinical signs are highly variable and imaging, using radiography, requires special equipment. Specific treatment for back pain can only be performed after identification of the site of pain and nature of the injury. It is these problems that make thermography a valuable tool in the identification of back problems. The objectives of clinical examination of the horse's back are to determine if back pain is present, the site or sites of pain, and the potential lesions for the pain. A number of confusing factors can make the diagnosis more difficult, specifically the effect of tack (saddles) and rider on the horse. Thermography aids each of these areas [3]. However, before any clinical discussion can be made an understanding of the instrumentation and how it works and the principles of use and the physiology studied must be reviewed.

Instrumentation

Thermographic instrumentation, in the past, has been divided into contacting and non-contacting.

- Contacting thermography
  - Contacting thermography utilizes liquid crystals in a deformable base [4,5]. The crystals change shape according to the temperature that contacts them, and as they do they reflect a different colour of light. Therefore, the colour of a crystal represents a specific temperature. In order to use this technology for medical purposes, the liquid crystals are embedded into a flexible and durable latex sheet. This method has fallen out of favour because of numerous inherent problems in applying the technology. Because of this, non-contacting thermography is the method of choice.
- Non-contacting thermography
  - Two different technologies exist, cooled and uncooled. Cooled technology utilizes a detector of infrared radiation to measure temperature [6–8]. In addition, a series of focusing and scanning mirrors are used to systematically measure an entire field of view. The camera/detector is usually coupled to a cathode-ray tube and the intensity of the detected radiation is converted to an electrical signal. This signal is displayed on the cathode-ray tube as a black and white (grey scale)

Equine Neck and Back Pathology: Diagnosis and Treatment, Second Edition. Edited by Frances M.D. Henson.
© 2018 John Wiley & Sons, Ltd. Published 2018 by John Wiley & Sons, Ltd.

image of the object. The radiation intensity is directly proportional to the grey scale. Through the use of microchips, the black and white image can be made into a coloured image of the thermal picture (thermogram) – hence a classic thermogram. Because of the heat generated by the camera the detector must be cooled to prevent interference from the machine heat. The complexity of the camera and the need to connect the camera to a computer makes this technology inconveniently portable.

The other technology available is uncooled technology. This technology employs a type of focal plane array that, simply put, means that the infrared radiation is focused and measured on a series of detectors. These cameras have no moving parts and are contained in instruments the size of a hand-held flashlight.

There are several factors to consider before purchasing a thermographic camera. Among the most important factors is the spectral range. For medical use, the range of 8 to 14 µm is ideal because this is the peak emissivity of skin. From a practical standpoint, there is also less environmental artefact at this range. The author prefers real-time thermography versus still thermography because real-time eliminates any problems with motion, real-time also makes thermographic assessment more dynamic in that the operator can immediately observe change and real-time allows for faster imaging. Sensitivity refers to the amount of temperature difference that can be detected. Cooled units can differentiate within 0.01 °C whereas most uncooled units can differentiate 0.08 °C; although cooled is more sensitive, it is not applicable to veterinary thermography where 0.3 °C is as sensitive as we need.

The final factor is portability and durability. In equine medicine, an instrument needs to withstand the rigors of daily use and it must be easy to carry. Relative to cooled units portability usually means increased cost. Also,

because of the detectors these units are usually more fragile. Uncooled cameras, utilizing the focal array technology, are very portable and durable because of no moving parts.

Principles of Use

Heat is perpetually generated by the body and is dissipated through the skin by radiation, convection, conduction or evaporation [8]. Because of this, skin temperature is generally 5 °C (9 °F) cooler than body core temperature (37 °C). Skin derives its heat from the local circulation and tissue metabolism [9]. Tissue metabolism is generally constant; therefore variation in skin temperature is usually due to changes in local tissue perfusion. Normally, veins are warmer than arteries because they are draining metabolically active areas. Superficial veins will heat the skin more than superficial arteries and venous drainage from tissues or organs with a high metabolic rate will be warmer than venous drainage from normal tissues.

The circulatory pattern and the relative blood flow dictate the thermal pattern, which is the basis for thermographic interpretation [8]. The normal thermal pattern of any area can be predicted on the basis of its vascularity and surface contour. Skin overlying muscle is also subject to a temperature increase during muscle activity. Based on these findings, some generalizations can be made regarding the thermal patterns of a horse: the midline will generally be warmer [6,8], which includes the back, the chest, between the rear legs and along the ventral midline. Heat over the legs tends to follow the routes of the major vessels, with the cephalic vein in front and the saphenous vein in the rear.

The thermal pattern of the back is warmest down the midline from withers to tail. There is a corresponding warm area from tuber coxae to tuber coxae. There will be isothermic bands of decreasing temperature on either side of the midline. In the lumbar area the isothermic bands are colder than they are over the thoracic area. The croup has a 'T'pattern with a warm isothermic band from across the tuber coxae and down the midline. The areas over the gluteal are isothermic cold zones.

Injured or diseased tissues will invariably have an altered circulation [8]. One of the cardinal signs of inflammation is heat, which is due to increased circulation. Thermographically, the 'hot spot' associated with the localized inflammation will generally be seen in the skin directly overlying the injury [4,10]. However, diseased tissues may in fact have a reduced blood supply either due to swelling, thrombosis of vessels, or infarction of tissues [5,11,12]. With such lesions the area of decreased heat is usually surrounded by increased thermal emissions, probably due to shunting of blood.

Use in Veterinary Medicine

In order to produce reliable thermographic images the following factors need to be controlled: motion, extraneous radiant energy, ambient temperature and artefacts.

- Motion
  - Motion can be controlled by immobilizing the horse in stocks or using a qualified handler. The use of real-time thermography decreases the need for complete immobilization. Chemical restraining agents to keep the horse from moving should be avoided because these drugs affect the peripheral circulation and cardiovascular systems, which could cause false thermal patterns to be produced; however, the author has not encountered this.
- Extraneous radiant energy
  - To reduce the effects of extraneous radiant energy, thermography should be performed under cover shielded from the sun [8]. Preferably, thermography should be done in darkness or low-level lighting. Ideally, the ambient temperature should be in the range of 20 °C (68 °F), but any temperature as long as

the horse is not sweating is acceptable. Heat loss from sweating does not occur below 30 °C (86 °F), as radiation and convection are responsible for heat loss below that temperature. Very cold environmental temperatures may cause vasoconstriction of the lower legs and interfere with imaging. In these cases, low-level exercise to stimulate vasodilatation is necessary. The thermographic area ideally should have a steady, uniform airflow so that erroneous cooling does not occur. Practically, the horse should be kept from drafts. Likewise, the horse should be allowed time to acclimate to the environment or room where thermography is performed. Typically, 10–15 minutes is adequate when going from a warm temperature to a cool one. However, up to 2 hours may be necessary when going from a cool environment to a warm one. In these cases, the acclimation can be sped up with low-level exercise.

- Artefacts
  - Artefacts are extraneous sources on the skin that can cause irregular images. Among these are debris, scar tissue, hair length, liniments, leg wraps, blankets and other equipment [8]. To avoid artefacts, make sure all subjects are groomed and free of leg wraps, blankets or sheets for two hours whenever possible. Hair insulates the leg and blocks the emission of infrared radiation. However, as long as the hair is short and of uniform length, the thermal image produced is accurate. The skin should always be evaluated for changes in hair length that may cause false 'hot spots' in the thermogram.

Multiple thermographic images of a suspect area should be made [13,14]. The area in question should be evaluated from at least two directions approximately 90° apart, to determine if a 'hot spot' is consistently present. The horse's extremities should be examined from 4 directions (circumferentially) [8]. Significant areas of inflammation will appear over the same spot on each replicate thermogram.

These facts have been reiterated in Guidelines for Veterinary Infrared Thermography prepared by The American Academy of Thermology (aatthermology.org). In addition, the Guidelines recommend the infrared camera should have a minimal detector resolution of at least 320 by 240 pixels.

There are at least three ways in which thermography can be utilized in equine veterinary practice [11]:

- **A diagnostic tool**
  - In these cases, thermography is a physiologic imaging method where a 1 °C difference between two anatomically symmetrical regions indicates that a region of inflammation and a decrease in temperature is as important as an increase in temperature. The image will identify an area of interest to pursue with an anatomic imaging method such as ultrasonography and/or radiography. The author finds that temperature differences as little as 0.3 °C are significant.
- **To enhance the physical examination**
  - In this case, thermography is used to identify changes in heat and therefore locate 'areas of suspicion'. Thermographic cameras are easily 10 times more sensitive that the hand in determining temperature differences. This method simply helps identify asymmetry and then the practitioner must utilize the information to determine the actual cause and significance of the temperature difference.
- **In a wellness program**
  - In this method, horses in training are followed on a routine basis, once weekly. Thermographic changes will occur 2 weeks prior to clinical changes. In these cases, thermography can be used to identify subclinical problems and then training alterations can be made so that injury may be avoided altogether.

Clinical Thermography

Thermography has been used to identify 6 different back injuries, over-riding dorsal spinous processes (ORDSPs, kissing spines), dorsal spinous ligament injuries, muscle pain, withers injuries, sacroiliac problems and saddle fit problems [2]. In order to obtain a readable thermogram of the back, one must get high enough behind the horse to get a full view of the back. To be 90° to the back is ideal but not always possible, but less than 60° is not high enough to produce a good thermogram of the back. An alternative is to stand the horse under a reflective mirror and capture the back image through the horse's reflection.

The author uses 2 different thermal images to assess the back, one a thoracolumbar view and the second a croup view (Figure 11.1). The thoracolumbar view shows the withers and the sacrum and is especially good for looking at the mid back. The croup view is best for evaluating the sacroiliac region. The thermal pattern is the most important aspect of assessing the thermogram of the back. It must be remembered that thermography establishes the location of a possible problem; it does not characterize the lesion. However, we will show that there are certain patterns that have been seen consistently with particular back problems.

The normal back pattern is: the warmest areas are down the midline, cooling slightly in the lumbar region and then a warm cross from *tuber coxae* to *tuber coxae* and over the *tuber sacrale*, then same warmth down the middle of the croup (Figure 11.2). The warm area has symmetric isothermic bands on either side. Any variation of this pattern is either due to an artefact (thin hair, rubbed area) or pathologic process. If the lesion occurs along the midline of the thoracolumbar area, radiographs of the thoracolumbar spine is indicated. If the lesion occurs off the midline or in the croup region, we usually image the area with ultrasonography.

ORDSPs has been associated with any one of three different thermal patterns [15].

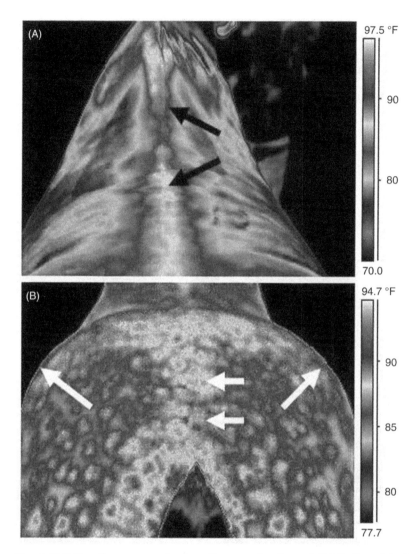

Figure 11.1 Two thermograms to show the normal pattern of distribution of body surface temperature. (A) Thermogram of the thoracolumbar region of the back of a normal horse; the midline is the warmest area (yellow stripe) (black arrows). (B) Thermogram of the lumbosacral and gluteal region of the back of a normal horse; the warmest area (yellow) is along the midline and from tuber coxae to tuber coxae (white arrows). (*For a colour version of this figure, see the colour plate section.*)

- Pattern 1: horses showed a 'hot streak' perpendicular to the thoracic spine (Figure 11.2A).
- Pattern 2: horses showed a 'cold streak' perpendicular to the thoracic spine (Figure 11.2B).
- Pattern 3 (the most common): horses showed a combination 'hot spot'–'cold streak' pattern over the back (Figure 11.2C).

Our practice has evaluated 95 cases of ORDSPs over 3 years. In these cases the sensitivity of thermography for the over-riding spinous process was 99%; however, the specificity was only 75%. This results in a positive predictive value of 94%. Compared to the positive predictive value of palpable pain in the thoracolumbar area for kissing spines, which is 74%, thermography performs well.

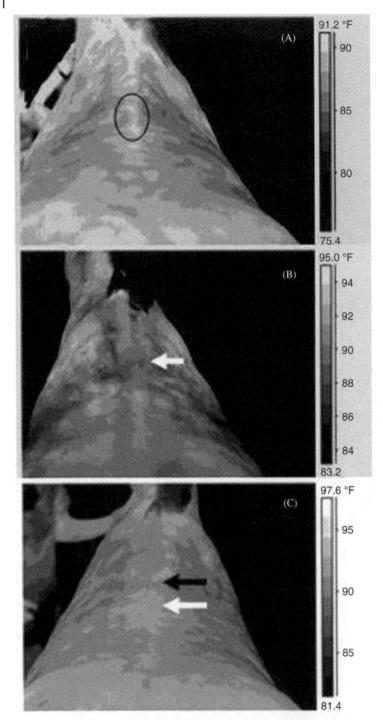

Figure 11.2 Three thermograms to show the pattern of distribution of body surface temperature in horses with over-riding dorsal spinous processes. (A) A horse with over-riding dorsal spinous processes showing the 'hot spot' (circle). (B) A horse with over-riding dorsal spinous processes showing the 'cold streak' (white arrow). (C) A horse with over-riding dorsal spinous processes showing the "hot" (black arrow)–"cold" (white arrow) pattern.

In contrast, injuries to the supraspinous ligament or dorsal sacroiliac ligament injuries have not presented with this type of identifiable pattern [2]. Thermography changes associated with these injuries have been abnormal thoracolumbar thermal images. The specific changes may be increased heat, decreased heat or simply an abnormal back thermogram. Following the identification of an abnormal thermogram, ultrasonography is used to identify the lesion (Chapter 13).

Muscle injuries of the thoracolumbar region likewise do not have characteristic thermograms [2]. Typically, however, the thermal patterns will show either 'hot spots' or 'cold spots' off the midline (Figure 11.3). It is in these regions that we have concentrated on ultrasonography to determine if muscle lesions can be seen. Withers injuries have all shown "hot spots" in the area of the withers but nothing more characteristic than that. The croup muscles will show some specific changes [12].

Sacroiliac region thermography has shown several different patterns [2]. The most common pattern is a cold area centred over the region of the *tuber sacrale* (Figure 11.4). This finding of cold is hypothesized to be due to lack of normal movement in the sacroiliac region. This lack of movement can be either due to primary pathology or secondary to other causes of the horse not moving normally through the pelvic region. This has been corroborated by our clinical findings as well. Specifically, we find only about half the horses exhibiting this thermal pattern actually show pain in the sacroiliac area. In addition, sonographic evaluation reveals pathology in only

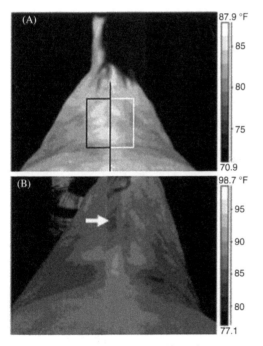

Figure 11.3 Two thermograms to show the pattern of distribution of body surface temperature in horses with suspected muscle pathology. (A) A horse with increased heat over muscle. The black line signifies midline, black box is the region of 'heat' on the left side and the white box is the corresponding "cooler" area on the right. (B) A horse with a 'cold area' over the epaxial muscle just left of the midline (white arrow).

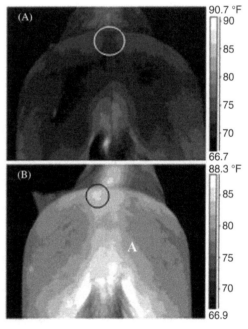

Figure 11.4 Two thermograms to show the pattern of distribution of body surface temperature in horses with suspected sacroiliac pathology. (A) A horse showing the 'cold spot' (white circle) over the tuber sacrale, indicating possible sacroiliac disease. (B) A horse showing the 'hot spot' (black circle) over the left tuber sacrale, indicating possible sacroiliac disease.

about half the cases and this pathology usually looks chronic in nature.

We have seen either thinning of the cross-sectional diameter of the dorsal sacroiliac ligaments or in a few cases thickening of the ligaments. In these cases with the cold area, generally, if there is pain in the area, we will ultrasonographically examine the sacroiliac region. On the other hand, if there is no pain or the horse moves normally through the pelvis we look for other causes for loss of back mobility. Pathology is seen much more commonly if the area over the *tuber sacrale* is hot or there is a hot spot centred over one tuber sacrale or the other (Figure 11.4). The pathology varies from hypoechoic areas within the dorsal sacral ligaments to generalized oedema in the region. This thermographic pattern is almost always associated with either pain or marked stiffness in the sacroiliac region.

Saddle fit thermography is very interesting and requires multiple examinations [3]. Thermography is an imaging modality that offers objective insight into saddle fit but has multiple other veterinary applications. In evaluating the dynamic interaction between the saddle and the horse's back, thermography will show not only the heat generated in contact areas on the saddle (Figure 11.5) but also the physiologic effects of the saddle on the horse's back (Figure 11.5). A consistent technique provides the most useful information. Our protocol is to perform a baseline thermographic examination of the horse's back. Then the horse is saddled over a simple cotton pad with the girth as tight as it would be for riding. Then the horse is lunged for at least 20 minutes. The horse should be exercised at its normal gaits (walk, trot, canter), paying attention to divide the lunging time equally in both directions. The saddle is then removed and the panels of the saddle are assessed thermographically. The most important criterion is thermal symmetry. After the saddle, the back is reassessed. Again thermal symmetry is important. Most commonly because of the heat generated by the saddle, the horse's midline is now colder than the other structures under the saddle. In addition, the

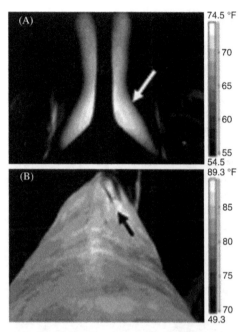

Figure 11.5 Two thermograms to show the pattern of distribution of body surface temperature in horses associated with the saddle. (A) A thermogram of the panels of a saddle; the right side of the saddle shows more heat (white arrow). (B) A thermogram of the horse where the saddle had been. The black arrow shows increased heat, correlating with the same region as the saddle in (A).

examiner is looking for focal hot spots, particularly along the spine, or hot or cold spots over the musculature. These abnormalities indicate problems caused by the saddle. The assessment is then repeated after a similar exercise session with the rider mounted. This evaluation allows consideration of the effect of the rider on the horse's back.

Conclusions

As our technological capabilities for equine practice increase and improvements are made in imaging the biologic organism, our ability to make accurate diagnoses continues to improve. It is important to understand that no imaging techniques can replace or be used in lieu of the physical examination. Rather, all imaging techniques only enhance the database established by the physical examination, and each imaging modality offers unique specific information. Similarly, each imaging modality correspondingly has its own limitations.

Thermography is a physiologic imaging modality [11]. Thermography provides information about tissue physiology: specifically it gives insight into the circulation. Thermography provides information as to the location of injury or disease as well as viability of the tissue. However, it does not provide information as to the specific nature of the problem. This must be reserved for an anatomic imaging modality that identifies the structure of the tissues in question.

Radiography generally evaluates changes in bone. Identifications of these changes are used to determine injuries to bone. Unfortunately, excepting fractures, most radiographic changes in bone often take 10–14 days to become evident [11,16]. Further, many of the bone changes are often permanent, so it can be difficult to determine if a change, especially a chronic change, is the cause of pain and lameness.

Thermography essentially images inflammation, which usually implies pain [6,8]. In this respect, thermography can directly help to determine if a radiographic change is associated with inflammation, and therefore the possible cause of lameness.

Thermography and ultrasonography are complementary. Whereas thermography may be used to locate an injury, ultrasonography evaluates the injured structure's morphology and the size and shape of the injury. Ultrasonography can be used to follow the healing, but thermography evaluates 'when' the inflammatory process is resolved [5,11].

Thermography is a practical aid in the clinical evaluation of the equine patient. It is of particular help in the assessment of the horse's back. This modality specifically increases the accuracy of diagnosis. Thermography is an excellent adjunct to clinical examination, as well as being complementary to other imaging techniques such as radiology, ultrasonography and scintigraphy.

References

1 British Equine Veterinary Association Survey of equine disease. *Veterinary Record*, 1965; **77**:528–538.

2 Turner, T.A. Back problems in horses. In: *Proceedings of the Annual Convention of the American Association of Equine Practitioners*, New Orleans, 2003.

3 Turner, T.A. How to assess saddle fit in horses. In: *Annual Convention of the American Association of Equine Practitioners*, Denver, CO, 2004.

4 Hall, J. et al. Correlation between contact thermography and ultrasonography in the evaluation of experimentally-induced superficial flexor tendinitis. In: *Annual Meeting of the American Association of Equine Practitioners*, New Orleans, 1987.

5 Townsend, H.G.G. et al. Relationship between spinal biomechanics and pathological changes in the equine thoracolumbar spine. *Equine Veterinary Journal* 1986; **18**:107–112.

6 Purohit, R.C. and McCoy, M.D. Thermography in the diagnosis of inflammatory processes in the horse. *American Journal of Veterinary Research* 1980; **41**:1167–1174.

7 Purohit, R.C., McCoy, M.D. and Bergfeld, W.A. Thermographic diagnosis of Horner's syndrome in the horse. *American Journal of Veterinary Research* 1980; **41**:1180–1182.

8 Turner, T.A., Purohit, R.C. and Fessler, J.F. Thermography: A review in equine medicie. *Compendium of Continuing Education* 1986; **8**:855–861.

9 Love, T.J. Thermography as an indicator of blood perfusion. *Annals of the New York Academy of Sciences* 1980; **335**:429–437.

10 Bowman, K.F. et al. Thermographic evaluation of corticosteroids efficacy in amphotericin B induced arthritis in ponies. *American Journal of Veterinary Research* 1983; **44**:51–66.

11 Turner, T.A. Diagnostic thermography. In: Kraft, S.L. and Roberts, G.D. (eds), *Veterinary Clinics of North America: Equine Practice*. Philadelphia, PA: Saunders, 2001, pp. 95–114.

12 Turner, T.A. Hindlimb muscle strain as a cause of lameness in horses. *Proceedings of the Annual Meeting of the American Association of Equine Practitioners* 1989; **34**:281.

13 Weinstein, S.A. and Weinstein, G. A clinical comparison of cervical thermography with EMG, CT scanning, myelography and surgical procedures in 500 patients. *Proceedings of the Academy of Neuromuscular Thermography* 1985; **2**:44–47.

14 Weinstein, S.A. and Weinstein, G. A review of 500 patients with low back complaints; comparison of five clinically-accepted diagnostic modalities. *Proceedings of the Academy of Neuromuscular Thermography*, 1985; **2**:40–43.

15 Turner, T.A. Back soreness in horses. *Proceedings of the American Association of Equine Practitioners* 2003; **49**:71–74.

16 Stromberg, B. The use of thermography in equine orthopedics. *Journal of Veterinary Radiology* 1974; **15**:94–97.

12

Neck Pathology

Richard Hepburn

Introduction

The clinical presentation of cervical spinal pathology can be broadly split into neurological disease (spinal compression, intervertebral nerve compression) and neck pain (altered head–neck position or movement, cervical lameness).

Potential aetiologies include developmental malformation, degenerative disease, and infectious, neoplastic and traumatic diseases.

An understanding of cervical anatomy and the relationship between the vertebra and the spinal cord is vital to understanding cervical spinal ataxia. As discussed in Chapter 6, clinical examination of neck disease should include a complete neurological examination as subtle ataxia may be present continuously whereas mechanical pain is often intermittent and positional. Recently there has been an increasing appreciation of the importance of pathologic change to the cervical articular process joints, both as a cause of spinal compression and of mechanical neck pain. This pathology can occur in conjunction with vertebral malformation in young horses with spinal ataxia, or with instability and muscular pain in older horses; in both cases treatment can be very successful. Whilst diseases of the vertebral body, intercentral joint, nuchal ligament and soft tissues of the neck are less common, it is important that the clinician be able to identify their clinical signs and assess the relevance of the results of diagnostic imaging when making a diagnosis.

Functional Anatomy

As discussed in Chapter 1, the horse has 7 cervical vertebra (C1–C7) and 8 cervical spinal segments (C7–T1 being the 8th). The cranial two vertebrae have distinct appearances: the atlas (C1) has no body or articular process and cranially articulates with the occipital via paired atlanto-occipital joints. The axis (C2) is made up of the dens, head, body, dorsal spine and caudal epiphysis. It articulates with the atlas via paired atlanto-axial joints. The 3rd to 7th cervical vertebrae have a consistent appearance (Figures 12.1 and 12.2). C2–T1 articulate with one another via paired synovial articular process joints (APJs, also known as interneural joints) and the fibrocartilagenous intercentral articulation (Chapter 1). The APJs are oval in shape with multiple outpouches and are contiguous with the elastic ligamentum flavum that spans the dorsal half of the vertebral canal linking adjacent vertebral arches. The cervical intervertebral discs are composed entirely of fibrocartilage and are continuous with the dorsal longitudinal ligament that forms the ventral floor of the vertebral canal and joins the adjacent vertebral bodies. The intervertebral foramen represents the space between the articular process of the cranial vertebra and the vertebral body of the caudal vertebra. The vertebral canal is not round; rather it has a flat base and a peaked top [1]. There is individual variation in the space between the bony vertebral margin and the dura mater.

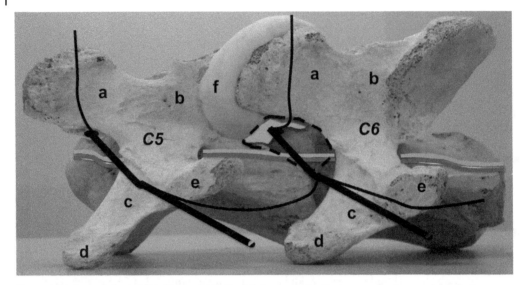

Figure 12.1 Lateral view of C5–C6, cranial to the left (a = cranial articular process, b = caudal articular process, c = transverse process, d = cranial tubercle, e = caudal tubercle, f = articular process joint in light grey. Black = segmental spinal nerves, dark grey = paravertebral blood vessels, light grey = paravertebral sympathetic nerve, black dotted line defines intervertebral foramen). (*For a colour version of this figure, see the colour plate section.*)

Each cervical segment of the equine spinal cord is relatively much longer than in small animals [2].

The vertebral arch and APJs oppose the dorsal and lateral funiculi of the white matter of the spinal cord, which contains ascending sensory proprioceptive neurons (spinocerebellar, spinocuneocerebellar tracts) and descending upper motor neurons (corticospinal, rubrospinal and reticulospinal tracts)

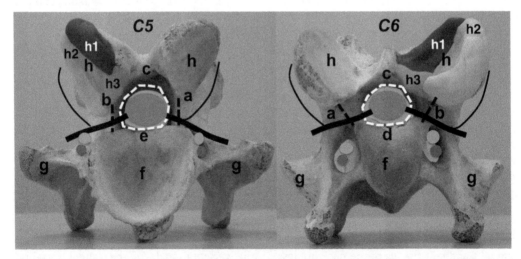

Figure 12.2 Cranial view of C5 (left) and caudal view of C6 (right) (a = right articular process, b = left articular process, c = vertebral arch, d = cranial epiphysis, e = caudal epiphysis, f = margins of intercentral joint, g = transverse process, h = articular surface of articular process joint, with h1/h2/h3/white denoting the joint outpouches, black solid line = segmental spinal nerves, grey = spinal cord, white dotted line = vertebral canal, black dotted line = intervertebral foramen, dark grey sphere = paravertebral blood vessels, light grey sphere = paravertebral sympathetic nerve). (*For a colour version of this figure, see the colour plate section.*)

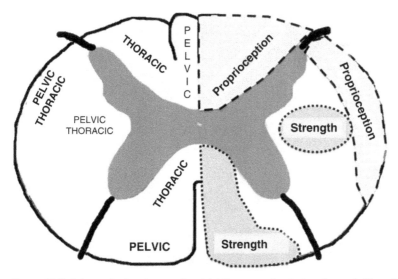

Figure 12.3 Schematic showing on the right the approximate locations of afferent sensory proprioceptive tracts and descending upper motor neuron tracts and on the left the location of tracts innervating either the pelvic or thoracic limb.

(Chapter 3) [3,4] (Figure 12.3). The cervical segmental nerves exit the intervertebral foramina and contain dorsal and ventral root nerve branches (Figures 12.1 and 12.2), which respectively contain sensory afferent somatic and proprioceptive neurons [4] and somatic efferent and visceral efferent lower motor neurons. The vertebral sympathetic nerve runs adjacent to the vertebral artery within the paravertebral foramina and provides local autonomic innervation [2]. The cutaneous trunci and coli reflexes have segmental sensory input via the dorsal root nerves; their motor pathways include ventral spinal nerves and the lateral thoracic nerve, which originates from the ventral branch of the segmental spinal nerves of C8–T1 [5].

The cervical vertebrae form an S-shape with a kyphotic shape cranially and a lordotic shape caudally (see Figure 9.2). The atlantooccipital joint allows flexion and extension and some lateral motion, and is responsible for 32% of the range of dorsoventral neck motion. The atlantoaxial joint enables the atlas and head to rotate extensively about the axis, accounting for 77% of this [6–8]. Adjacent cervical vertebrae articulate in all three planes, with the greatest lateral motion at C6–C7 and

the greatest dorsoventral motion at C3–C4. The cervicothoracic junction essentially acts as a hinge facilitating movement of the entire neck. Flexion of the neck leads to a functional reduction in vertebral canal size, predominantly affecting the dorso- and ventrolateral margins, and reduces intervertebral foramina dimensions.

The muscles of the neck have two roles (Figure 1.5 and 12.4):

1) *Provide dynamic segmental stability.* For example, the perivertebral muscles (*m. multifidus, m. longus colli*) span up to three vertebrae, directly inserting on to the articular and transverse processes.
2) *Provide antigravity support and neck motion.* The superficial muscles (*m. semispinalis, m. spinalis, m. splenius*) sit ventrally and laterally to the nuchal ligament and insert on to their dorsal and dorsolateral surfaces.

The nuchal ligament has two components (Figure 12.4): the bilobed funicular part that runs from the occiput to the dorsal spines of the whither and the lamellar part that runs from the ventral surface of the funicular

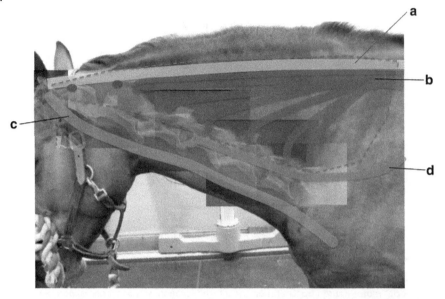

Figure 12.4 Relevant structures within the cervical region, overlayed with laterolateral radiographs of the cervical spine and caudal skull (a = nuchal ligament, funicular part, b = nuchal ligament, lamellar part, circles = nuchal bursae, c = brachiocephalicus muscle, d = spinalis muscle, area within dotted line = semispinalis and splenius muscles). (*For a colour version of this figure, see the colour plate section.*)

ligament to insert on the dorsal surface of C2 to T5. The atlantal bursa is interposed between the funicular nuchal ligament and the dorsal arch of the atlas, with a second bursa sometimes found in a similar position above C2.

Neck Pain

Mechanical neck pain describes an inability to display a normal range of neck motion and should be considered distinctly from spinal ataxia. The basic mechanisms causing primary neck pain in the horse, where the clinical presentation is variable and non-specific, are incompletely understood. Often the rider complains of neck stiffness, poor bending when working in a circle, or even violent throwing of the head, but these signs are not specific to neck pain [6]. In severe cases the horse may be unable to lower the neck to graze, necessitating a 'giraffe-like' stance.

Neck flexibility should be assessed from side to side and up and down. Many horses resist forced manipulation, and many ignore feed incentives, or merely move to get to them.

Positioning the opposite side of the trunk against a wall can help, with the incentive positioned initially at the elbow, then the mid thorax and finally the stifle [8]. The clinician needs to distinguish between the horse properly flexing the neck and inappropriate twisting of the head on the neck. As neck pain is often positional, observing for an altered neck carriage or stiffness whilst the horse moves in hand, on the lunge and when ridden can be helpful.

Cervical Neurological Disease

Most neurological disease related to the cervical vertebrae is compressive in nature, with cervical vertebral compressive myelopathy (CVCM) seen most commonly. Less common causes are vertebral fractures, cervical vertebral epidural haematomas, vertebral subluxation, neoplasia, osteomyelitis and discospondylitis. Direct contamination of the subdural/subarachnoid space is rare, with resultant physical damage to the spinal cord or stimulation of a local inflammatory response.

Neurological Consequences of Spinal Compression

Compression can lead to both functional and physical neuronal alteration [9]. Functional alteration represents clinically relevant transient changes in neuronal activity without histologic damage and could occur where compression is intermittent or is yet to reach the threshold at which rapid physical neuronal degeneration occurs [10]. Physical alteration is seen histologically as neuronal swelling and Wallerian degeneration [9], which is greatest at the site of compression but is also present in ascending white matter tracts cranial and descending tracts caudal to the compression site [10]. Initially the peripheral regions of the white matter are damaged (dorsal spinocerebellar tracts) and then gradually deeper layers (rostral spinocerebellar tracts) are involved (Figure 12.3). Neuroanatomically this explains why cervical spinal cord compression produces more severe hindlimb ataxia than forelimb [11].

Radiographic Considerations with Cervical Spinal Compression

As discussed in Chapter 7, in a horse with neurological deficits that localise to the cervical spine, the aim of radiography is to identify potential sites of spinal compression and to define the origin of that compression to an extent that either a treatment plan can be formulated or appropriate further diagnostics suggested. In the majority of cases the need is to distinguish compression due to either vertebral malformation or disease of the articular process joints, or both:

1) *Vertebral malformation.* This author recommends two stages to assessing the adequacy of the vertebral canal. The first step is to derive intravertebral minimum saggital ratios (MSRs) and apply a relevant significance cut-off: <0.52 for C2–C3 to C5–C6; <0.56 for C6–C7 [12]. These cut-offs have a sensitivity and specificity of 89% within a population of predominantly <4-year-old horses, and so should be interpreted with caution in older horses. Intervertebral MSRs are potentially useful, and a cut-off of <0.485 has been suggested [13]; however, this author cautions the use of this specific value as it was derived from a very small sample set. Instead the intervertebral MSR should be measured at all articulations, with the lowest value articulation being the one of interest. This author also recommends examining any articulations with an abnormal MSR for qualitative evidence of vertebral malformation: dorsal lamina extension, caudal epiphyseal flare, vertebral instability (Figure 12.5) [14].

Figure 12.5 Laterolateral plain radiograph of C2–C3 in an ataxic 18-month-old foal, showing a low minimum sagittal ratio, vertebral subluxation, caudal epiphyseal flare (dotted line) and dorsal laminar extension (dashed line).

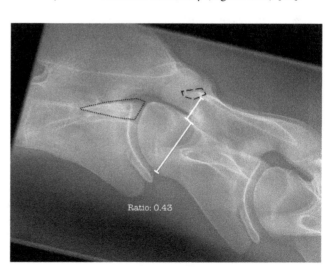

Ratio: 0.43

2) *Articular process joint disease.* High-quality laterolateral radiographs of the occipit to T1 should be obtained and images that show rotation should be repeated as this will artefactually reduce intervertebral foramina size and increase APJ size [15,16]. Arthropathy and irregular radiographic enlargement of the margins of the APJs should be assessed using a novel grading scheme [17]. Anecdotally APJ enlargement has been described as a normal variation in mature horses [6], but this has only been shown to occur at C5–C6 [17]. The nature of the association between clinical disease and radiographic grade at a particular articulation is currently unclear [13]. This diagnostic problem is compounded in areas where non-compressive disease such as equine protozoal myeloencephalitis is common. Preliminary analysis of the appearance of individual cervical articulations in 188 horses with spinal ataxia, in a region free of EPM, demonstrated a significantly increased incidence of ventral osteophytosis (Hepburn and Butler, unpublished data), suggesting that ventral osteophytosis could be a more useful radiographic predictor of neurologically significant APJ/LF disease. In this population C6–C7 was the most commonly implicated articulation. Oblique lateral views of the caudal cervical articulations (C5–T1) should be taken if arthropathy is found, and are particularly important in cases where there is asymmetry of the neurological deficits or where possible spinal outflow compression is suspected.

Clinical Conditions

Cervical Vertebral Compressive Myelopathy

Cervical vertebral compressive myelopathy (CVCM) [18,19] describes multilimb ataxia and paresis due to extradural spinal cord compression caused by any combination of vertebral malformation, disease of the APJs and ligamentum flavum, and vertebral instability. This condition has been reported from C2–3 to C7–T1 and is distinct from occipitoatlantoaxial malformation. The term CVCM has replaced the myriad of historic terms for cervical spinal compression, such as Wobbler syndrome or cervical stenosis. There are two main pathologic processes responsible for CVCM:

1) *Vertebral malformation.* In skeletally immature horses high soluble carbohydrate diets are associated with intermittent high serum insulin and low serum thyroxine levels, resulting in cartilage proliferation and retention without maturation. This proliferation causes cranioventral extension of the dorsal laminar of the cranial margin of the vertebral arch and caudodorsal flaring of the caudal epiphysis of the vertebral body. These changes increase repetitive loading strain of the ligamentum flavum dorsally and the dorsal longitudinal ligament ventrally, causing them to thicken, which in turn leads to vertebral instability and further osteochondral change. Retention of the cartilage matrix at the insertion site of the LF occurs in young horses with spinal ataxia, but not in controls [20].

2) *APJ and ligamentum flavum disease.* The histological degeneration of APJs and the ligamentum flavum is similar in both osteoarthritis and osteochondrosis [9,20–22]. In osteoarthritis moderate fraying and fibrillation of articular cartilage, villous proliferation of the synovial membrane, joint capsule hypertrophy and production of new bone at the articular margins occurs [20,21]. Lesions of osteochondrosis are more varied, with profound malformation and instability of the APJs, OC dissecans, subchondral bone cysts and extradural synovial cysts described [20,21,23]. In both aetiologies the LF becomes increasingly rigid due to hypertrophy, fibrovascular proliferation and thickening of the contiguous joint capsule, and sclerosis and enlargement of the

fibrocartilagenous attachment with the dorsal lamina. Haemorrhage within the LF and necrosis of marginal fat also occur. In older horses the most likely pathophysiology is articulation stress, particularly repeated flexion–extension and torsion [24], which may also worsen the osteochondrosis seen in younger horses.

Neurological examination of a CVCM case demonstrates deficits that neuroanatomically localize to the cervical spine: forelimb hypermetria and hindlimb spasticity that may be exaggerated during backing up and hill walking; forelimb pivoting and hindlimb circumduction during tight circling; and weakness and uncontrolled distal limb pronation during tail pulling whilst walking. Muscle atrophy, localised to the dorsal midline and rump, is variably present. The median grade of ataxia is 2/5 in the thoracic limb and 3/5 in the pelvic limb [25], with concurrent grade 2–3/5 pelvic limb lower motor neuron paresis. Neurological asymmetry is common, but this is often not associated with any specific pathologic asymmetry. Cutaneous colli hyperreflexia can be seen as an exaggerated skin-prick response over the neck base compared to the trunk; if conscious resentment is shown then hyperaesthesia is also present. Skin sensation changes are significantly associated with APJ osteophytosis, but also found more commonly in cases of acute onset [25,26]. Mechanical neck pain or stiffness is variably present – in this author's experience it is uncommon and inconsistent. The median duration of clinical signs prior to diagnosis is 28 days (range 1–730), with a history of tripping and stumbling, particularly downhill, and altered performance (unbalanced, refusing to jump, weak behind, 'clumsy') [26,27]. A single bout of shoulder/neck trauma may have occurred days to years previously.

Two broad types of CVCM are reported [18,19]:

1) *Type 1* describes a developmental disease where compression is predominantly caused by vertebral malformation. Soft tissue compression from osteochondrosis changes within the APJ and ligamentum flavum can also be present. It primarily affects young (3–18 months), well-fed rapidly growing horses. It has been reported in most light and draught breeds, and is most common in thoroughbreds, possibly warmbloods and in geldings. Typically cases present with acute onset ataxia, paresis and gait changes. Recent trauma may be associated with the onset of neurological signs, or the horse may have been mildly ataxic prior to the episode of trauma. In older young horses (2–4 years) progressive disease occurs over a period of weeks to months, before the gait abnormalities become obvious enough to warrant neurological examination. Owners often describe these horses as being 'a free mover' or 'late developers'.

2) *Type 2* refers to compression solely due to osteoarthritis of the APJ and ligamentum flavum, and predominantly occurs in older horses (8–25 years old at onset), geldings and warmbloods; with C5–C6 and C6–C7 most commonly identified [17,26]. Typically cases have chronic progressive onset of ataxia, paresis and gait change over 1 month.

This author believes that this two-type system has limitations as it does not focus on the cause of spinal compression, which is ultimately what will define treatment options. Instead this author recommends considering CVCM based upon the origin of the compression:

1) Young horses with vertebral canal malformation as the sole cause of compression.
2) Young horses with APJ disease as the sole cause of spinal compression.
3) Young horses with vertebral canal malformation and concurrent APJ disease.
4) Older horses with APJ/LF disease as the sole cause of spinal compression.

This derivation highlights the appreciation that spinal compression can occur *without* evidence of vertebral canal malformation [9,13,21,28], *i.e. it is possible for younger horses to have spinal compression solely due to APJ pathology*. This is vital to interpretation of cervical radiographs, as alteration in minimum saggital ratios will not occur with APJ compression alone. In this author's experience the differences between young horses with sole APJ pathology from those with concurrent vertebral canal malformation are: sole APJ disease tends to occur in older animals (3–6 years); it causes neurological gait deficits that are less severe and more similar in presentation to those seen in type 2 CVCM horses; muscle atrophy is less obvious; and the onset of disease is more insidious and less progressive than those with concurrent canal malformation.

Diagnosis of CVCM first requires suitable neurological deficits that localise to the cervical spinal cord, with or without signs of spinal segment nerve compression. If the horse is located in an area where equine protozoal myeloencephalitis is prevalent then appropriate diagnostic measures should be taken to exclude it: currently for *Sarcocystis neurona* the SnSAG2,4/3 ELISA serum:CSF ratio and for *Neospora hughesii* the NhSAG ELISA serum:CSF ratio (Martin Furr, personal communication, ACVIM Consensus update). The results of cervical radiography should then be considered in the light of the patient's signalment, history and presentation. *For instance: a 15-year-old successful competition horse with recent onset progressive multilimb ataxia in which cervical radiography demonstrates low minimum saggital ratios and enlarged APJs is more likely to have compression due to APJ disease (as this occurs more commonly in older horses) than the vertebral malformation suggested by low MSRs (this is a developmental condition)*. In order to make an effective diagnosis of CVCM this author recommends the use of specific decision criteria, with all diagnostic test results analysed in series and in parallel:

1) *Young horse with vertebral malformation as a sole cause of spinal compression*. The intravertebral MSR is below the articulation cut-off at 1 + articulation and qualitative evidence of vertebral malformation is found associated with these specific articulation(s). These cases are typically aged <18 months, although they can occur up to 4 years of age.

2) *Young horse with APJ disease as a sole cause of spinal compression*. Normal intravertenbral MSRs are found at all cervical articulations; there is no qualitative evidence of vertebral malformation. Abnormal APJ appearance at 1+ articulation; oblique lateral radiographs should be taken to assess for developmental APJ asymmetry.

3) *Young horse with vertebral malformation and APJ disease as potential causes of spinal compression*. The intravertebral MSR is below the articulation cut-off at 1+ articulation; qualitative evidence of vertebral malformation is found associated with these specific articulation(s). Abnormal APJ appearance at 1+ articulation; oblique lateral radiographs should be taken to assess for developmental APJ asymmetry. In this scenario it is not possible to define which pathology is responsible for the spinal compression; myelography under general anaesthesia is the next diagnostic step. These cases are typically aged 3–6 years.

4) *Older horses with APJ disease as sole cause of spinal compression*. Normal intravertenbral MSRs are found at all cervical articulations; there is no qualitative evidence of vertebral malformation. Abnormal APJ appearance at 1+ articulation; oblique lateral radiographs should be taken if there are asymmetric neurological deficits or cutaneous colli hyperaesthesia. If an abnormal MSR is found then its relevance should be discussed along with the potential for myelography.

Cervical myelography under general anaesthesia can be used to better describe the location and nature of spinal compression. Specific decision criteria should be used to identify compression during extension and flexion at individual articulations [29]. When concurrent APJ changes and a narrow MSR are found at a single articulation, it may be possible, though technically challenging, to assign relative significance to dorsoventral compression (from vertebral canal malformation) versus dorsolateral compression (from APJ pathology) by attempting oblique lateral projections. Scintigraphy of CVCM is of little value as clinically normal horses have increased radiopharmaceutical uptake in the APJs of C5–C7, reflecting the increased mobility of these joints and making scintigraphy relatively insensitive and non-specific [30]. Computed tomography (CT) has the potential to image the cervical spine in three dimensions in superior anatomical detail to plain radiography, as discussed in Chapter 9, but has significant patient handling and technical difficulties (Figures 12.6 and 12.7). CT myelography could be similarly useful but limitations to positioning will necessitate different decision criteria to those used in plain myelography. Anatomical considerations essentially make magnetic resonance imaging of the cervical spine impossible in live adult horses [9,31,32]. A large variation

in the outline of APJs, caused by the irregularity of the insertions of the epaxial muscles, is found on transcutaneous ultrasonography, making identification of osteophytosis or APJ enlargement difficult [33]. Electromyography has not been studied in cervical ataxia, but transcranial magnetic stimulation has shown significantly different evoked motor responses in cases of CVCM when compared to normal horses [34]. This could be a useful ancillary test to differentiate between mild ataxia and lameness. Thermography has no utility in CVCM.

Management of CVCM in young horses has two stages. In the immediate period following acute onset of neurological disease the aim is to reduce neuronal cell swelling and oedema formation. This author recommends the use of intravenous mannitol, DMSO, vitamin E and strict box rest. The next stage of therapy is to minimize further cyclical spinal cord compression, which can be achieved by medical or surgical means, depending on the age at presentation. In cases <12 months old with recent onset ataxia due to vertebral malformation a 'paced diet' program can be followed [35], which aims to alter vertebral growth patterns. Total daily dietary intake is

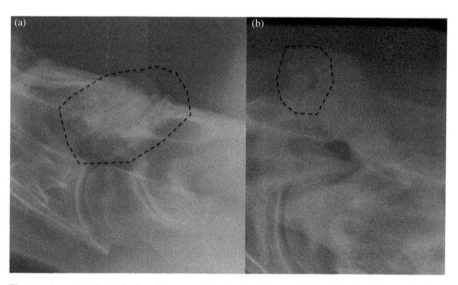

Figure 12.6 Laterolateral (a) and oblique lateral (b) radiographs of C6–C7 in a 5-year-old horse with CVCM due to articular process joint (APJ) osteochondrosis. Marginal osteophytes are seen dorsally in (a) and cranially in (b).

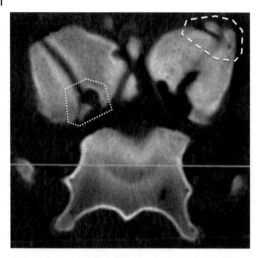

Figure 12.7 Bone window transverse section CT image of C6–C7 from the same horse showing marginal osteophytes and a bone cyst dorsally on the right articular process joint (APJ) (dashed line) and ventrallyon the left APJ (dotted line).

75% of 2% of body weight (readjusted monthly) and the diet is based upon high-quality roughage and fat. Vitamin E supplementation is also given. Strict box rest is required, and so this approach is not universally suitable. Neurological examination should be repeated monthly and cervical radiographs every 3 months. With professional supervision neurological resolution can occur over a 3–18 month period, although further study is required to better define efficacy.

Surgical treatment of type 1 CVCM (vertebral malformation as the sole cause of compression) involves vertebral interbody fusion, which is most appropriate in a young horse (1–2 years old) with recent onset grade 2/5 neurological deficits and myelographic confirmation of a single site of compression due to vertebral malformation alone at either C3–C4 or C4–C5. Approximately 60% of vertebral interbody fusion cases have a 2-grade neurological improvement over a 12-month period, with approximately 50% of cases returning to their prior function [36,37]. The complication rate is high and a significant number of cases are euthanased. There is also

concern about the future safety of riding a horse with a cervical implant and current recommendation is not to jump these horses.

When treating spinal compression associated with APJ osteoarthritis (type 2 CVCM) the response to NSAIDs and reduced exercise or rest is poor [6]. Instead intra-articular administration of corticosteroid under ultrasound guidance is recommended, although there is little published evidence of its efficacy. A study of 33 sport horses with spinal ataxia attributable to CVCM, in addition to 26 with other cervical diseases (neck pain, obscure lameness), reported that overall 32% returned to full function and 39% improved [38]. The overall effect was of variable duration (<1 month to 5 years). It is difficult to draw conclusions from this study as the number with ataxia was small, the diagnostic criteria were poorly defined, the response was owner assessed and the treatment was variable. Preliminary analysis of a larger population of horses aged >8 years with spinal ataxia, that fulfill this author's APJ/LF disease inclusion criteria has shown a >80% positive response rate (defined as all limbs neurological grade ≤1/5) (Hepburn, unpublished data). All horses received either triamcinolone acetonide (8 mg/joint, 16 mg maximum dose) or methyl-prednisolone acetate (40 mg/joint, 160 mg maximum dose), with follow-up neurological examination performed at 1, 4 and 12 months. Neurological resolution occurred over 1–4 months and lasted for 1–5 years. Repeated radiography of affected APJs >12 months after treatment did not show significant progression of the osteoarthritis. Application of the same approach to a smaller population of horses aged 4–8 years (young horses with sole APJ compression or those where a low MSR was excluded by normal myelography) has shown a >60% positive response rate, with a duration of response lasting between 1 and 8 years (Hepburn, unpublished data). The reduced response rate in younger horses with sole APJ/LF compression reflects the variety and increased severity of pathological changes that occurs in osteochondrosis.

Cervical APJ Injection Technique

The horse should be sedated and a $10\,cm^2$ area dorsal to the transverse process of the affected vertebra clipped and prepared aseptically. A microconvex or phased array probe (6–10 MHz, 6–10 cm depth) is ideal as the small footprint facilitates easy needle placement; the probe itself should be placed inside a sterile glove that has been filled with a small amount of acoustic gel. A standardised ultrasound image aids orientation – this author always positions the probe reference dorsal, with the screen reference to the right, and holds the probe in a transverse orientation. The probe is placed 6–8 cm dorsal to the palpable transverse process, angled 10–20 degrees downwards and slightly cranially, and then moved ventrally until the APJ margins are imaged as 2 crescent-shaped hyperechoic contours, which cast acoustic shadows, separated by the anechoic joint space (Figure 12.8). With the joint space in the middle of the screen, the depth of the joint should be noted (typically about 4–5 cm). The probe is then held in a fixed position and a 12.5 cm 18G spinal needle is inserted approximately 1 cm dorsal to the probe, with its long axis parallel to the long axis of the probe, at a downward angle so that the needle crosses the centre of the ultrasound image at the depth of the joint. The needle is then advanced towards and into the joint. If repositioning is required it can be confusing as the skin acts as a pivot: to move the tip of the needle dorsally, the hub should be moved ventrally and vice versa. This approach is accurate, with 89% injections being either intra-articular or intracapsular, with a further 9% within 1 mm of the APJ capsule [39]. Injection should be directly visualised as hyperechoic, sparkling within the joint space.

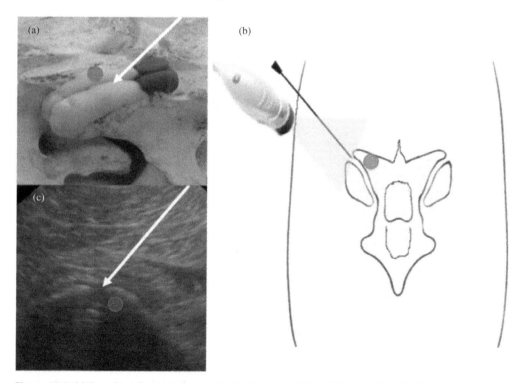

Figure 12.8 (a) Dorsolateral aspect of cervical articular process joint (APJ), cranial to left, showing the APJ pouches (white, light grey, dark grey). (b) Schematic diagram showing the position of ultrasound probe and spinal needle relative to the skin surface and vertebral cross-section. (c) Ultrasound image of the dorsolateral aspect of an APJ, dorsal to right, with a white arrow representing the needle approach. In all images the sphere signifies the caudal articular process of the cranial vertebral, which is located dorsally to the joint space. (*For a colour version of this figure, see the colour plate section.*)

Cervical APJ Osteoarthritis

Cervical APJ osteoarthritis can produce non-specific signs of mechanical neck pain such as an abnormal, often lowered head–neck carriage, stiffness and reduced voluntary lateroflexion during ridden exercise or during manipulation. A complete neurological examination should be performed, although in this author's experience most cases do not have concurrent deficits suggestive of spinal compression. Rarely forelimb lameness that does not abolish with local perineural or intrathecal anaesthesia may be present, often showing rotational abduction of the limb during the cranial stride phase. In a series of 129 cases of neck pain, over 60% had cervical APJ osteoarthritis, with C6–C7 most frequently affected and the majority of horses aged 6–15 years (Sells, personal communication). A syndrome of episodic, transient, marked neck pain, stiffness and lowered head carriage is also reported [6]. In between episodes these horses are often completely normal, although mild ataxia may be present. In this author's experience a history of bucking or running away and cutaneous hypereflexia may be reported. Radiographic enlargement of the caudal APJs is often found, which raises the possibility of cervical radiculopathy being present (Figure 12.9) [40]. In general mechanical pain due to cervical APJ OA should be treated identically to CVCM due to APJ OA. In this author's experience these cases can initially respond very favourably, but the duration of response is variable and can be short (2–3 months), particularly if APJ asymmetry is found on oblique lateral radiographs. A more positive effect can occur if regular physiotherapy of the neck muscles is performed.

Occipitoatlantoaxial Malformation

Occipitoatlantoaxial malformation (OAAM) is uncommon, with Arab foals up to 1 year most frequently diagnosed. Affected cases

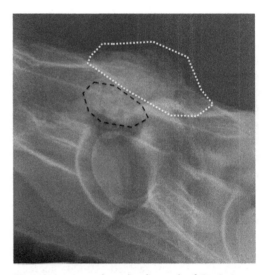

Figure 12.9 Laterolateral radiograph of C5–C6 in a horse with neck pain showing marked dorsal osteophytosis (white dotted line) and ventral irregularity (dashed black line) of the articular process joint.

can be still-born, be ataxic at birth or show progressive multilimb ataxia, paresis and altered head–neck carriage. Cutaneous cervical hypalgesia can also occur. A malformed atlas and axis can be palpated, sometimes with a clicking sound, with reduced mobility of the cranial neck, especially the atlanto-occipital joint. Occasional cases can present with just a stiff extended neck and normal neurologic function. Laterolateral radiographs of the skull base to C2–C3 are diagnostic, showing fusion of the occiput and atlas, hypoplasia of the dens and atlas, and varying subluxation and scoliosis. Four subtypes of OAAM are seen: (i) occipital bone-like modification of the atlas and atlas-like modification of the axis (Figure 12.10), (ii) two atlases, (iii) asymmetric atlantoaxial fusion, (iv) non-specific asymmetric malformation [41]. No therapy is indicated and the condition is fatal. As the disease is likely to be inheritable the same family lines should be avoided. Chronic, healed atlanto-occipital injury can radiographically resemble OAAM, but with a different signalment and presentation.

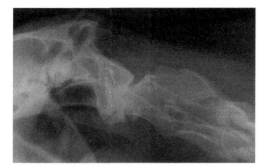

Figure 12.10 Plain laterolateral radiograph of the skull base and cranial cervical vertebra of a case occipitoatlanoaxial malformation showing an occipital bone-like modification of the atlas and atlas-like modification of the axis.

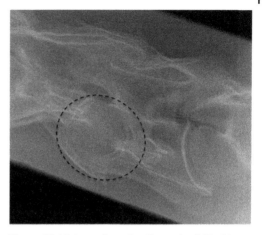

Figure 12.11 Laterolateral radiograph of C5–C6 showing complete ankylosis of the intercentral joint (dotted line) due to chronic discospondylitis in a 12-year-old horse with a history of chronic neck stiffness and low grade pain.

Discospondylitis

Discospondylitis is rare in the horse, the sites typically affected being C3–C4, C6–C7 and C7–T1 [42]. Clinically it is more likely to present as severe mechanical neck pain, reduced neck mobility or intermittent forelimb lameness. When spinal compression does occur the neurological deficits are non-specific. Diagnosis is typically made radiographically, where a loss of normal opacity of the cranial and caudal vertebral endplates, and alteration of the intercentral joint space is seen (Figure 12.11). Concurrent APJ enlargement can be found, reflecting instability across the articulation.

Cervical Vertebral Fractures

Cervical vertebral fractures are usually traumatic: rotational or headlong falls at speed, falling sideways on to the neck base or pulling back whilst tied up. In adults the vertebral body or arch of C3–C6 and the articular processes or APJs of C5–C7 are most commonly affected [22]. Vertebral body fractures may also involve the adjacent intervertebral disc and dorsal longitudinal ligament [6]. In foals, atlas and axis fractures are also common, typically through the separate ossification centre of the dens (odontoid peg). This can also

fracture in adults (Figure 12.12) [43]. In all cases clinical signs are immediate and include focal guarding pain, neck stiffness, abnormal neck position/inability to move the neck, muscle contracture and focal sweating; soft tissue swelling is not always present. Spinal ataxia is often not present, but when it is can be of variable severity and duration. Thoracic limb lameness may also be present, as can persistent pawing. Diagnosis is confirmed with lateral–lateral, oblique lateral or dorsoventral radiographs. In young horses it is important not to confuse physes and separate ossification centres with fragments. Acute treatment is identical to acute onset type 1 CVCM. Food and water should be offered from an elevated position, hay should be loose to limit excessive neck movement, and cross-tying is not recommended due to the risk of pulling back. Foals with midcervical fractures can be stabilised in a neck cast or with a neck cradle; this is contraindicated with fractures of C1–C2 or C6–C7 as it will encourage fracture movement. It is difficult to give an accurate prognosis, but most vertebral body and articular process fractures heal within 6–9 months, with a good prognosis for return to athletic function. Repeat neurological examination and radiography every 6 weeks

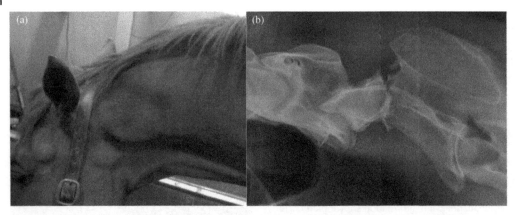

Figure 12.12 (a) A case of acute onset lowered head–neck carriage with an abnormal dorsal position of the dorsal process of C2 and guarding pain on palpation. (b) Laterolateral radiograph of C1–C2 showing a fracture of the dens and cranial body of C2 with dorsal displacement of the body of the axis and atlantoaxial subluxation.

is recommended. If ataxia persists or significant focal muscle atrophy develops, then the prognosis is poor; this is often associated with callus formation and resultant neuronal compression.

Cervical Vertebral Epidural Haematomas

Cervical vertebral epidural hematomas are most commonly associated with trauma originating from the ventral internal plexus, spinal branch of the vertebral artery or the intervertebral vein [44]. The hematoma typically occurs asymmetrically in the caudal cervical region and is confined within the vertebral canal between the dura mater and the ventral aspect of the articular process. Ataxia and paresis affecting all 4 limbs and potentially neck pain occur. Diagnosis is difficult as survey radiographs are usually normal, as is lumbosacral CSF analysis. Myelography or CT can demonstrate the site of compression, but not its cause. Presumptive diagnosis is by exclusion and relies on history, clinical signs and negative radiography. Treatment involves supportive care and recovery is typically prompt and complete unless callus formation occurs due to concurrent periosteal damage when the prognosis is guarded.

Vertebral Subluxation

Subluxation of C5–C6 or C6–C7 is an unusual cause of mild to moderate hindlimb ataxia, dysmetria and paresis in adults; in younger horses C3–C4 is the most common articulation [6,16]. Lateral–lateral radiographs typically show dorsal displacement of the head of C6 or C7 and subluxation of the associated intercentral joint; APJ enlargement and asymmetry is often found. Occasionally the subluxation occurs in a ventral direction. This condition carries a poor prognosis, although if the origin of the lesion is APJ OA, intra-articular corticosteroid medication could be beneficial, but the effect is often transient.

Vertebral Neoplasia

Vertebral lymphoma, melanoma, fibrosarcoma, myeloma and hemangiosarcoma have all been described at the level of the vertebral canal to cause spinal cord compression [45]. Cases are usually advanced when diagnosed, with neurological signs dependent upon location and degree of compression or vertebral weakness/instability. Associated soft tissue swelling or pain, or evidence of spinal outflow compression, may also be present. Depending upon the origin of the mass

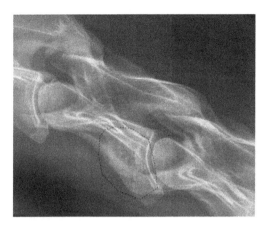

Figure 12.13 Laterolateral projection of C3-C4 showing an irregular appearance of the caudal epiphysis and ventral vertebral body of C3 due to multicentric lymphoma (dotted line); neoplasms were also found within the thorax.

osteolysis of the vertebral body an irregular radiolucency may be found radiographically (Figure 12.13). Cervical myelography may identify extradural compression, scintigraphy may show increased bone turnover at the lesion margin, but CT is probably most useful. Chemotherapy is rarely available or affordable and would likely require some measure of intervertebral stabilisation.

Vertebral Osteomyelitis

Vertebral osteomyelitis rarely occurs, but is more common in younger animals secondary to haematogenous spread to physeal growth plates [46]. Bacterial infection results in destruction, remodelling and instability of the vertebra, and may extend to abscessation within the paravertebral tissues. Various pathogens have been isolated: in adults – *Aspergillus* spp., *Mycobacterium bovis*; in foals – *Rhodococcus equi*, *Klebsiella* spp., *Streptococcus* spp., *Escherichia coli* and *Actinobacillus* spp. Fever, pain and stiffness over the affected vertebrae often precede development of neurological deficits typical of spinal compression. Radiographic signs include osteoproliferative change, osteolysis, sclerosis and associated soft tissue swelling; however,

osteomyelitis may not be radiographically evident until 2–8 weeks after onset of clinical signs when up to 50% of the vertebra has undergone demineralisation. Nuclear scintigraphy or CT should be used to identify early cases. Aggressive long-term broad spectrum antimicrobial therapy is required. In adults the combination of penicillin G and enrofloxacin or chloarmphenicol is recommended; in foals a macrolide or chloarmphenicol. Surgical debridement is advisable, though not often possible. As the diagnosis is rarely made until the infective process has extended peridurally, the condition carries a grave prognosis.

Apparent Muscle Pain

In general the relevance of localised muscle soreness within the neck to gait change or poor performance is unclear. Pain at the insertion of brachicephalicus at the base of the neck can cause abnormal lifting of the head–neck during limb protraction and a shortened cranial stride phase when the horse is ridden in walk. These signs are abolished with physiotherapy or acupuncture [6].

Nuchal Ligament Insertional Desmopathy

Chondroid metaplasia, dystrophic mineralisation and new bone formation on the nuchal ligament insertion on the occiput is a common incidental finding in warmbloods (up to 85%), but not in thoroughbreds (5%) [47].

Insertional desmopathy of the nuchal ligament or tendinopathy of the insertion of the semispinalis muscle typically occurs after local trauma (especially pulling back when tied), but can also occur as a repetitive strain injury after excessive lunging whilst restricted by side reins or draw reins [6,47,48]. Affected cases are usually not painful to palpation, but resent head–neck ventroflexion when lunged and/or ridden and are described as resistant against the reins and may shake their heads or rear. Radiography reveals new bone formation that can extend ventrally and dorsally beyond the insertion on the occiput, but this may not differ from that seen incidentally. Ultrasonography of the ligament is challenging and hard to interpret. CT is the most sensitive means of detecting potentially significant lesions in either the nuchal ligament or semispinalis tendon, but diagnosis relies upon a positive response to local anaesthetic infiltration with the horse reassessed after 15–30 minutes. Long-term treatment consists of repeated local infiltration of corticosteroid and local anaesthetic, and modification to training (off the bit, in a straight line). Shock wave therapy and acupuncture can also be beneficial.

Return to full work occurs in 50–70% of cases over an 8–10 week period [48,49].

Nuchal Bursitis

Traumatic infection and non-infections inflammation of the nuchal bursae is a rare cause of neck stiffness and abnormal head–neck posture [50]. Palpation demonstrates painful focal soft tissue swelling dorsal to C1–C2. Increased fluid within the bursa and a thickened sheath are seen ultrasonographically. Surgical debridement can produce complete resolution.

References

1 Schmidburg, I., Pagger, H., Zsoldos, R.R. et al. Movement associated reduction of spatial capacity of the equine cervical vertebral canal. *Veterinary Journal* 2012, July; **192**(3):525–528.

2 Mayhew, I.G. The equine spinal cord in health and disease 1: The healthy spinal cord. In: *Annual Convention of the AAEP*, 1999, pp. 67–84.

3 King, A.S. *Physiological and Clinical Anatomy of the Domestic Mammals*, Vol. 1: *Central Nervous System*, 2nd edn. Oxford: Oxford University Press, 1993.

4 Auer, J.A. and Mackay, R.J. Chapter 49: Anatomy and physiology of the nervous system. In: *Equine Surgery*, 4th edn. Elsevier Inc., 2012, pp. 665–676.

5 De Lahunta, A. and Glass, E.N. Large animal spinal cord disease. *Veterinary Neuroanatomy and Clinical Neurology*. Missouri: Elsevier Ltd, 2009, pp. 285–318.

6 Dyson, S.J. Lesions of the equine neck resulting in lameness or poor performance. *The Veterinary Clinics of North America: Equine Practice* 2011, December; **27**(3):417–437.

7 Zsoldos, R.R., Groesel, M., Kotschwar, A. et al. A preliminary modelling study on the equine cervical spine with inverse

kinematics at walk. *Equine Veterinary Journal* 2010, December; **42**(38):516–522.

8 Clayton, H., Kaiser, L., Lavagnino, M. and Stubbs, N. Evaluation of intersegmental vertebral motion during performance of dynamic mobilization exercises in cervical lateral bending in horses. *American Journal of Veterinary Research* 2012; **73**(8):1153–1159.

9 Mitchell, C.W., Nykamp, S.G., Foster, R., Cruz, R. and Montieth, G. The use of magnetic resonance imaging in evaluating horses with spinal ataxia. *Veterinary Radiology and Ultrasound: The official journal of the American College of Veterinary Radiology and the International Veterinary Radiology Association* 2012, May 25; **53**(6):613–620.

10 Yovich, J.V., LeCouteur, R.A., Gould, D.H. and Couteljr, R.A.L. Chronic cervical compressive myelopathy in horses: Clinical correlations with spinal cord alterations. *Australian Veterinary Journal* 1991, October; **68**(10):326–334.

11 Van Biervliet, J. An evidence-based approach to clinical questions in the practice of equine neurology. *The Veterinary Clinics of North America: Equine Practice* 2007, August; **23**(2): 317–328.

12 Moore, B.R., Reed, S.M., Biller, D.S., Kohn, C.W. and Weisbrode, S.E. Assessment of vertebral canal diameter and bony malformations of the cervical part of the spine in horses with cervical stenotic myelopathy. *American Journal of Veterinary Research* 1994, January; **55**(1): 5–13.

13 Hahn, C.N., Handel, I., Green, S.L., Bronsvoort, M.B. and Mayhew, I.G. Assessment of the utility of using intra- and intervertebral minimum sagittal diameter ratios in the diagnosis of cervical vertebral malformation in horses. *Veterinary Radiology and Ultrasound* 2008, January 10; **49**(1):1–6.

14 Mayhew, I.G., Donawick, W.J., Green, S.L. et al. Diagnosis and prediction of cervical vertebral malformation in Thoroughbred foals based on semi-quantitative radiographic indicators. *Equine Veterinary Journal* 1993; **25**(5):435–440.

15 Withers, J., Voute, L., Hammond, G. and Lischer, C. Radiographic anatomy of the articular process joints of the caudal cervical vertebrae in the horse on lateral and oblique projections. *Equine Veterinary Journal* 2009; **41**(9):895–902.

16 Butler, J.B., Colles, C., Dyson, S., Kold, S. and Poulos, P. *The Spine. Clinical Radiology of the Horse*. Chichester, West Sussex: Wiley-Blackwell, 2008, pp. 505–539.

17 Down, S.S. and Henson, F.M.D. Radiographic retrospective study of the caudal cervical articular process joints in the horse. *Equine Veterinary Journal* 2009, July 5; **41**(6):518–524.

18 Peters, D.F. and Rombach, N. Neck pain and stiffness. In: *Robinson's Current Therapy in Equine Medicine*, 7th edn. St Loius, MO: Elsevier, 2015, pp. 97–100.

19 Van Biervliet, J., Mayhew, J. and De Lahunta, A. Cervical vertebral compressive myelopathy: Diagnosis. *Clinical Techniques in Equine Practice* 2006, March; **5**(1):54–59.

20 Powers, B.E., Stashak, T.S., Nixon, A.J., Yovich. J.V. and Norrdin, R.W. Pathology of the vertebral column of horses with cervical static stenosis. *Veterinary Pathology* 1986, July1; **23**(4):392–399.

21 Trostle, S.S., Dubielzig, R.R. and Beck, K.A. Examination of frozen cross sections of cervical spinal intersegments in nine horses with cervical vertebral malformation: Lesions associated with spinal cord compression. *Journal of Veterinary Diagnostic Investigation* 1993, July 1; **5**(3):423–431.

22 Nixon, A.J. Fractures of the vertebrae. In: *Equine Fracture Repair*. Philadelphia, PA: W.B. Saunders, 1996, pp. 299–312.

23 Fisher, L.F., Bowman, K.F. and Macharg, M.A. Spinal ataxia in a horse caused by a synovial cyst. *Veterinary Pathology* 1981; **18**:407–410.

24 Laynon, L. and Rubin, C.T. Static vs dynamic loads as an influence on bone remodelling. *Journal of Biomechanics* 1984; **17**:897–905.

25 Levine, J., Scrivani, P., Divers, T. et al. Multicenter case-control study of signalment, diagnostic features, and outcome associated with cervical vertebral malformation–malarticulation in horses. *Journal of the American Veterinary Medical Association* 2010; **237**(7):812–822.

26 Levine, J.M., Adam, E., MacKay, R.J. et al. Confirmed and presumptive cervical vertebral compressive myelopathy in older horses: a retrospective study (1992–2004). *Journal of Veterinary Internal Medicine* 2007; **21**(4):812–819.

27 Maher, O., Aleman, M., Puchalsk, I.S. and Snyder, J.R. Sport horses with neurologic deficits and cervical vertebral osteoarthrosis presenting within one year of prepurchase examination: 18 cases (2000–2007). XIV Congress of the Italian Society of Equine Practitioners (SIVE) and Veterinary European Equine Meeting (FEEVA), 2008.

28 Stewart, R., Reed, S.M. and Weisbrode, S.E. Frequency and severity of osteochondrosis in horses with cervical stenotic myelopathy. *American Journal of Veterinary Research* 1991; **52**:873–879.

29 Van Biervliet, J., Scrivani, P.V., Divers, T.J. et al. Evaluation of decision criteria for detection of spinal cord compression based on cervical myelography in horses: 38 cases (1981–2001). *Equine Veterinary Journal* 2004, January; **36**(1):14–20.

30 Didierlaurent, D., Contremoulins, V., Denoix, J.-M. and Audigie, F. Scintigraphic pattern of uptake of [99m]Technetium by the cervical vertebrae of sound horses. *Veterinary Record* 2009; **164**:809–813.

31 Claridge, H., Piercy, R., Parry, A. and Weller, R. The 3D anatomy of the cervical articular process joints in the horse and their topographical relationship to the spinal cord. *Equine Veterinary Journal* 2010; **42**(8):726–731.

32 Sleutjens, J., Voorhout, G., Van Der Kolk, J.H., Wijnberg, I.D. and Back, W. The effect of *ex vivo* flexion and extension on intervertebral foramina dimensions in the equine cervical spine. *Equine Veterinary Journal* 2010, November; Suppl., **42** (38):425–430.

33 Berg, L.C., Nielsen, J. V., Thoefner, M.B. and Thomsen, P.D. Ultrasonography of the equine cervical region: a descriptive study in eight horses. *Equine Veterinary Journal* 2003, November 5; **35**(7):647–655.

34 Nollet, H., Van Ham, L., Dewulf, J., Vanderstraeten, G. and Deprez, P. Standardization of transcranial magnetic stimulation in the horse. *The Veterinary Journal* 2003, November; **166**(3):244–250.

35 Mayhew, I.G. Milne Lecture 1999 II: The diseased spinal cord. In: *Proceedings of AAEP Convention*, 1999; **45**:67–84.

36 Walmsley, J.P. Surgical treatment of crevical spinal cord compression in horses: A European experience. *Equine Veterinary Education* 2005; **17**(1):39–43.

37 Moore, B.R., Reed, S.M. and Robertson, J.T. Surgical treatment of cervical stenotic myelopathy in horses: 73 cases (1983–1992). *Journal of the American Veterinary Medical Association* 1993, July; **203**(1):108–112.

38 Birmingham, S.S.W., Reed, S.M., Mattoon, J.S. and Saville, W.J. Qualitative assessment of corticosteroid cervical articular facet injection in symptomatic horses. *Equine Veterinary Education* 2010, February 12; **22**(2):77–82.

39 Nielsen, J.V., Berg, L.C., Thoefnert, M.B. and Thomsen, P.D. Accuracy of ultrasound-guided intra-articular injection of cervical facet joints in horses: A cadaveric study. *Equine Veterinary Journal* 2003, November; **35**(7):657–661.

40 Rubinstein, S. and Pool, J. A systematic review of the diagnostic accuracy of provocative tests of the neck for diagnosing cervical radiculopathy. *European Spine Journal* 2007; 307–319.

41 Furr, M. Congential malformation of the nervous system. In: *Equine Neurology*, 2nd edn. Ames, OH: John Wiley & Sons Inc., 2015, pp. 401–405.

42 Meehan, L., Dyson, S. and Murray, R. Radiographic and scintigraphic evaluation of spondylosis in the equine thoracolumbar spine: A retrospective study. *Equine Veterinary Journal* 2009, November 5; **41**(8):800–807.

43 Vos, N.J., Pollock, P.J., Harty, M. et al. Fractures of the cervical vertebral odontoid in four horses and one pony. *Veterinary Record* 2008; **162**:116–119.

44 Gold, J.R., Divers, T.J., Miller, A.J. et al. Cervical vertebral spinal hematomas in 4 horses. *Journal of Veterinary Internal Medicine* 2008; **22**:481–485.

45 Raes, E.V., Durie, I., Wegge, B. et al. Imaging findings of a haemangiosarcoma in a cervical vertebra of a horse. *Equine Veterinary Education* 2012, March 15; **26**:548–551.

46 Giguere, S. and Lavoie, J.P. *Rhodococcus equi* vertebral osteomyelitis in 3 Quarter Horse colts. *Equine Veterinary Journal* 1994; **26**(1):74–77.

47 Dyson, S.J. The cervical spine and soft tissues of the neck. In: Ross M.W. and Dyson, S.J. (eds.), In: *Diagnosis and Management of Lameness in the Horse*,

2nd edn. Missouri: W.B. Saunders, 2010, pp. 606–616.

48 Nowak, M. Die Insertiondesmopathie des Nackenstrangursprungs beim Pferd. Diagnostik, differential Diagnostik. In: *Proceedings of the 7th Congress on Equine Medicine and Surgery*, Geneva, 2001.

49 McClure, S,. and Weinberger, T. Extracorporeal shock wave therapy: Clinical applications and regulation. *Clinical Techniques in Equine Practice* 2003; **2**:358–367.

50 Garcia-Lopez, J., Jenei, T., Chope, K. et al. Diagnosis and management of cranial and caudal nuchal bursitis in four horses. *Journal of the American Veterinary Medical Association* 2010; **237**:823–839.

13

Back Pathology

Adam Driver, Frances M.D. Henson, Jessica A. Kidd,
Luis P. Lamas and Rob Pilsworth

13.1 Traumatic damage

Adam Driver and Rob Pilsworth

General principles

In many cases of pathological change in the skeleton of the equine athlete, predictable patterns of the site and nature of the pathology have been documented [1]. This is because many of the conditions that we encounter in our equine athletes are stress injuries produced by a focal accumulation of micro-damage as a result of cyclical loading or over-loading at specific sites. These sites are predetermined by the anatomy of the horse and the discipline that the horse is used for, which subjects certain areas to an increased likelihood of damage. In contrast, in traumatic damage to the spine and pelvis, these rules do not apply. The combination of the weight of the horse and the speed at which it was travelling, together with whatever inciting cause produces the traumatic damage, can lead to a bewilderingly complex array of injuries that can occur alone or in combination, e.g. after a fall a horse can sustain fractures to one, or several, elements of the pelvis, depending on how the horse falls and on to what it falls. Distinct clinical entities are therefore often merged and can be a diagnostic challenge.

Fracture of the Dorsal Spinous Processes (DSP) of the Thoracic Vertebrae (Fractured Withers)

Presentation and Clinical Signs

This injury almost always follows the horse rearing up over backwards and landing on the withers. There is usually a reluctance to walk, with the horse planting all four feet, similar to the presentation of a horse with quadrilateral acute laminitis. Great pain is usually exhibited initially with sweating and boarding of the entire musculature associated with the thoracolumbar spine. The head is usually held in hyperextension and the neck held rigid, in the horse's attempt to avoid movement of the nuchal ligament. Almost always several dorsal DSPs fracture together and the entire segment of 'freed' thoracic spines, along with the muscular insertions, is pulled to one side or the other of the midline. This normally results in a deviation of the line of the spine when viewed from the rear. This is sometimes more easily appreciated by palpation, by running the finger tips gently along the tips of the DSPs, than by visualisation, because the initial associated soft tissue swelling may obscure the spinal deviation.

The displacement of the fractured wither to one side also allows the proximal scapula on the contralateral side to protrude dorsally

Equine Neck and Back Pathology: Diagnosis and Treatment, Second Edition. Edited by Frances M.D. Henson.
© 2018 John Wiley & Sons, Ltd. Published 2018 by John Wiley & Sons, Ltd.

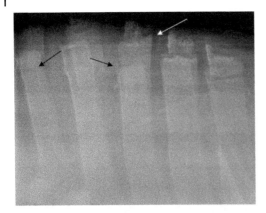

Figure 13.1 A lateromedial radiograph of the withers region (T5–T9) showing fracture and displacement of the thoracic dorsal spinous processes (four fractures are apparent in this radiograph). The normal separate centres of ossification (white arrow) should not be mistaken for fractures of the tip of the process (black arrow). This case shows the considerable overriding of the fracture, which results in 'sinking' of the contour of the wither.

more than is normal. This should not be confused with a specific injury to the scapula, and is merely the result of displacement of the fractured segment of spine.

Diagnostic Imaging

A radiographic examination of the withers region is recommended to confirm the diagnosis. The radiographs will show fracture and displacement of the DSPs and are usually diagnostic (Figure 13.1). In most cases of fractured DSPs, nuclear scintigraphy is probably not indicated. As discussed in Chapter 8, care should be taken not to overinterpret the normal separate centres of ossification seen in the DSPs of all horses.

Treatment and Prognosis

The treatment of fractured DSPs consists of administration of analgesics and non-steroidal anti-inflammatory drugs (NSAIDs) in the initial shock-like state. The horse should then be confined to the stable for at least 4 weeks to allow the fractured segment of the spine to stabilise in its new position. In the initial period, the horse will be unwilling to lower the head. Feed, hay and water should therefore be provided in elevated mangers. The temperature of the horse should be monitored daily, but, as the concurrent use of NSAIDs can artificially suppress pyrexia, occasional blood samples should be taken to guard against the possible development of pleuropneumonia. The risk factors for pleuropneumonia have been documented to increase as a result of impaired drainage of bronchial secretions, which follows continued elevation of the head and neck [2].

The prognosis for return to full function is usually good, but the horse will require care with saddling because of possible traumatic impingement between the front of the saddle and the new position of the withers. The apparent asymmetry often becomes less marked with time as the acute swelling subsides. In rare instances, the parent bone of one or more of the fractured DSPs can erode its way through the intervening tissues and ulcerate the skin. Should this occur, surgical treatment for removal of this spiculated sharp piece of bone will be necessary to avoid the development of chronic discharging fistula and infection of the associated site.

Fractures of the Thoracolumbar Vertebral Column

Fractures of the vertebral column include fractures of the articular facet joints and fractures of the vertebral body and laminae. Each of these are considered in turn.

Fractures of the Articular Facet Joints

Presentation and Clinical Signs
Clinically horses present with localised marked muscle spasm, guarding, reluctance to flex the back and severe pain when the back is manipulated. A mild scoliosis towards the affected side may be present when the horse is observed from behind.

Diagnosis

The diagnosis of articular facet joint fractures has, historically, been a difficult challenge. However, with the advent of nuclear scintigraphy, the fractures can be readily seen within the spine. The fractures result in focal moderate-to-marked, increased radiopharmaceutical uptake at the site of the articular facet joint. This is in the dorsal region of the vertebral body, similar to the position where vertebral laminar stress fractures are seen in racehorses (discussed later in this chapter). Once a lesion is suspected, radiography can be targeted at the site of the lesion. Specialist dorsomedial–ventrolateral oblique (DMVLO) projections, highlighting the facet joints, can also be beneficial in demonstrating fractures (Chapter 8). Ultrasonography may be helpful in some cases. In the acute phase, ultrasonography may visualise incongruity of the bone surface at the fracture site when performed diligently. In the chronic phase callus formation will be visible around the joint.

Treatment and Prognosis

The treatment of a fractured articular facet is conservative. This conservative therapy comprises box rest for a period of 4–6 weeks, together with the administration of NSAIDs at least for the first 2 weeks. If the fracture is diagnosed in the chronic phase, with arthropathy or ankylosis of the facet joint, periarticular injection with corticosteroids may be beneficial, along with supportive therapy for epaxial muscular spasm and altered exercise. Overall, however, the prognosis for return to exercise is guarded at best.

Fractures of the Vertebral Body and Laminae

Presentation and Clinical Signs

The horse presenting with vertebral body fractures will have clinical signs dependent on the degree of spinal cord compression and neurological compromise. Vertebral body fractures can cause a range of presentations, including cases in which no neurological changes are seen and the horse demonstrates severe back pain, to cases in which minor nervous damage

is caused, leading to neurogenic atrophy of the epaxial musculature. In severe cases spinal cord damage leads to complete recumbency or 'dog sitting' (hindlimb paralysis with functional forelimbs), with paralysis and loss of deep pain response in the hind limbs. It must also be noted that the clinical signs can change with time depending on the ongoing swelling or haemorrhage around and in the spinal cord. Vertebral fractures are often a result of high-speed falls or impact with static objects, leading to the initial examination often being performed in difficult surroundings.

Diagnosis

A thorough clinical and neurological examination is essential to determine the severity and prognosis of the trauma. It should be remembered that, in any traumatic incident, the neurological signs seen could be associated with cranial trauma, so the entire nervous system should be evaluated, including the cranial nerves. The examinations should aim to determine the site of the lesion and the severity. By evaluating the presenting upper motor neuron (UMN) and lower motor neuron (LMN) signs the location of the lesion can be identified. UMN signs include mild weakness and ataxia, spastic bladder paralysis and hypermetria, and hyperreflexia. LMN signs include marked weakness or paresis, flaccid paralysis of the bladder, hyporeflexia and, over a short period of time, marked neurogenic muscle atrophy. The spine can be divided into regions producing characteristic signs (summarised in Table 13.1).

Lesions between C6 and T2 produce LMN signs in the frontlimbs and UMN signs in the hindlimbs, with spastic urinary incontinence. Lesions between T3 and L3 produce UMN signs in the hindlimbs, spastic bladder incontinence, normal front limbs, and with time possible neurogenic atrophy of the muscles of the back in that region. Lesions between L4 and S2 produce LMN signs in the hindlimbs, flaccid bladder paralysis, loss of anal sphincter tone and reflex and tail tone, and normal front limbs. The proprioceptive system should also be evaluated during the

Table 13.1 A summary of the clinical signs of traumatic damage at different sites of the spinal column. LMN, lower motor neuron; UMN, upper motor neuron.

Site of damage	Clinical signs of damage
C6–T2	Front legs – LMN signs Hind legs – UMN signs Spastic urinary incontinence
T3–L3	Front legs – normal Hind legs – UMN signs Spastic bladder incontinence
L4–S2	Front legs – normal Hind legs – LMN Flaccid bladder paralysis, loss of anal sphincter tone and reflex and tail tone

Table 13.2 Drugs that may be used in the treatment of vertebral fractures and their recommended dosages.

Drug	Recommended dosage
Dexamethasone	Up to 0.2 mg/kg i.v.
Methylprednisolone sodium succinate	2–4 mg/kg
Flunixin meglumine	1 mg/kg i.v.
Mannitol	1 g/kg (20% solution over 20 min)
Dimethylsulphoxide	1 g/kg (10% solution twice a day)

neurological examination, to help determine the severity of the lesion. Mild compression will produce placement deficits and ataxia, the same as UMN signs. Moderate compression can result in paresis or paralysis of voluntary movements and reflexes, and a loss of skin sensation. Severe compression or transection will lead to a loss of deep pain sensation.

Once the lesion has been localised, and if the horse retains enough motor neuron and proprioceptive control to be moved, radiography is the imaging modality of choice to determine the fracture configuration and help determine the prognosis and treatment plan. Sometimes, however, although a vertebral fracture is suspected the diagnosis will only be made postmortem.

In cases of severe fracture dislocation of the spine, e.g. after collision with a motor vehicle or a very severe fall in competition, the veterinarian is often presented with a recumbent horse, in a difficult situation. The full neurological examination is difficult in these circumstances. A pragmatic approach has to take into account the welfare of the horse and the needs of the situation, if, for example, on a public road or in a competition arena. Any horse that, after a known fall or collision, is fully conscious, but remains recumbent and has made no attempt to rise for more than an hour, with associated hemi- or tetraplegia, can be considered a justifiable case for euthanasia, even in the absence of a definitive diagnosis [3].

Treatment and Prognosis

Treatment is aimed at aggressive anti-inflammatory and antioxidant therapy (summarised in Table 13.2). This will include corticosteroid and NSAIDs such as dexamethasone (up to 0.2 mg/kg i.v.) or methylprednisolone sodium succinate (2–4 mg/kg i.v.) and flunixin meglumine (1 mg/kg i.v.). Mannitol use has also been proposed to reduce vasogenic oedema (1 g/kg maximum dose given as a 20% solution over 20 minutes). Antioxidative therapy includes dimethylsulphoxide (DMSO) (1 g/kg as a 10% solution twice a day) and vitamins E and C supplementation. Strict box rest and maintaining the horse in a quiet environment are essential. In most cases traumatic fracture of the back holds a poor-to-hopeless prognosis, however, with most fractures proving fatal.

Pelvic Factures

Fractures of the Tuber Coxae

Presentation and Clinical Signs

Fractured *tubera coxae* often follow a history of impact with an inanimate object, usually a door frame, or after a fall on to a hard surface [4]. In the racehorse these can present as an acute fracture after hard work, but probably as the end-stage of stress pathology at the site rather than after trauma [5].

Complete fractures of the *tuber coxae* present with marked asymmetry of the bony prominences of the pelvis, with the fractured *tuber coxae* normally displaced ventrally and cranially into the sublumbar fossa. This displacement is due to the continued, unopposed contraction of the muscles that originate on the *tuber coxae*: the external abdominal oblique, superficial gluteal and *tensor fasciae latae*. This cranioventral displacement gives the condition its colloquial name of 'knocked-down hip'.

Clinically, a fractured *tuber coxae* causes a moderate-to-marked lameness, with gross asymmetry of the *tuber coxae*, as noted previously, giving a pathognomonic presentation. Crepitus and swelling may also be present at the site of the fracture, along with a moderate-to-marked pain response to palpation.

Diagnosis

Further diagnostic tests are not often required to diagnose the fracture, but the remainder of the pelvic girdle should be fully assessed, particularly if the inciting incident is unknown or if the incident consisted of a high-speed fall, because further fractures may also be present. Ultrasound examination is the modality of choice to assess the integrity of the remainder of the pelvic girdle, and can also be used to confirm the primary diagnosis (Figure 13.2).

Treatment and Prognosis

Treatment for a fractured *tuber coxae* consists of box rest for 8–12 weeks to allow for stabilisation of the fracture pieces in their new positions. The main complications that can occur include progression to a compound fracture if the sharp bone margins from the fracture bed penetrate the skin, leading to infection and potential sequestration of the fracture fragment if the blood supply is compromised. In these cases surgical débridement

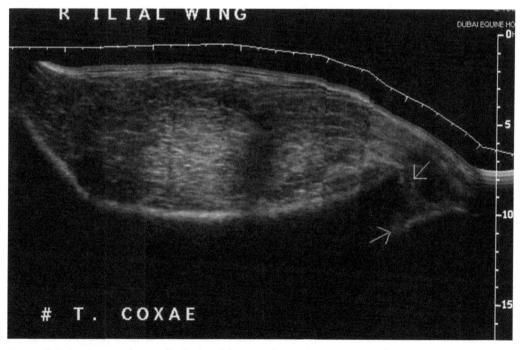

Figure 13.2 An ultrasound scan of a displaced fracture of the tuber coxae. Note the clear gap (white arrows) between the iliac surface and the displaced bone fragment.

of infected or necrotic bone may be required, along with antibiotic therapy and management of the discharging lesion.

The prognosis for return to exercise is guarded, with an expected mechanical restriction of the stride length due to the occurrence of altered pelvis conformation. However, despite this expected impairment, many racehorses with this injury return to full competitive athletic function in that discipline after healing, so the prognosis depends to some extent on the expected and acceptable level of gait impairment after recovery.

Fractures of the Ilial Wing and Shaft

Presentation and Clinical Signs

Ilial wing fractures are most common in the racehorse because this is a predilection site for stress fracture, but can also result from a fall at high speed. Due to the traumatic nature of the latter fractures, they can occur in any configuration. Fractures are most commonly unilateral but can be bilateral. Horses present with marked or non-weight-bearing lameness on the affected side, and will show signs of marked pain, including spasm of and sweating over the gluteal musculature, a hunched-up appearance and a reluctance to move or bear weight. There is frequently asymmetry of the *tuber sacrale*, with the affected side displacing ventrally if the fracture is complete and at its base. If the fracture is at the base of the shaft or extends from the wing into the shaft, there is a particularly high risk for laceration of the internal iliac artery, leading to the horse presenting in hypovolaemic shock, often with swelling of the upper thigh region as the blood is forced through the fascial planes. In these cases the horse will sometimes exsanguinate rapidly.

Ilial shaft fractures can occur in isolation or as part of a complex fracture of the pelvis. In the authors' experience these fractures hold a greater risk for laceration of an internal iliac artery and exsanguination of the horse than the ilial wing fracture described above. The horse will present with marked lameness or be non-weight bearing, with spasm of the gluteal

muscles, similar to an ilial wing fracture. If the fracture is complete, the ipsilateral *tuber coxae* may appear ventrally displaced compared with the contralateral side. Frequently there is also crepitus or distinct 'clicking' as the horse shifts weight with complete fractures. A rectal examination may allow the clinician to palpate the fracture site and associated haemorrhage on the axial margin of the shaft.

Diagnosis

Ultrasonography is the imaging modality of choice for confirmation of diagnosis [6,7]. The normal ilial wing has a continuous, smooth, hyperechoic, curving bone margin when scanned through the gluteal muscle mass. A fracture will present as a discontinuity or 'step' in the hyperechoic bone margin (Figure 13.3), frequently with an area of anechoic/hypoechoic haemorrhage around the site, with disruption of the overlying, normal, hypoechoic/echogenic, striated muscular pattern. The wing should be scanned in both a longitudinal and a transverse plane, paying particularly close attention to the caudal margin, which

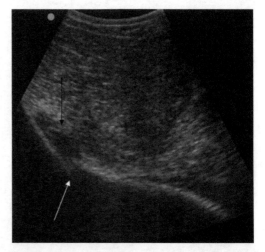

Figure 13.3 An ultrasound scan of an ilial wing fracture. Displaced fractures such as these show an easily demonstrated abrupt 'step' in the surface of the ilium (white arrow), often associated with an area of hypoechogenicity resulting from haemorrhage within the muscle (black arrow).

is often the only site that will present with an incongruity in incomplete fractures. Caution should be observed when interpreting acoustic shadowing caused by focal neurovascular bundles or fascial plane intersections that will extend to the wing margin and cause a focal anechoic spot, creating a false-positive finding. Linear, curvilinear or microconvex probes with a frequency range from 3 MHz to 5 MHz are all suitable for examining the ilial wing.

Ultrasonography of the shaft can be technically more difficult to perform than examination of the ilial wing and a thorough knowledge of the structural anatomy of the pelvis is required. It is essential that the probe be aligned parallel to the shaft; otherwise obliquity can create false 'steps' in the shaft, which may be misdiagnosed as fractures. The shaft should be examined over its entire length, from the base at the ilial wing to the raised cup of the acetabulum at the coxofemoral joint. Similar to the shaft, the fracture site will present as a disruption or 'step' in the normal, smooth, sharply defined, hyperechoic bone margin, with hypoechoic/anechoic haemorrhage in the surrounding soft tissues. Ultrasound examinations can often give a false-negative result in the acute phase, when the fracture is incomplete. At postmortem examination a common configuration of these fractures is such that the cranial exit point of the fracture is on the ventral aspect of the shaft, at the junction with the iliac wing, and the fracture line extends along the shaft, similar to the splitting of a log along its length. It will be appreciated that, as only the dorsal aspect of the shaft can be evaluated with ultrasonography, the fracture cannot be identified until complete collapse or displacement occurs.

Nuclear scintigraphy may be useful in confirming a diagnosis of a fractured ilial wing or shaft, particularly in some shaft fractures when ultrasonographic evaluation is inconclusive (Chapter 9), but it should not be performed until 5–7 days after the inciting incident to minimise the risk of false-negative results. These false-negative results (i.e. failure to diagnose the fractures) are probably a result of attenuation of the gamma radiation due to the overlying muscle mass or disruption of the blood supply to the fracture site limiting supply of radiopharmaceuticals to the bone after the acute fracture. Depending on the severity of lameness and stability at the fracture site, it may not be possible to transport a horse to a scintigraphy facility safely.

Prognosis and Treatment
Treatment, as with all pelvic fractures, is conservative, with box rest for a minimum of 8–12 weeks. Many authors also recommend cross-tying of the horse during the first 3- to 4-week period, until the fracture site is stable, to prevent laceration of the internal iliac artery. Managing the cross-tied horse is essential to a successful outcome. The horse should be untied at least four times a day to feed from the ground. The rectal temperature should be monitored twice daily or, if NSAIDs are being administered, routine haematology testing performed every 48 hours, to ensure early detection of any developing pleuropneumonia. The contralateral limb should be closely monitored for signs of laminitis if the horse is non-weight bearing or severely lame on the fractured side, and appropriate support therapy including deep bedding or bedding on sand, aspirin (20 mg/kg p.o. twice daily) and acepromazine (0.02–0.04 mg/kg i.m. or p.o. twice daily). Frog support such as Styrofoam pad or sole support material should also be applied, but this is frequently not possible in the acute phase of the fracture. Pain relief for the horse must be balanced between allowing the horse to remain comfortable and minimising morbidity, while maintaining the inherent protective mechanisms of pain. All four limbs will require careful bandaging to minimise the degree of distal limb oedema, and these bandages should be changed twice daily. The horse should be placed in as quiet a stable as possible and should be able to see what is happening in its surrounding environment so that it is not startled or surprised. There should always be a piece of twine between the headcollar and each shank connecting the

horse to the overhead rope or wall rings, to prevent the horse from throttling itself if it decides to lie down.

The prognosis for uncomplicated ilial wing fractures is good for a return to racing. Fractures of the ilial shaft hold a guarded-to-poor prognosis for a return to racing, not only due to the increased risk of exsanguination but also because the increased pain associated with these fractures increases the risk of contralateral laminitis and other complications such as contracture of *biceps femoris, semimembranous* and *semitendinous*, and upward fixation of the patella.

Fractures of the Ischium and *Tuber Ischii*

Presentation and Clinical Signs

These fractures occur predominantly from falling over backwards or reversing into inanimate objects at speed. The horse has a marked-to-severe unilateral lameness, with pain and progressive swelling over the affected *tuber ischii.* Fractures within the ischium itself are rarer and often present with minimal external clinical signs, so presenting a greater diagnostic challenge. Occasionally, in displaced fractures there may be laceration of the internal pudendal or obturator blood vessels, which can lead to haemorrhage and progressive swelling of the caudal thigh and ultimately death, but this is less common than in ilial shaft or wing fractures. Clinically there is pain to palpation of the affected tuber ischii and, if the fracture is complete, asymmetry between the *tubera ischii.* There is frequently a marked reduction in the cranial phase of the stride of the limb on the affected side.

Diagnosis

Diagnostic techniques that are useful in the diagnosis of these fractures include ultrasonography, nuclear scintigraphy and radiography. Ultrasonography of the ischium is a greater technical challenge than that of the ilial wing (Figure 13.4). False-negative findings often occur due to the fracture being incomplete or non-displaced. Nuclear scintigraphy can be a useful technique to

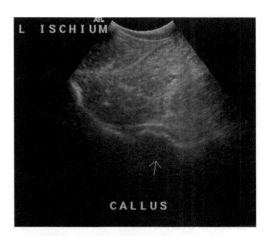

Figure 13.4 An ultrasound scan of the surface of the ischium. The irregular contour is the result of callus (white arrow) over the site of a healing, non-displaced, ischial fracture.

demonstrate a fracture not visible using ultrasonography (Figure 13.5), but again can produce false-negative results for up to 2 weeks after the inciting incident. Radiography requires a high-power generator to produce the exposure factors required to obtain a diagnostic image. However, it can be a valuable tool to confirm the diagnosis (Figure 13.6) and determine the prognosis, especially if the fracture is within the body of the ischium and may involve the caudal aspect of the coxofemoral joint.

Treatment and Prognosis

Treatment is based on box rest for 4 weeks followed by gradually increasing daily hand walking for a further 4 weeks. These cases are normally left loose in the stable and not tied up. The prognosis for return to competition is fair for simple fractures of the tuber ischii, although, if there has been displacement of the fracture fragment, there may be long-term mechanical restriction of the stride length. The prognosis for complete fractures of the ischium are dependent on the involvement of the coxofemoral joint and generally hold a guarded prognosis, with those extending into the joint having a grave prognosis.

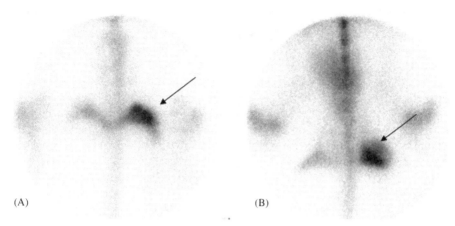

(A)   (B)

Figure 13.5 Nuclear scintigrams of an ischial fracture: (A) caudocranial view of the caudal pelvis; (B) dorsoventral view of the caudal pelvis. The black arrows show an area of increased radionuclide uptake in the tuber ischii on both views. This fracture was not visible after ultrasonographic examination in the acute stage, as is often the case with traumatic impaction fracture in this site. The horse reared and fell in the stable 2 weeks previously and was lame subsequently.

Pubic Fractures

Presentation and Clinical Signs
Fracture of the pubis in isolation is an infrequent occurrence but normally follows a fall or the horse slipping and spread-eagling the hind legs. Horses affected with pubic fractures tend to stand in a 'hunched-up' manner and often have the tail raised. They may walk with a very short protraction, indicative of severe pain and bilateral hindlimb lameness. This can mimic the signs of severe exercise-induced rhabdomyolysis. There may be associated swelling of the vulva and perineal region in the female. There is usually an unwillingness to move after a standstill.

Diagnosis
In these cases radiography is impractical because only radiography under general anaesthesia will produce diagnostic images of the region, and the risks of fracture displacement involved with general anaesthesia are usually considered too great to proceed. Nuclear scintigraphy can be useful if the appropriate images are acquired. Nuclear scintigrams obtained in the usual dorsoventral manner rarely identify the fracture because of the screening effect of the overlying spine and musculature, and the small bone

mass of the pubis (and hence origin of signal) causes significant attenuation of the signal. However, a caudal view, obtained with the camera face parallel to the posterior surface of the thighs, with the tail gently pulled to one side, gives excellent visualisation of fractures of the pubis, which appear as an intense area of increased radiopharmaceutical uptake in the midline between the femora. Rectal examination can also be rewarding. The symphysis pubis should be palpated with the horse standing fully weight bearing, and then the horse rocked gently from side to side by an assistant while the hand remains over the pubic symphysis. Motion of one hemipelvis in relation to the other is often appreciated in conjunction with crepitus at the site.

Fractures and Dislocation of the Coxofemoral Joint

Presentation and Clinical Signs
Fractures of the coxofemoral joint are often a result of the horse slipping and falling on a hard surface or 'doing the splits'. The horse will present with a non-weight-bearing lameness for both fracture and dislocation. In the dislocated joint the femoral head is usually displaced dorsally and cranially, and as a result the leg may appear shortened, the stifle

rotated outwards more than the contralateral limb and the greater trochanters may not be symmetrical, although these changes can be difficult to assess. These horses may also have upward fixation of the patella due to the altered position of the femur to the quadriceps muscle mass. In horses that have landed on their side and fractured the acetabular cup by punching the femoral head inwards, there can be few signs except severe pain. A rectal examination may identify swelling or sharp bone edges around the dorsal axial surface of the acetabulum, but often it is the ventral portion of the cup that is fractured, which cannot be palpated. If the horse is able to move then crepitus may be appreciated either externally or during the rectal examination. As with all pelvic fractures there is marked-to-severe muscle spasm and guarding with marked pain, which may be mistaken for severe exertional rhabdomyolysis.

Diagnosis

Diagnostic imaging techniques that may be used in these cases include ultrasonography, nuclear scintigraphy and radiography. Ultrasonography can be disappointing as many of the fracture configurations are not accessible for scanning. However, most commonly with dislocated coxofemoral joints or comminuted fractures, there will be a loss of the normal relationship between the femoral head and dorsal acetabular rim or it may not be possible to identify the joint at all due to shadowing from the greater trochanter. If the joint is intact, distension of the joint may be identifiable. Rectal ultrasonography may also be beneficial in identifying callus or incontinuities on the axial margin of the acetabulm. Nuclear scintigraphy can also be disappointing in these cases, particularly if performed close to the inciting incident, as discussed above. Generally there should be a minimum delay of 5–7 days and preferably 14 days before performing the scan. The most common positive finding is a localised moderate-to-marked increased radiopharmaceutical uptake around the joint. Oblique, dorsal and caudal views may be required to definitively determine that the uptake is actually associated with the joint. Radiography, as with fractures of the *tuber ischii*, requires a high-power generator, but can be very useful in identifying fractures. The use of an oblique lateral view in the standing horse has proved useful [8] (see Figure 13.6) in identifying traumatic injury to the coxofemoral joint. The main limitation of radiography and scintigraphy is the necessity to move the horse, which is often not possible, due to a persistent non-weight-bearing lameness.

Treatment and Prognosis

The prognosis for dislocation or fracture of the coxofemoral joint in the adult horse is grave in most cases. General anaesthesia and reduction of the dislocation have been described, but in most cases reduction is not achieved or is unstable, and dislocation recurs on recovery or shortly afterwards. Fractures of the coxofemoral joint, even if stable and non-displaced, will ultimately lead to significant osteoarthritis of the joint and permanent lameness.

Multiple, Complex, Comminuted Fractures of the Pelvis

Presentation and Clinical Signs

Obviously any combination of fractures of the pelvis can occur if sufficient trauma is imparted to the horse. Severe fractures involving the acetabulum and iliac shaft after a fall may result in the horse remaining recumbent and apparently being unable to rise. This is presumably because of the severe pain, in addition to instability of the coxofemoral joint on the affected side. These fractures will often be associated with intense haemorrhage and a shock-like state may ensue. The horse may attempt and attain the 'dog-sit' position only to fall back down to the ground. The signs can mimic those of a spinal fracture with partial or total transection of the spinal cord, but careful examination of tone in the limbs and tail may show the normal spinal reflexes to be intact, although in 'shocked' horses this is sometimes not the case. Rectal examination in a recumbent horse in distress is dangerous and

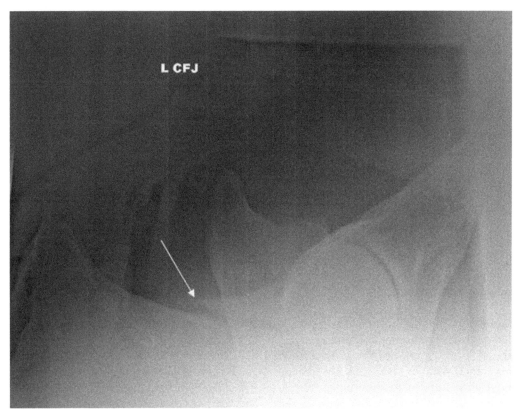

Figure 13.6 A radiograph demonstrating a fracture of the tuber ischii. This radiograph is obtained by using a standing oblique radiographic projection. Here a fracture of the ischium (white arrow) is seen extending into the coxofemoral joint.

should not be attempted, and it is sometimes impossible to make an antemortem diagnosis. If severe unilateral fracture is present, the horse may well be able to rise if rolled over on to the other side and this should be attempted, with care, before consideration of euthanasia [3].

Where the horse is able to rise, it will show a severe unilateral or bilateral hindlimb lameness and unwillingness to move. Combinations of one or more of the clinical signs described in the previous section may be present, which will aid in the assessment of viability of treatment.

Diagnosis

The diagnosis of a complicated fracture is made using a combination of clinical signs, radiography, nuclear scintigraphy and ultrasonography.

Treatment and Prognosis

The basic principles of treatment of pelvic fracture have been described in detail [5] and in an earlier section in this chapter. Essentially, the treatment is almost always conservative, with box rest for a minimum of 8–12 weeks, with a recommended period of 3–4 weeks cross-tying of the horse. As previously stated, careful thought should be given to the likely end-result of treatment in cases of severe or multiple pelvic fracture at the outset.

Sacral Fractures

Presentation and Clinical Signs

These can occur either alone or in combination with fractures to one or both iliac wings. As a result of the important nerves that exit from the spine in this region, the sacral fracture can be accompanied by a variable set of neurological symptoms (Chapter 3). Fractures situated cranially in the sacrum may cause nerve root injuries of the entire cauda equina, which may have symptoms in the pelvic limbs, as well as the normal cauda equina complex of urinary incontinence, flaccid paralysis of the anal ring and paralysis of the tail. Fractures situated more caudally often involve only symptoms involving urination, defecation and loss of skin tone around the perineum, in association with flaccid paralysis of the tail. In the mare the flaccid paralysis of the vulva can cause abrupt and marked pneumovagina, which can be distressing to the horse and produce an excitable fear-response behaviour. Urinary dribbling will be noted and rectal examination often reveals faecal accumulation within the rectum.

Diagnosis

Horses affected with complete displaced fracture of the sacrum have a characteristic appearance with an abrupt angle change visible just caudal to the tuber sacrale (Figure 13.7) and apparent hollowing of the

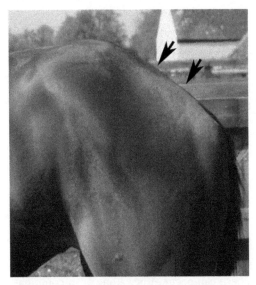

Figure 13.7 A photograph of a horse showing the pathognomonic clinical appearance of a sacral fracture, i.e. the abrupt abnormal angle change caudal to the tubera sacrale (black arrows).

caudal pelvis and coccygeal region. Radiographic confirmation of sacral fracture is difficult and not without significant radiation hazard. More specific information can be obtained from a nuclear scintigraphic examination of this site where images taken from the lateral, dorsal and caudal perspectives will give complete information for the site and severity of the injury. Rectal examination, both manual and together with ultrasonography using a rectal probe, can also be used to assess a sacral fracture, but great care should be taken as the rectum often 'balloons' and becomes atonic as a result of the neurogenic damage incurred. Ultrasound examination of the sacrum has been described [9]. Localised hyperaesthesia or pruritus has been reported following non-displaced fractures of the sacrum, which have healed and in which subsequent callus formation has presumably exerted pressure on nerves [10]. The formation of callus and scar tissue after a fracture may lead to the development of cauda equina syndrome some time after the original inciting incident. Damage to the nerve roots innervating skeletal muscle also results in very rapid, often very focal, neurogenic muscle atrophy, which will result in marked depressions in the contour of the quarters adjacent to the sacrum.

Treatment and Prognosis

Horses affected with the cauda equina syndrome must have supportive care. If the bladder is paralysed it will need to be emptied three times daily by catheter or an in-dwelling catheter left in situ. If the rectum is ballooned and atonic, as is often the case, manual evacuation of faeces will be required. This in itself is not without risk given the lack of tone in the rectal wall. Antibiotic cover with trimethoprim sulphonamide combinations is advisable given the urine stasis that will be present in the bladder. The urine soaking of the hindlimbs will lead to scalding of the skin if barrier creams and meticulous hygiene are not used. The tail can become very excoriated because of constant soaking with urine and faeces, and may require subsequent amputation. However, this is often best left until it is obvious whether the horse will recover some degree of function and not require permanent nursing care.

The medical treatment of sacral fractures has been well summarised [11]. Initially this consists of treatment to diminish inflammatory changes around the nerves such as intravenous DMSO drips and the use of corticosteroids and NSAIDs can be helpful from the acute injury to approximately 14 days after injury. At this stage, it is considered that the inflammatory effect on the nerves will have diminished and, if neurological symptoms persist after this time, they are likely to be the result of partial or complete transection of the nerves rather than neuropraxia. In this situation axon re-growth is reported to occur at approximately 1 mm/day and the practicality of salvaging the horse depends on the length of the nerve that has to re-grow. It has been suggested that, if there is no improvement in the condition after 2 months from the date of the original injury, nerve damage may be permanent, requiring long-term intensive care [11]. Surgical decompression of the sacrum has been described as a treatment for a chronic sacral fracture that led to permanent pruritus on the croup. In this description the tail was also amputated and the horse made a complete recovery [10].

The prognosis is obviously dependent on the site and severity of the sacral fracture, in conjunction with the willingness of the connections of the horse to undertake prolonged intensive and expensive medical care to allow recovery.

Coccygeal Fractures

Presentation and Clinical Signs

These fractures can follow the horse rearing up and landing on the posterior aspect of the coccyx and can occur together with ischial fractures. Usually there is some degree of flaccid paralysis of the tail and an area of hyperaesthesia immediately proximal to the fracture site where the horse is extremely resistant to manual palpation. In the filly the tail may become soaked in urine because of the horse's inability to raise the tail during urination, and remedial steps have to be taken to avoid scalding in this situation. The horse may appear agitated and ill at ease and may mimic the signs of exercise-induced rhabdomyolysis or colic. Fractures can occur at any site but the most common is Cy1–2.

Diagnosis

Radiography of the coccyx is relatively easily carried out. The tail hairs can be used to extend the coccygeal vertebrae horizontally so that they can be imaged in the standing lateral position. Nuclear scintigraphy may be helpful and indicated in cases of suspected incomplete fracture if there is a specific pain response to palpation.

The innervation of the coccygeal muscles is derived from the coccygeal nerves. There are normally five pairs of these, the dorsal and ventral branches of which anastomose to run as nerve trunks immediately adjacent to the vertebrae on either side of the tail. Obviously the specific site and severity of injury will determine the degree of atonia and lack of sensation in the tail. The apparent flaccid paralysis may resolve fairly speedily if there is no involvement of the sacrum, and is often the result of neuropraxia after acute swelling rather than complete transection of the nerves.

Treatment and Prognosis

As long as there has not been complete severance of the nerves the horse normally regains control of the tail within a period of 2–6 weeks once the swelling and pressure changes subside. If the nerves are severed, full function may take much longer to return and some degree of dysfunction become permanent. Healing is often accompanied with a subsequent malangulation of the coccygeal vertebrae, but this does not appear to interfere with the horse's athletic function in many cases and the prognosis is usually favourable.

13.2 Over Riding Dorsal Spinous Processes ('Kissing Spines')

Frances M.D. Henson and Jessica Kidd

Anatomy of the Dorsal Spinous Processes

As discussed in Chapter 2, a typical thoracic vertebra is made up of a vertebral body, a vertebral arch and vertebral processes. The vertebral processes include the dorsal spinous processes (DSPs), the transverse processes (TPs) and the articular processes (APs). The DSPs project dorsally and are believed to serve an important function as levers for the soft tissue attachments of the vertebral column.

Each DSP arises from a separate vertebra and therefore each has its own theoretical space above the vertebra. In the normal horse, there is a gap between each DSP, visible on lateromedial radiography. The size of the 'normal' gap is more than 5–7 mm. However, in many cases the DSPs do not have separate space in the back, but make contact with adjacent vertebra – impinging or overriding dorsal spinous processes (ORDSPs). In severe cases of overcrowding the DSPs overlap. When two DSPs are sufficiently close together, a false joint will eventually form between the two bones in order to stabilise the interface (Figure 13.8).

Incidence

DSP impingement has affected animals of the equine species for many, many years with the condition even being found in the extinct *Equus occidentalis* [12]. In more recent times Jeffcott reported that impingement of the DSPs was the most common cause of back pain in horses [13], and this is certainly the authors' clinical impression. However, it must be emphasised that the demonstration of an anatomical abnormality does not necessarily mean that this is the cause of back pain in an individual and ORDSPs can be found in many athletic and performance horses with no clinical signs of back pain. Indeed the question 'Where is the source of pain in cases of ORDSPs?' is frequently posed. Some horses have ORDSPs throughout their athletic careers, with no obvious clinical signs of back pain. Indeed, in many cases the ORDSPs simply form painless false joints at the sites of impingement. Clearly not enough is known at the current time about the pathogenesis of the pain in this condition.

The formation of false joints between some affected DSPs is, presumably, a response by the bones to their unexpected proximity. These false joints involve the remodelling of both cranial and caudal DSPs, often in a very marked fashion. This remodelling usually takes the form of a flattening and widening of the opposing bony

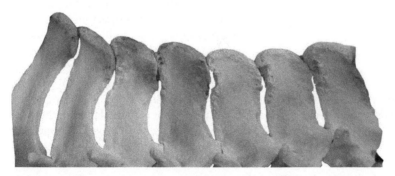

Figure 13.8 A postmortem specimen of the thoracic vertebrae T11–T16. There are overriding DSPs in all the bones. Note the marked remodelling at the sites of overriding T12–T16.

edges of the DSPs. Histologically, the false joints are cartilaginous.

Although the true incidence of pain arising from ORDSPs in the horse population is not known, the anatomical abnormality itself is extremely common. The anatomical incidence of ORDSPs has been described radiographically and postmortem. Postmortem studies have reported an incidence of between 86% and 92% [14,15], whereas radiographic surveys have reported the incidence of ORDSPs as 34% (normal horses) and 33% (horses with a history of thoracolumbar pain) [13,16]. There is a difference in incidence of ORDSPs in different breeds; the thoroughbred has a higher incidence of ORDSPs, possibly due to the shape of the summits of the DSPs (thoroughbreds have a markedly beak-shaped summit to the DSPs) and in horses undertaking different athletic endeavours. Jumping horses and dressage horses are reported to have the highest incidence of lesions.

Pathogenesis

ORDSPs may arise by a number of different mechanisms. In the simplest case the horse simply has a thoracolumbar spine that has the DSPs closer together than another individual; e.g. horses that are 'short backed' (Chapter 6) have to fit the same number of vertebrae and their DSPs into a smaller length than a 'long-backed' horse, and the ORDSPs will occur due to a crowding of the DSPs into the space provided. In other cases, the horse will have an apparently normal length of back, but the DSPs themselves are more markedly 'beak shaped', meaning that there is an increased chance of a DSP contacting the DSP immediately adjacent to it.

ORDSPs can also theoretically arise when the back undergoes excessive dorsiflexion (e.g. as potentially occurs in jumping horses) or spinal manoeuvres (e.g. as occurs in high-quality dressage horses). However, biomechanical studies have shown no evidence for increased movement in the T13–T18 region compared with other parts of the thoracolumbar spine and so this explanation may not be correct. Another hypothesis is that the weight of a saddle and rider causes a downward force on the T13–T18 area, consequently forcing the DSPs in this region to become close together. However, given that ORDSPs have been described in unbroken/unridden horses and horses that compete in athletic but non-ridden disciplines (driving, trotting races), this too seems unlikely.

Site of Pathology

Although all thoracic and lumbar vertebrae have DSPs, ORDSPs do not occur with similar frequency in the different areas of the thoracolumbar spine. They are almost unknown in the cranial withers region and are most commonly seen between T13 and T18 [16,17]. In 1979 Jeffcott [16] reported that soft tissue pathology in the back tended to occur in the cranial and caudal parts of the spine, whereas ORDSPs were centred around the midpoint of the back. The reason for this distribution is not known. It may merely be a function of the anatomy of the horse, in that this is the site that has less space per DSP in all horses. As stated above, this does not seem to be a site of increased movement that may cause the DSPs to move closer together, nor is it likely that rider weight has an effect.

History

Horses can present with ORDSPs at any age. In non-racing competition horses, there seem to be three categories of presentation: young animals (3–4 years) that exhibit clinical signs of back pain when broken in and first ridden, young competition animals (6–9 years) that fail to train on as expected and are found to be suffering from ORDSPs and older horses (10+ years) that have been competing satisfactorily and then begin to suffer back pain, apparently from ORDSPs. Any breed and sex can be affected, although thoroughbred geldings have been reported to be overrepresented in some case series [16].

Clinical Signs

As discussed in Chapter 6, there is a very broad spectrum of clinical signs pertaining to back pain and back pain due to ORDSPs presents in a similar fashion. The clinical signs of ORDSPs, in the authors' opinion, cover the entire spectrum of signs of back pain in the horse. In some horses there are apparently no clinical signs at the time of the examination (even though ORDSPs are clearly demonstrable using diagnostic imaging), whereas in other horses extreme reactions are demonstrated.

Clinical signs may include difficulty in posturing to urinate or defecate, or reluctance to lie down in the box. Some horses resent having rugs placed or dislike being groomed. Some find it difficult to be shod because they find it difficult to lift the hindlimbs or bearing their weight on one hindlimb for the other foot to be shod. Many horses are said to be 'cold backed', which means that they collapse downwards or occasionally buck when mounted or ridden and many of these horses may have clinical back pain that eases with exercise. Opinion is divided between clinicians, but some feel that back pain can also cause a hindlimb lameness and rarely a forelimb lameness. Generally, the hindlimb lamenesses associated with back pain are usually bilateral and of a low to moderate grade or may simply appear as an alteration to the hindlimb gait. If a horse has an appreciable unilateral lameness it is unlikely to have back pain as its primary concern. Some owners report that the horse simply is not interested in their work anymore or that they do not feel 'quite right' when ridden. The clinical signs are often significantly worse when the horse is being ridden and if an owner presents a horse with signs that are exacerbated by being ridden or only observable under saddle, axial skeleton issues should be borne in mind. Some horses show a reluctance to jump,

which may include refusing jumping completely or jumping with a very hollow back or an abnormal head carriage.

Clinical Examination

For the purposes of this chapter the authors are assuming that a basic examination will take place, as described in Chapter 6. The aim of the following section is to highlight any particular aspects of the clinical examination of horses with ORDSPs that are of importance.

A visual inspection of the horse is performed first. Assessment should be made as to whether the horse has a 'short-backed' appearance, indicating that a crowding of DSPs may be occurring. The musculature of the thoracolumbar spine should be visually assessed for evidence of atrophy or swelling. In cases of chronic back pathology and pain (and not exclusive to ODSPs), atrophy of *longissimus dorsi* is often noted, leading to the summits of the DSPs becoming almost visually apparent in some animals.

Once the horse has been visually examined, palpation of the dorsal midline of the back should be performed to identify the presence of any heat, pain and swelling, and to assess the flexibility of the spine. This is ideally performed in stocks, in which the horse cannot evade the movements required during the examination.

During the clinical examination for ORDSPs particular attention must be paid to the presence of any obvious areas of pathology in the midline region. As regards dynamic tests of back soundness, one of the most consistent clinical signs of ORDSPs is a reluctance towards/resistance to dorsiflexion of the spine (dipping). In some cases a marked response to this test will be seen, with the horse sinking to the floor. Often this reluctance to dorsiflex the back is accompanied by marked spasm of *longissimus dorsi* and/or a show of anxiety or bad behaviour from the horse. However, in some cases, particularly when the back pain is severe, the horse may not move the back at all in response to thoracic pressure, i.e. the dorsiflexion response will be absent. This gives the clinical impression of 'guarding' the painful site. The horse will often, however, appear anxious and unsettled during the application of the pressure.

Following an examination at rest the horse should be assessed in-hand at walk, trot and canter in straight lines and on the lunge. Ideally the horse should also be seen ridden with its normal jockey or another suitably experienced rider. Caution must be exercised before asking anyone to ride a horse that is known, by the veterinary surgeon, to be a danger to the rider or people on the ground.

Some horses with ODSPs have other areas of pathology, most commonly in their hindlimbs or pelvis. These sources of pain should also be identified if possible for several reasons. Treatment of ODSPs may be unsuccessful in the short or long term if there are other causes of pain or lameness that have not been identified. In the older horse who develops clinical signs of ODSPs in what may have been a previously quiescent back, another cause of pain or lameness may have been the reason the back has become clinically active.

Diagnosis

Once back pain is established the clinical diagnosis of ORDSPs should be made in two stages. First, any anatomical evidence of ORDSPs must be demonstrated and, second, the functional evidence of pain arising from ORDSPs must be demonstrated. As a large number of horses will have anatomical evidence of ORDSPs, as discussed above [18], with no signs of pain, the proof of functional pain is the most important diagnostic step.

Diagnosis of Anatomical Abnormalities

The anatomical abnormality of ORDSPs can be demonstrated by radiography, nuclear scintigraphy and ultrasonography.

The Use of Radiography in the Diagnosis of ORDSPs

The ease with which ORDSPs can be identified on lateromedial radiographs is both a diagnostic blessing and curse. It is a blessing because it means that lesions can be easily seen and clearly demonstrated. Conversely, it is a curse because this is often the only site that is investigated diagnostically by some practitioners, who wrongly interpret changes at this site as indicative of clinical pathology and do not go on to look for any other cause of pain. This leads to an incorrect diagnosis and, worse, in some cases, a needless and unsuccessful surgical procedure.

On radiography, DSPs are usually seen to be separate from their neighbours, with no evidence of remodelling or sclerosis on their cranial and caudal borders. When ORDSPs occur a number of radiographic abnormalities can be seen (Figure 13.9A). These include DSPs that are simply touching, DSPs that have sclerosis of their cranial and caudal borders and DSPs that have radiolucencies on their cranial and/or caudal borders (Figure 13.9B). In severe cases, marked remodelling is seen. These radiographic changes have been described by a

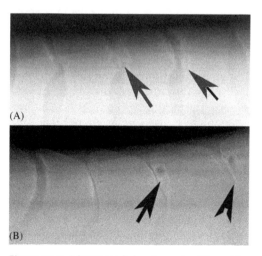

Figure 13.9 A lateromedial radiograph of the mid-thoracic region showing contact between adjacent DSPs. In A there is overlapping of adjacent DSPs (arrows) and in B there is lysis of the bone at sites of over-riding DSPs.

number of authors and grading systems introduced (Chapter 8); however, there is no evidence that the grade of the changes correlates with clinical pain.

It is useful to place radiodense markers along the back, which correspond to small clip marks in the haircoat. This makes anatomical localization of affected sites easier.

The Use of Nuclear Scintigraphy in the Diagnosis of ORDSPs

As described in Chapter 9, a nuclear scintigraphic examination can be very useful in the identification of active ORDSPs. Nuclear scintigraphy works on the principle that the radiolabel will bind to areas of remodelling bone. Therefore, physiological or pathological sites of osteoclast/osteoblast activity will be identified. Nuclear scintigraphy is, therefore, a sensitive indicator of active bone remodelling in the DSPs. However, it must be appreciated that active bone remodelling is *not synonymous with pain* [19]. Some horses with demonstrable pain arising from ORDSPs may have minimal increase in radionuclide uptake on a nuclear scintigraphic examination of this site, whereas other horses with focal areas of increased radionuclide uptake in the DSPs may show no signs of back pain.

On nuclear scintigraphy ORDSPs are detected by the presence of a focal increase in radionuclide uptake in the summits of the DSPs; this increase can be small but still clinically significant (Figure 9.7). Nuclear scintigraphy is also very useful to the veterinarian because it provides information on the presence of bone remodelling at sites other than the DSPs within the back and pelvis, e.g. the scintigraphic examination may reveal focal areas of increased radionuclide uptake in the DSPs but it may also reveal increased radionuclide uptake in, for example, the articular facets of the thoracic vertebrae [18,20]. This is important not only from the diagnostic aspect of the case but also from the treatment aspect, e.g. surgical treatment of ORDSPs is not recommended

by some in the presence of other concurrent back pathology [17].

The Use of Ultrasonography in the Diagnosis of ORDSPs

As discussed in Chapter 10, ultrasonography can be useful in the diagnosis of ORDSPs. It can be used to identify the summits of the DSPs on longitudinal section and to ascertain the distance between the DSPs. It can identify the presence of remodelling at the summits between the bones and can provide evidence of overlapping DSPs, as well as cases in which the supraspinous ligament is involved. The technique of ultrasonography of this site is detailed in Chapter 10. Ultrasonography can also be very useful in the diagnosis of active ORDSPs because it can be used to identify the spaces between the DSPs for placement of diagnostic analgesia.

Diagnostic Local Analgesic

Although the techniques described above can provide information about the presence of ORDSPs they do not provide proof that the ORDSPs are causing the clinical signs of back pain. To prove this, diagnostic analgesia of the affected ORDSPs is performed. Before placement of the local analgesia the clinical signs exhibited by the horse must be established. Thus, the horse must be examined in a reproducible manner, often including ridden exercise. The horse is then injected with local anaesthetic and the horse re-examined exactly as it was before the injection at 10 and at 30 minutes post-injection. The clinician and rider/handler, where appropriate, must then decide if there has been a positive response to the analgesia.

Anaesthesia of the DSPs can be achieved in a number of ways. Ideally, in order to avoid false-positive results due to diffusion of the local anaesthetic away from the DSPS, a small volume should be accurately placed between the affected DSPs. However, by virtue of the fact that these bones are overriding, it follows that the gap that should be the target of the anaesthetic is not present, so it is not possible, in such cases, to inject into the interspinous space. An infiltration of the soft tissues around the interspinous space is all that can be reasonably achieved.

The exact site can be identified radiographically and radio-opaque markers placed on the skin to provide landmarks for subsequent injection, as described above. Alternatively, ultrasound can identify the areas of ORDSPs. Once the anatomical site(s) has been chosen and the area prepared in a sterile manner, the local anaesthetic infiltration should be performed by injecting 5–10 ml of mepivacaine either side of the suspected lesion to a depth of approximately 5 cm. It is usual to provide analgesia to all of the affected DSP spaces at the same time for diagnostic purposes, rather than try to isolate any particular lesion.

Theoretically this infiltration technique could desensitise other structures in the region. The supraspinous ligament may well be anaesthetised, but a detailed ultrasound examination of the ligament can identify and rule out lesions of supraspinous ligament desmitis. Epaxial muscle analgesia may also occur, but it is considered that such focal anagesia would be unlikely to significantly affect injuries to such large structures as long as the horse is assessed in a timely manner after the block is performed. Similarly, placement of the local anaesthetic too deep may lead to inadvertent analgesia of the articular facets of the vertebrae. Pathology at this site should, however, be ruled out on radiographic and nuclear scintigraphic examination.

Treatment

Once a diagnosis of ORDSPs has been made, treatment should be instituted. A number of different treatment options are available including conservative/medical and surgery. Few detailed comparisons between treatment modalities have been reported; however, one comparison between medical and surgical treatment of ORDSPs was made by Pettersson

et al. [21]. These authors showed that surgical treatment was associated with a better outcome (72% return to former function compared with 22% for those undergoing non-surgical treatment).

Conservative and Medical Treatment

Conservative treatment of ORDSPs includes rest, physiotherapy and anti-inflammatory medication. Case selection for conservative treatment is relatively straightforward. It is usual to treat most cases of proven ORDSPs conservatively/medically in the first instance, unless there are specific indicators to the contrary. It is also advisable to be patient with conservative/medical therapy in those older horses who have clearly had anatomical ORDSPs for some considerable time, but who are only now showing acute signs of back pain. In these animals it is reasonable to assume that they have exacerbated a usually quiescent region and the aim of therapy here is to reduce inflammation and allow the horse to return to its non-painful state.

The aim of rest in the management of ORDSPs is to reduce the inflammation associated with the bone contact, bone remodelling and soft tissue damage. As we know that, given time, ORDSPs form a non-painful false joint, theoretically many horses should have the capability to progress to this state. However, not all horses/owners/trainers have the time and/or inclination to undertake prolonged rest. Rest to reduce inflammation alone should be of sufficient length to be beneficial (between 3 and 9 months rest may be necessary). It is recommended that this rest be combined with oral, systemic, non-steroidal anti-inflammatory drugs (NSAIDs) in order to reduce inflammation at the sites of contact. Physiotherapy and rehabilitation therapy can also be helpful in these cases with exercises such as repeated ventroflexion exercises aimed at 'opening up' the back (Chapters 16 and 17).

More direct medical treatment of ORDSPs is also widely used, particularly in competition horses that are required to continue performing. Intralesional medication may be anti-inflammatory (e.g. corticosteroids) or analgesic (e.g. Sarapin injection). Corticosteroids are a potent anti-inflammatory and can be injected between DSPs or adjacent to ORDSPs if the interspinous space is no longer present. The dose of corticosteroid used depends on the number of DSPs affected and the drug used. A number of different drug doses have been reported including 10 mg triamcinolone or 40–60 mg methylprednisolone acetate or 0.5–1.0 mg flumethasone or 1.5–2.5 mg dexamethasone per space [17,19]. In competition horses the rules of the organisation under which the horse competes must be observed regarding drug withdrawal times.

An alternative to corticosteroid treatment is the use of intralesional Sarapin, a sterile aqueous solution of soluble salts of the volatile bases from *Sarraceniaceae* species (pitcher plant). Sarapin is believed to exert its action by blocking pain from the affected site by an, as yet, unknown mechanism. It is administered in a similar fashion to the corticosteroids described above. It is reported to provide long-term analgesia in some horses, but is not, however, licensed for such use.

In addition to these intralesional medications other treatment techniques have been described. The use of mesotherapy to treat back pain is well established in Europe. Mesotherapy relies on the principle of inhibition of nerves carrying painful information from the deep structures within a spinal segment by the stimulation of nerves from more superficial structures. Mesotherapy is performed by administering multiple intradermal injections of saline/corticosteroid/local anaesthetic at the level of the lesion and caudal to it [19]. This therapy is reported to be very beneficial in some patients. Acupuncture may exert an effect in a similar way.

Extracorporeal shock wave therapy (SWT) may also be beneficial in treating cases of ORDSPs. SWT uses high-energy ultrasonic acoustic radiation to impart energy into tissues under treatment. In horses it is used particularly in the treatment of ligamentous insertion pathology, e.g. proximal suspensory desmitis. However, it is believed to have analgesic properties and may help to provide analgesia to sites of pain. The exact mechanism by which SWT works is not known; however, a number of theories have been discussed, including the idea that microtrauma caused by repeated shock waves in the affected area induces neovascularisation and promotes an environment more conducive for healing. In the treatment of ORDSPs it is recommended that the horse repeat three treatments with SWT, 7–10 days apart on three occasions before being reassessed for an improvement.

Surgical Treatment

The standard surgical treatment of ORDSPs is based on the removal of DSPs that have been identified to be causing a clinical problem using the diagnostic procedures described above. This procedure was first described by Roberts [22], and later by a number of other authors. More recently, a less invasive surgical procedure, desmotomy of the interspinous ligament, has also been described [23]. When considering surgical treatment of ORDSPs, *case selection is extremely important to the success of this surgery*. It is vital to be certain that the back pain is arising from those DSPs to be treated and that there is no evidence of concurrent pathology, or, if there is, the fact that the concurrent condition may decrease the overall effectiveness of surgery has been discussed with the owner. The presence of, for example, articular facet disease is considered by some to be a contraindication for surgery.

The indications for surgery are cases in which conservative/medical therapy has not worked and cases that would be considered to benefit from immediate surgical relief. There is no evidence in the literature that the prognosis after surgery is affected by the chronicity of the disease process.

Surgical Techniques

The original method of surgical removal of ORDSPs described removal of the affected bony portions by an open approach under general anaesthesia. However, an open standing technique and an endoscopic technique of DSP removal have also been described. At the current time the open, general anaesthetic surgical technique is most widely used.

Open Method under General Anaesthetic

Before anaesthesia the DSPs that are to be resected are marked using radio-opaque skin markers under radiographic guidance. The aim of the surgery is to remove as few DSPs as possible; thus if there are two or three DSPs in close apposition only one is removed; if there are four DSPs in apposition only two are removed.

The horse is anaesthetised and placed in lateral recumbency. Care must be taken in positioning the horse because it is extremely important to ensure that the spine is straight and free from rotation and that the skin surface of the dorsum is on the edge of the operating table. This positioning facilitates access to the soft tissues ventral to the DSP in surgery. The skin is clipped and prepared for aseptic surgery. Two approaches to the DSPs can be used. The authors prefer a midline incision made through the skin, subcutis and supraspinous ligament, although an incision just lateral to the DSPs has also been described [17]. (A slight modification to these techniques is the use of localised small incisions directly over the affected DSP, through which it is removed.)

Whichever technique is used the incision should be long enough to include one DSP cranial and one DSP caudal to the DSPs to be resected. The soft tissue attachments to the DSPs (supraspinous and interspinous ligaments and multifidus muscles primarily) are bluntly dissected away from the bone to a depth of 5–8 cm. The surrounding musculature is then held back from the surgical site using large retractors (hand-held or self-retaining depending on surgeon preference). The DSPs to be removed are then resected using a hand-held oscillating saw. It is important to ensure that not just the easily accessible summits are resected – palpation of the surgical site will allow identification of the areas of overriding and remodelling, and the surgeon should aim to ensure a minimum gap of 5 mm between the remaining bodies of each DSP [6]. Before closure it is often recommended that the top 5–10 mm of the adjacent, remaining DSPs be removed with the oscillating saw in order to prevent a large, step-like change in the contour of the back after surgery, or that the edges of the remaining DSPs be beveled for the same reason. The surgical incision is closed in routine fashion, including closure of the supraspinous ligament. It is recommended that the incision be protected in the initial postoperative period by a stent bandage sewn in place.

Endoscopic Method under General Anaesthesia

Endoscopic resection of the DSPs has been described by Desbrosse et al. [24]. This surgery is performed under a general anaesthetic with the horse in lateral recumbency. The affected portion of the ORDSP is identified endoscopically and removed with rongeurs and burrs. This surgical procedure has the advantage of being minimally invasive and may well prove to be the method of choice for resection in the future.

Ostectomy in the Standing, Sedated Horse

Subtotal ostectomy of dorsal spinous processes in sedated horses has also been described [25–27]. This procedure is performed in the standing horse. Analgesia of the region is provided by local infiltration of local anaesthetic solution (40–60 ml per site) around the affected DSPs and surrounding soft tissues to a depth of approximately 10 cm. The affected portion of the ODSP is identified and removed with an oscillating saw. This surgical procedure has the advantage of avoiding a general anaesthetic and its inherent risks and expenses, and is reported to reduce haemorrhage at the surgical site. It is feasible in most patients other than those who, even though heavily sedated, will not allow the local anesthetic solution to be injected at the start of surgery and thus will require treatment under anaesthesia.

Surgical Complications and Bone Reactions after Resection of ORDSPs

There are few significant complications of surgical resection of ORDSPs. The most common complications are wound infection with/without wound breakdown (reported as between 3.5% and 20% [21,28]. Swelling and seroma formation at the surgical site are also reported. In the authors' experience wound infection, although not common, can be persistent and require long courses of antibiotics and local treatment to treat it.

Longer-term consequences of surgical resection of ORDSPs are remodelling of the remaining, adjacent vertebrae, although this is considered to be reduced in subtotal ostectomy. In addition, there is new bone formation at the surgical site, although this is not of clinical consequence. The superficial cosmetic outcome can be excellent, with horses capable of return to a showing career if required. It is as yet unknown how the removal of portions of DSPs affects the overall biomechanics of the back, including the articular facets.

Interspinous Ligament (ISL) Desmotomy

Transection of the interspinous ligament between ORDSPs in the standing horse has been described [23]. This surgery is recommended to be used with a modified physical therapy programme to encourage spinal ventroflexion and build epaxial muscle strength. The initial description of this surgical technique reported good success and this technique is less expensive and requires less time away from ridden exercise than more traditional osteotomy treatments. The exact mechanism underlying the improvements in back pain are not known; the surgery may function as a neurectomy and is difficult to perform in cases with active impingement and false joint formation. However, a DSP resection can still be performed in cases in which the ISL desmotomy has not been effective. Until more outcome data are published, the true value of this technique remains unclear.

Surgical Outcome

Surgical treatment for ORDSPs has a favourable outcome. In one large series of 215 horses 72% of horses were reported to return to full use, with the treatment being curative. In the authors' experience this operation is extremely successful *if performed on genuine cases of ORDSPs.* However, given the limitations of the diagnostic techniques available to equine clinicians when compared with other species (no MRI or CT scanners for use on the backs of horses), there must be many cases that have concurrent pathology, which we just cannot locate at the current time. It is these individuals that will not respond well to surgical treatment.

Conclusion

ORDSPs are the most common anatomical abnormality reported in the horse with back pain; however, it must be remembered that a diagnosis of ORDSPs cannot be made on diagnostic imaging alone. Functional evidence of pain must be proven. ORDSPs can be successfully managed medically, but should this not prove successful an excellent surgical option for therapy can be offered.

13.3 Miscellaneous Osseous Pathology

Frances M.D. Henson

Introduction

In addition to the pathological conditions that are commonly reported in the back and pelvis, a number of other clinical entities are seen infrequently. These include:

- Anatomical abnormalities
- Degenerative conditions

- Infectious conditions
- Stress fractures
- Neoplasia
- Miscellaneous

Anatomical Abnormalities

From time to time the veterinarian will be presented with a horse that appears to have an anatomical abnormality of the back or pelvis. Often these will be foals or young horses that have congenital defects; in other cases the condition is apparently acquired. A number of different anatomical abnormalities of the equine back are recognised including lordosis, kyphosis, scoliosis and vertebral malformation [29]; abnormalities of the pelvis are rarely reported. The incidence of structural abnormalities is relatively low; Jeffcott [13] reported that these abnormalities accounted for 2.9% of a series of 443 horses that presented with thoracolumbar pathology.

Lordosis

Lordosis of the back is seen as a significant dipping of the back in the thoracolumbar region. The back of the horse follows a natural dip just after the withers but is then roughly horizontal, rising gently to the tuber sacrale. In cases of lordosis, however, this dip is exaggerated. Lordosis can be considered to be primary – when the horse is born with this condition or acquires it in early life – or secondary. To some extent older horses all develop secondary lordosis with age, acquiring a dipped back conformation over time, but it is more common in some breeds. In the American Saddlebred lordosis is present in 5% of horses [30] and has been associated with the inheritance of a recessive gene [31].

The diagnosis of lordosis is made on the clinical signs. Radiography of the thoracolumbar region may be useful to identify whether or not the abnormality is due to malformation of the vertebrae. There is no treatment for lordosis; some horses with mild lordosis can be useful riding animals, although others

cannot be fitted for saddles and/or are unable to weight bear comfortably.

Kyphosis

Kyphosis of the back is seen as a rising or upward arching of the back in the thoracolumbar region. As discussed above, the back of the horse rises gently to the tuber sacrale. In cases of kyphosis, however, this rising is exaggerated into a definite upward arch. This is usually most visually apparent in the lumbar region and can be difficult to identify in the cranial thoracic region.

As with lordosis, kyphosis may be considered a primary or a secondary condition. In the primary condition the kyphosis is present at birth or apparent in early life and can be considered congenital. It has also been reported to be associated with scoliosis (lateral deviation of the spine, see below) [31–33]. In most of these congenital cases it is due to malformations in the vertebral column, such as the presence of hemivertebrae [34]. Kyphosis has been reported to occur secondary to back trauma (e.g. fractured thoracic vertebrae [35]) and in some horses with bilateral hindlimb pain, particularly young horses – anecdotally, and in the author's experience, particularly those with stifle pain. This kyphosis disappears when the lameness has been treated.

The diagnosis of kyphosis is made on the clinical signs. Radiography of the thoracolumbar region may be useful to identify whether the abnormality is due to malformation of the vertebrae, vertebral fracture or other vertebral trauma. In addition, in cases of secondary kyphosis careful attention should be paid to whether or not hindlimb lameness is present. There is no treatment for primary kyphosis; most horses with mild-to-moderate kyphosis can be useful riding animals.

Scoliosis

Scoliosis of the back is seen as a deviation of the vertebral column from the midline when the horse is viewed from above (Figure 9.18). Primary scoliosis is reported in foals and young horses, often associated with vertebral body hypoplasia and hemivertebrae [36]. The diagnosis of scoliosis is made on clinical signs and radiography is very useful to determine whether or not the scoliosis is accompanied by vertebral body malformations, which are usually present. There is no specific treatment for scoliosis in the horse, although therapeutic manipulation may be of benefit in mild acquired cases [37].

Degenerative Conditions

Degenerative conditions are relatively common in the equine spine. These conditions include osteoarthritis of the articular facets of the thoracolumbar spine, ventral spondylosis and discospondylosis.

Osteoarthritis of the Synovial Intervertebral Facet Joints ('Articular Facets')

Osteoarthritis (OA) occurs at a number of sites in the equine back. Of these sites, OA of the articular facets of the thoracic and lumbar spine is quite commonly identified as a possible source of back pain, with articular facet pathology being most commonly diagnosed in the caudal thoracic/thoracolumbar spine at more than one anatomical location [38,39].

Articular facet disease is not straightforward. First, little is known about the normal ageing of the equine spine and how the articular facets in 'normal' horses change over time. Jeffcott [40] states that OA at this site is common in older horses, but that it is probably not clinically significant. Indeed, in the few studies that have been reported, the incidence of articular facet joint changes is high; e.g. in one postmortem study of thoroughbred racehorses, Haussler et al. [41] reported that 97% of the horses examined had a degree of lumbar vertebrae articular facet degeneration. Although the incidence of articular facet changes is high, the clinical significance of OA at this site is not fully understood, so the veterinarian must be

cautious about assuming that the presence of visible articular facet OA automatically means that this is the cause of the back pain in the horse. However, articular facet lesions are more consistently associated with back pain than ORDSPs, in both the author's experience and the experiences of others [19].

Denoix [42] reports that articular facet pathology in the lumbar vertebrae and the thoracolumbar junction is one of the most common spinal conditions associated with back pain. In humans, OA of the articular facets, ankylosing spondylitis and rheumatoid arthritis are all considered to be significant sources of back pain. At present it can be concluded that insufficient is published in the literature about this pathology and its clinical significance in the horse to be able to conclusively predict whether or not the presence or absence of articular facet degeneration is significant. However, clinically it is considered that evidence of articular facet degeneration is a significant finding in horses with back pain, especially when both radiographic evidence and scintigraphic evidence are available, indicating active remodelling at the site.

Diagnosis of Articular Facet OA

It is reasonable to assume that articular facet OA is more likely in the middle-aged to older horse as is true with all arthritic/degenerative disease in the horse. The clinical signs of articular facet OA are varied and not pathognomic. Most cases will present with a history of mild-to-moderate chronic back pain and poor performance. It is rare, in the author's experience, for these horses to show marked and dramatic signs of back pain. In many individuals, that animal will still be competing at the level at which it is expected to be, but with a reduction in results/placings/scorings. These signs are all typical of a low-grade, chronic back problem.

On clinical examination horses with articular facet OA show classic clinical signs of back pain, which will lead the clinician to suspect that there is genuine back pathology. OA of the facets is then diagnosed using nuclear scintigraphy, radiography and ultrasonography. However, although demonstration of pathological changes at the facets is straightforward, proving that they are the source of the pain remains virtually impossible.

A nuclear scintigraphic examination of the back is particularly useful in the diagnosis of articular facet OA because it will reveal the presence of increased radionuclide uptake over the affected articular process(es) and can provide valuable information on bone remodelling in both the thoracic spine and the lumbar spine. Uptake associated with OA at this site is usually mild to moderate in intensity and may be difficult to detect above the background uptake at this site. This mild uptake is in marked contrast to the high uptake seen at this site in, for example, lamina stress fractures.

A radiographic examination is essential for the diagnosis of articular facet OA. Dorsomedial–20° ventrolateral–oblique (DM20°VLO) views are recommended in order to visualise the articular facets (Chapter 8). Normal articular facets are readily identified on the ventrolateral–dorsomedial–oblique (VLDMO) views. In the thoracic region the facets are seen as 'L'-shaped joints, described as having a cranial oblique branch and a caudal vertical branch [19]. In the thoracolumbar junction and the lumbar region the joint spaces become more linear and are seen to run at an angle of 40° to the horizontal.

Radiographic changes associated with OA in the articular facets include loss of the joint space, sclerosis around the joint and new bone formation associated with the joint (Chapter 8). More detailed radiographic changes associated with facet OA and grading systems have been described [42]. However, it must be appreciated that identification of basic sclerosis around the articular facet and identification of new bone formation may be all that is possible in the standing horse with most X-ray machines in most clinics.

In addition to nuclear scintigraphy and radiography, ultrasonography can be helpful in the diagnosis of articular facet OA.

Transverse ultrasonography of the articular facets can produce good images of the region (Chapter 10). Although technically tricky, this ultrasonography may be useful in identifying dorsal new bone formation at the site, particularly in cases in which nuclear scintigraphy/radiography has identified a potential problem.

Although it is relatively straightforward to obtain diagnostic imaging evidence of OA in the articular facets, the interpretation of the findings can be difficult. Ideally, as at other sites of pain arising from OA in the horse, the response to local anaesthesia at the site should be ascertained before ascribing clinical significance to a lesion. Injections of local analgesia into the articular facets of the thoracic and lumbar spine have been described [43,44]. However, it is not an easy technique. The difficulties of using local anaesthetic to diagnose OA of the facet joints include the technical difficulty of the injection, although use of ultrasonographic guidance can be very helpful. However, placement of the anaesthetic actually into the joint is at best an approximation in most cases and should be interpreted as such. Other difficulties with the technique include the risk of local anaesthetic diffusing from the site of the injection to the spinal cord or outflow nerves. Such diffusion carries with it the risk of temporary paresis of the patient.

Treatment of Articular Facet OA

General treatment

Once a diagnosis of articular facet degeneration has been made treatment options must be considered. Unfortunately, there is no absolute specific treatment for this condition and it is often considered that management of the clinical signs is the most that can be achieved. To reduce the pain arising from the pathology, general therapies involve resting the horse to reduce the load and movement on the joint or in extreme cases retirement of the horse from the activities that may be exacerbating the condition. The use of systemic nonsteroidal anti-inflammatory drugs (NSAIDs) to reduce the inflammation around the joint is of merit in this condition, as it is in treating

OA at other sites in the horse. Physiotherapy and extracorporeal shock wave therapy have also been suggested to be efficacious, although there are no published data available on the effect of these treatment modalities for articular facet OA.

Specific Treatment

Specific therapies that have been described to treat articular facet OA include corticosteroids, Sarapin, tiludronate and mesotherapy.

Perilesional anti-inflammatory injections of corticosteroids, in a similar fashion to which OA would be treated elsewhere in the horse, have been described by a number of authors. Injection of the corticosteroids actually into the joints is very difficult, even under ultrasound guidance, although it can be done. Most clinicians inject into the multifidus muscle surrounding the articular facet, on either side of the horse, just 2 cm off the midline, preferably using ultrasound guidance. The injection should be performed under aseptic conditions and corticosteroids (to a total dose of 20 mg triamcinolone acetate or 140 mg methylprednisolone acetate per horse) administered. In competition horses, the rules of the governing council under which the horse is competing must be observed with regard to withdrawal times.

In addition to injecting corticosteroids, the use of perilesional injections of Sarapin is also common, based on the management of human lumbar facet joint pain in which it has been found that Sarapin can provide pain relief. Sarapin does have an advantage over corticosteroids in having no reported side effects in the horse. However, some clinicians have suggested that as multifidus contains proprioreceptive nerve endings that are important for vertebral movements, injections at this site are not recommended, although Sarapin is reported to have specific nociceptor effects. These specific effects are possibly based on an ammonium ion antagonism action, although the exact mechanism of action of Sarapin has not yet been elucidated.

The use of intravenous tiludronate (Tildren) has been advocated by one clinical research group [45], which reported promising results. This method of treatment certainly does have some logic because tiludronate is licensed for use in the treatment of OA at other sites in the horse, and this treatment may prove to be extremely useful in the management of this difficult disease in the future.

Finally, the use of mesotherapy to treat articular facet disease is well established in Europe and relies on the principle of inhibition of nerves carrying painful information from the deep structures within a spinal segment by the stimulation of nerves from more superficial structures. Thus mesotherapy is based on administering multiple intradermal injections of saline/corticosteroid/local anaesthetic at the level of the lesion and caudal to it. This therapy is reported to be very beneficial in some patients, with a substantial improvement expected in 7–14 days, lasting from 3 to 12 months.

Ventral Spondylosis

New bone formation on the ventral aspect of the vertebrae in the thoracolumbar region is termed 'vertebral spondylosis'. Although extremely common in humans and dogs, ventral spondylosis is considered to be relatively rare in the horse, with an incidence of around 3% reported [13,46]. Little is currently known about the pathogenesis and significance of ventral spondylosis in the horse and the interpretation of the clinical significance of the condition in the horse is extremely difficult. Indeed, even among experienced veterinarians dealing with a high caseload of horses with back pathology, there is currently no consensus opinion over the significance of the lesions. Some consider ventral spondylosis the condition to be clinically insignificant, and some highly significant, particularly if the lesion can be demonstrated to be currently active (see below).

Diagnosis

Ventral spondylosis does not present with any pathognomic signs. Clinical cases with ventral spondylosis have signs reported as reduced thoracolumbar mobility, *longissimus dorsi* spasm and back stiffness when ridden [46].

Ventral spondylosis is diagnosed on radiography and nuclear scintigraphy. Radiographically, ventral spondylosis is seen as a spectrum of severity of new bone formation ventrally on the vertebral body, associated with the disc space (Figure 9.8A). A grading system for new bone formation has been described [19]. In cases in which there is active new bone formation at the site, nuclear scintigraphy will show a focal area of increased radionuclide uptake associated with ventral aspect of the vertebral column (Figure 9.8B).

Although the diagnosis of ventral spondylosis is easy, given access to sufficiently powerful radiographic equipment and nuclear scintigraphy, there is, as yet, no method available for proving that it is the source of the back pain exhibited by the patient. Local analgesic techniques for this site are not described, so obtaining proof of the significance of the lesion is difficult. It is not unreasonable, however, in cases in which there are clear radiographic signs of ventral spondylosis and focal increased radionuclide uptake at the site and, in the absence of other back pathology, to consider ventral spondylosis as clinically significant. It has been proposed that ventral spondylosis is a progressive form of vertebral body OA [47,48] and that the spondylosis is painful only as the bony bridges form.

Treatment

There is no specific current treatment for ventral spondylosis in the horse. However, the general therapies that were discussed above for the management of articular facet OA are equally applicable. Rest, treatment with NSAIDs and physiotherapy should all be considered. Theoretically, on the basis that 'active' lesions are painful, once the spondylosis has formed the clinical signs should abate.

Discospondylosis

Again, compared with humans and dogs the incidence of discospondylosis is extremely low in the horse. It is likely, however, given the difficulty in diagnosing the condition, that subclinical cases are more frequent than currently recognised. In the horse it is considered that degenerative disc disease is extremely rare, but that disc degeneration secondary to external trauma may well occur. It has been proposed that trauma to the discs and associated structures, through falls and repeated, strenuous exercise, lead to progressive spondylosis associated with the disc.

The clinical signs of discospondylosis in the thoracolumbar spine are similar to those reported for discospondylitis (see below) but do not include the signs reflecting the infectious organism. The horse may show moderate-to-severe back pain and a variety of neurological signs. The diagnosis is achieved through radiography of the vertebral column, which should demonstrate the collapsed disc space and new bone formation depending on the anatomical site of the lesion. Nuclear scintigraphy is also useful in identifying any active bone remodelling associated with the pathology. However, the major diagnostic problem remains in the differentiation between infectious and non-infectious disc disease. There is no specific treatment for non-infectious discospondylosis in the horse at the current time.

Infections of the Back and Pelvis

Spondylitis/Discospondylitis

Infection in the back can be divided into infection within either the vertebrae (spondylitis/vertebral osteomyelitis) or the vertebrae and the intervertebral disc (vertebral discospondylitis). Both these conditions are rare in the horse, but often devastating when they occur. Spondylitis and discospondylitis are usually caused by haematogenous spread of organisms, usually bacteria. Both conditions are more common in foals in which there has been a failure of passive transfer. A number of organisms have been reported as being associated with spinal infections in the horse, including streptococci, staphylococci, mycobacteria, and *Rhodococcus* and *Aspergillus* species. Infective osteitis is extremely rare in the pelvis, although there have been isolated case reports, including infection of the pubic symphysis with *Rhodococcus equi* [49].

Diagnosis

The diagnosis of spondylitis can be very difficult because the clinical signs of osteomyelitis and discospondylitis are initially vague and can be quite variable. The early clinical signs of spinal infections are acute localised spinal pain and signs of systemic infection, which may progress until other systems become involved, i.e. neurological signs are seen, due to either direct spinal cord involvement or meningitis. The horse can present with a range of clinical signs including pyrexia, lethargy, and back stiffness with or without signs of nerve compression. Haematology may well indicate a leukophilia, neutrophilia and hyperfibrinogenaemia. If the infection is located close to the spinal column it may erode into the spinal canal and cerebrospinal fluid collection, and analysis may provide further evidence of an infectious process.

Diagnostic imaging may be very useful in identifying a lesion; radiographic views of the thoracic and lumbar spine may reveal evidence of infection. Radiographically, vertebral endplate lysis with sclerosis surrounding is seen, often associated with some ventral new bone formation [50], and in some cases the infection can be associated with a prolapsed disc [51]. Where available, nuclear scintigraphy should be employed in suspected cases because it is a very sensitive indicator of the bone remodelling caused by the infection. Nuclear scintigraphy will identify bone infection as a marked focal increase in radionuclide uptake.

Treatment

Unfortunately the treatment of spondylitis can be difficult and often unrewarding, particularly in cases in which neurological signs have occurred before a diagnosis has been made. Treatment relies on the use of long-term, high-dose antibiotics, anti-inflammatory drugs and supportive therapy where required [52].

Fistulous Withers

'Fistulous withers' is a rare condition that refers to chronic inflammation within the supraspinous bursa that runs over the summits of the DSPs in the withers region. Fistulous withers can be either primary or secondary. Primary cases are caused by inflammation, or parasitic or infectious diseases. In these cases initially the infection is within the bursa; however, over time the infected tissue ruptures and a draining fistula develops. In addition, primary fistulous withers can, in severe, chronic cases, lead to osteomyelitis and periostitis of the DSPs.

Brucella abortus and *Actinomyces bovis* are most commonly isolated from cases of fistulous withers [53]; however, in cases when the withers have become damaged by trauma other opportunistic organisms may be isolated. In addition *Onchocerca* species have been associated with the development of the condition.

Fistulous withers can also be seen secondary to trauma to the withers region, e.g. after a fracture of the DSPs of the cranial thoracic vertebrae.

Clinical Signs

The clinical signs of fistulous withers differ according to whether the lesion is open or closed. In earlier, closed cases the clinical signs are of a soft tissue swelling over the withers region that is usually associated with pain. In open cases there is an open, draining wound in the withers region, again usually with associated pain in the area. In some cases systemic illness is also present – depression, pyrexia and possible anorexia.

Diagnosis

The main diagnostic step to be taken is to ascertain whether the draining tract is due to a primary infection or whether there is some underlying condition leading to the formation of a draining tract, e.g. fractured withers. Aspiration of the fluid within the swelling is useful in closed lesions in order to identify the presence of an infectious agent. Radiography and nuclear scintigraphy can be used to rule out primary or secondary bony involvement and ultrasonography is also useful to determine the extent of the lesion and whether there are any, for example, foreign bodies within the lesion that may be causing the problem. Ultrasonography is also useful in more chronic cases in which the supraspinous ligament can also become infected.

In addition to the diagnostic steps outlined above, it is advisable to test whether the horse is seropositive for *Brucella abortus* because this is a zoonosis and subject to control measures in some countries.

Treatment

The treatment of fistulous withers can be very difficult and unrewarding. In simple cases medical therapy can be attempted. This usually consists of a long course of broad-spectrum antibiotics, e.g. trimethoprim/sulphonamide combinations [54], together with the use of NSAIDs and local anti-inflammatory measures such as hydrotherapy, hot packing and topical administration of dimethyl sulphoxide (DMSO). In unresponsive and/or severe cases, and cases in which there is bony involvement, surgical treatment may be necessary, which involves resection of the damaged tissue and excision of the DSPs of affected vertebrae.

Stress Fractures

Fractures of the back and pelvis are either traumatic, as discussed earlier in this chapter, or are part of a stress fracture pathology. Although traumatic fractures can occur in all types of horses, stress fractures are confined to those athletic horses undergoing strenuous and repetitive exercise and stress fractures of the back and pelvis are predominately reported in racehorses. There is a high prevalence of stress-induced pathology in racehorses, where 57% of the total fractures seen in racehorses are due to stress fractures [55].

Two sites of stress fracture of the back and pelvis are recognised: the vertebral lamina stress fracture and the pelvic stress fracture (discussed in 13.1).

Vertebral Lamina Stress Fracture

Vertebral lamina stress fractures (VLSFs) were first described by Hassler and Stover [56] in a postmortem survey of thoroughbred racehorses. A study into the pathophysiology of lumber vertebral fractures in the US has shown that overt lumbar vertebral fractures are the third most common cause of death of Quarter Horses in racing and that caudal lumbar fractures are likely to be progressions of pre-existing bone damage, i.e. part of the stress fracture complex [32]. VLSFs were reported to occur in the caudal part of the thoracic or lumbosacral spine and were seen in 50% of the horses examined. The site of the VLSFs is consistent between horses: they are found on the cranial aspect of the vertebra, near the junction of the articular process and the DSP, and they are continuous with the articular surface of the articular facet (Figure 15.6). These stress fractures usually continued on to the articular surface, leading to articular cartilage fissures and damage. VLSFs were found to be most common at L1, with a decrease in incidence either side of this segment [57].

Diagnosis

VLSFs can be diagnosed using nuclear scintigraphy, radiography and ultrasonography. A nuclear scintigraphic examination will reveal a very marked focal increase in radionuclide uptake at a very similar site to the articular facet, just dorsal to the vertebral bodies in the lumbar region. OA of the articular facets will also cause a focal increase in radionuclide uptake in this region, but the amount of uptake is marked in the VLSF and mild to moderate in the articular facet disease as a general rule. Radiography can be useful when the VLSF affects those vertebrae that can be imaged successfully (the thoracic vertebrae) and when the VLSF is associated with new bone formation at this site. However, it may not be possible to differentiate new bone formation caused by the VLSF from new bone formation resulting from OA of the articular facets in some cases.

Ultrasonography can also be used to identify new bone formation associated with VLSFs; however, the subtle fracture lines of the VLSF are not appreciable with ultrasonography in most cases and, again, it may not be possible to differentiate the changes from those associated with OA of the articular facets. Although it is clear that diagnostic imaging techniques do not differentiate clearly between stress fractures and OA at this site, the history and signalment of the horse should be very helpful in making the diagnosis.

Treatment
The treatment of VLSFs is, as with most stress fractures, rest. The horse should be put on to a reduced plane of exercise and the high intensity exercise stopped. However, as noted above, the progress of the lesion can be monitored scintigraphically.

Neoplasia

The incidence of neoplasia affecting the back and pelvis is extremely low in the horse. Primary osseous tumours are rare at any site in the equine skeleton and the vertebral column is an extremely unlikely site to find tumours, even in cases of skeletal neoplasia. Likewise the vertebral column and pelvis are unlikely sites to find secondary metastatic tumours. If a bone tumour is suspected, radiography and nuclear scintigraphy can be very useful to identify remodelling, new bone formation and bone lysis at the site of the tumour. At the current time the prognosis for neoplasia of the back and pelvis is very poor to hopeless, regardless of the tumour type.

Miscellaneous Conditions of the Vertebral Bodies

In addition to the conditions described above there are occasional case reports in the literature of unusual findings in the back and pelvis. These include incidental findings of vertebral body deformations (usually hemivertebrae), disc enthesiopathy (due to deformity of adjacent vertebrae) and dorsal bony extension of the vertebral fossa found in the caudal thoracic area. Most of these conditions are incidental findings postmortem and are not proven causes of back pain.

13.4 Pathology of the Supraspinous and Dorsal Sacroiliac Ligaments

Luis P. Lamas

Introduction

The spinal ligaments that have been most frequently associated with clinical signs of back pain are the supraspinous (SSL) and the dorsal sacroiliac ligaments (DSIL). Similar to many other conditions of the equine back, injuries to these structures often cause equivocal clinical signs, and defining the cause of the injury, the significance of any ligamentous damage detected and the best management of clinically proven cases of desmitis can be equally frustrating.

Supraspinous Ligament

The SSL is a strong fibrous ligament that inserts on the summits of the DSPs of the thoracolumbar vertebra and is the continuation of the more elastic nuchal ligament (Chapter 1). As it runs caudally it becomes progressively less extensible. It also is thicker in the cranial thoracic region and the lumbosacral area [58]. Important for the stabilizing function of this ligament are its multiple attachments to the tendinous portion of the *longissimus dorsi* muscles. It lies directly beneath the skin and a variable amount of subcutaneous adipose tissue. The ventral fibres of the ligament course downwards to become continuous with the interspinous ligament, which attaches to the cranial and caudal margins of adjacent DSPs.

Aetiology of Damage to the SSL

No controlled trials or models of injury to the SSL have been reported and therefore the aetiology of damage to the ligament is not known. However, there are a number of different ways in which SSL damage could occur:

- Tensile forces. The SSL will experience strain when tensile forces are applied. These forces increase during neck flexion and thoracolumbar ventroflexion [58]. Acute injures usually result from this type of strain.
- Direct compressive forces. Due to its proximity to the skin and saddle region the ligament is also under direct dorso-ventral compressive forces that can induce injury or remodelling of the ligament: this is especially relevant over the summits of the DSPs, where the SSL could theoretically become 'sandwiched' between the saddle and the bone.
- Enthesiopathies. Desmopathy may occur at the ligament insertion sites on the DSP where, in rare cases, avulsion fractures can occur.
- Pathology secondary to other conditions. For example, the SSL may become damaged in over-riding DSPs (ORDSP). Multiple sites of back pathology is a common clinical finding [59].

SSL injuries are reportedly more common at high levels of athletic activity, with most reports involving racehorses and show jumpers, although all types of horses may develop injuries to this structure [60]. A common presentation for these cases is a sudden change in behaviour during ridden exercise following a traumatic episode (e.g. fall, jump, stable cast). In less severe cases a reduction in performance or lameness might be the presenting complaint.

In the author's experience most cases of low grade or chronic SSL injury have a concurrent site of pathology elsewhere in the back. This suggests that biomechanical alterations following a primary pathology might lead to changes in ligament stresses leading to ligament damage. In the case of over-riding DSPs (ORDSPs) (see a previous section in this chapter), SSL damage occurs more commonly in the interspinous space where it is probably induced by the impingement and remodelling occurring in the region.

The importance of injuries to the SSL and its poor ability to heal may be overestimated. This opinion derives from the fact that induced injuries to the SSL and the disruption of its osseous and muscle insertions, as occurs during surgical resection of the DSPs, does not cause a recognised postoperative complication. This is despite massive trauma and disruption of the SSL during the procedure. Recently, a surgical procedure that involves transection of the SSL and the interspinous ligament at sites of impingement has been suggested to manage pain deriving from ORDSPs [23].

Clinical Signs

The clinical signs of injury to the SSL depend on the use of the horse and whether the injury is acute or chronic. In order to diagnose SSL desmitis a full clinical examination, lameness and back evaluation should be performed. The duration of clinical signs is usually long and cases often present after other management strategies have failed and localising signs have dissipated.

Acute Injuries

Acute injuries are usually accompanied by the cardinal signs of inflammation. Most cases are associated with an area of focal swelling on the dorsal midline; these can occur in any region of the back but are most common in the T15–T18 region. A variable degree of pain on palpation is usually present, but reactions may vary from horse to horse regardless of the severity of the lesion depending on the horse's temperament (Chapter 6). Local subcutaneous adipose tissue deposits or areas of fibrous tissue might cause a similar appearance to a swelling; these are non-painful but may cause a cosmetic blemish in show horses. Ultrasonography allows identification of these non-pathological changes.

A variable degree of unilateral or bilateral hindlimb lameness is occasionally present, although the relationship of this lameness to the SSL lesion is not known at the current time. This is usually exacerbated on soft surfaces and when the horse is lunged. Horses will resent tacking up and might have violent reactions similar to those seen on a 'cold back' horse. If no change in the horse's management has occurred in the same period as the onset of such clinical signs it is likely that this is pain related. A change in ownership or rider is often associated with a change in behaviour, and in these cases the presence of pain must be ruled out.

Chronic and Low Grade Injuries

Once rested and apparently recovered from acute injury, this ligament, like other similar structures in the body, does not recover to have the same physical properties as before injury. Thus the ligament is stiffer than before, leading to a higher chance of re-injury. A low grade pain response is often seen. Localizing signs might still be present and are usually associated with enlargement of the ligament due to fibrosis, but painful responses on palpation are not as evident as with acute injuries. Care should be taken to identify horses that have developed a hypersensitivity at the site of a previous injury.

Entheseopathies are often seen in association with other sources of back pathology. They often have little or no localising signs but pain on direct pressure on the summits of the DSPs might render a painful response. Many normal horses react to such a test, so this should be accompanied by diagnostic imaging of the area.

These injuries might have an insidious onset of clinical signs, are usually associated with hindlimb lameness and remain undiagnosed for long periods of time. Like other pathologies of the horse's back the presenting complaint is usually a reduction in performance. In the case of jumping horses an intermittent moderate to severe pain response following a jump might be seen.

Diagnosis

Ultrasound

Ultrasonographic evaluation is the most useful imaging modality for investigating SSL pathology. The technique of ultrasound of the SSL and the normal structure of the ligament is described in Chapter 10 (see Figure 13.10A). When SSL desmitis is suspected the SSL should be examined for the following ultrasonographic features: echogenicity, fibre pattern and size. It is considered that local thickenings of the ligament, alterations in echogenicity (hyperechoeic lesions (Figure 13.10B) and hypoechoeic lesions (Figure 13.10C)) and remodelling of the ligament are all indicators of pathology [61].

It has been suggested that thickening of the ligament and focal hyperechoeic lesions are typical of chronic lesions (Figure 13.10B), whilst hypoechogeneic images (Figure 13.10C) within the SSL are more indicative of acute lesions. However, an interesting study has found that variations to the normal echogenicity and pattern of the SSL can occur in the absence of back pain, and were not influenced by ridden exercise [62]. This demonstrates that changes to the normal ultrasonographic pattern correlate poorly with pain and a careful clinical examination (Chapter 6) is the key to an accurate diagnosis.

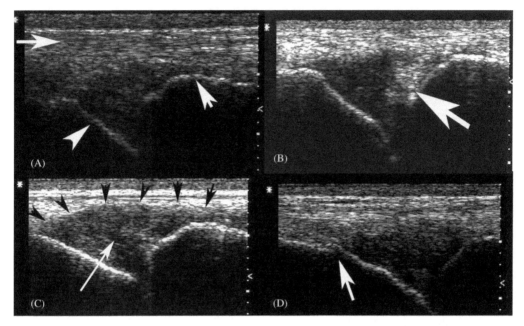

Figure 13.10 Ultrasonograms to show the ultrasonographic appearance of the supraspinous ligament (SSL) in longitudinal section. (A) The normal appearance of the ligament in longitudinal section. The ligament runs over the summits of the dorsal spinous processes (DSPs) (arrowheads) and is seen to be a horizontal structure. The fiber pattern is visible (arrow). (B) A hyperechoic lesion (whiter) within the supraspinous ligament (arrow) adjacent to a dorsal spinous process. (C) A hypoechoic lesion (blacker) within the supraspinous ligament (arrow). This hypoechoic lesion extends dorsally into the body of the supraspinous ligament (black arrowheads). (D) Enthesiopathy. The supraspinous ligament has been torn away from the summit of the dorsal spinous process and a small piece of bone has become detached (arrow).

Radiography

Lateral radiographs of the thoracolumbar spine should be a diagnostic step in all cases of suspected back pathology (Chapter 8). In the case of SSL desmitis, radiography can be useful in recognizing avulsion fractures that may have been detected on ultrasonography (Figure 13.10D), bone modelling and sclerosis of the dorsal margins of the DSPs that might be associated with SSL desmitis. Low exposures are used for this and, in the case of acute injuries, soft tissue exposures will reveal swelling of the affected area. Radiographic abnormalities present in the dorsal half of the DSPs justify ultrasonography of the SSL.

Nuclear Scintigraphy

An increase in radiopharmaceutical uptake at the site of insertions on to the DSP can occur in cases of entheseopathies. In cases of desmitis a diffuse radiopharmaceutical uptake pattern is sometimes seen on lateral views of the thoracolumbar spine. In acute cases where the horse is very painful to touch, this nuclear scintigraphy can be used to rule out fractures of the DSPs.

Thermography

Thermography can be very useful in the diagnosis of SSL injury (Chapter 11). In acute SSL the associated inflammation will cause an increase of skin temperature. As shown by Tunley and Henson, the imaging conditions should be carefully monitored to avoid artefacts [63]. The differences in temperature should be compared along the dorsal midline rather than to the surface temperature over the epaxial muscles, as there is a normal temperature difference between these two sites. Thermographic imaging only measures surface (skin) temperature, making it fairly non-specific.

Local Analgesia

Infiltration of local anaesthetic around the damaged area of a ligament can produce improvement in clinical signs. Approximately 5 ml of 2% mepivicaine (or lignocaine) are infiltrated on either side of the dorsal midline using a 1 inch 23 gauge needle. Injection directly into the SSL should be avoided. Evaluation under ridden exercise must be performed pre- and postanalgesia. Analgesia of a section of the supraspinous ligament is often unrewarding and non-specific as other structures in the area (e.g. dorsal spinous processes) can also be desensitised.

Management

Acute injuries

Like other acute injuries rest and anti-inflammatory therapy is paramount. In the first week following injury the horse should be box rested and systemic anti-inflammatory therapy (e.g. phenylbutazone at 2.2 mg/kg BID) initiated. Due to the superficial location of the SSL, topical anti-inflammatory therapy can be beneficial. In the first 24 hours cold therapy and topical application of a NSAID cream [64] will help resolve the acute inflammation. Feeding the horse from a hay net and a hanging water bucket will limit straining the ligament. Once pain on palpation is minimal regular hand walking should be encouraged. The change in clinical signs and the ultrasonographic appearance should be evaluated regularly in order to adjust the exercise level appropriately.

Once the clinical signs have resolved the aim should be to strengthen the epaxial muscles to provide more support to the spine [65]. This can be accomplished, for example, by walking and trotting on soft, sandy surfaces, swimming or walking in water up to the knees (Chapter 17). The total period of recovery can extend to a few months and care must be taken not to ride the horse too early as it may develop a 'cold back'. When ridden exercise is to resume, NSAIDs should be given to control any residual pain.

If clinical signs remain, it is recommended that further investigation is made once the inflammatory period has resolved (3–4 weeks postinjury).

Chronic Injuries

Apart from entheseopathies, chronic SSL pain should be managed with a paradoxical increase in exercise in order to increase muscle support to the thoracolumbar spine. A prolonged period (up to six months) might be required to accomplish full resolution of clinical signs. Ultrasonographic appearance may remain unchanged in the face of clinical improvement. If the horse has developed a significant behavioural response when being saddled a prolonged period of turnout might be necessary and rehabilitiation/retraining (Chapter 17) undertaken when the horse is brought back into work.

In the case of entheseopathies and the more persistent cases, local infiltration with corticosteroids can be useful. A total of 180 mg/500 kg of methyl prednisolone acetate should not be exceeded. Often two or three injections a couple of weeks apart are necessary before clinical improvement is seen.

Other Therapies

Extracorpoeal Shockwave Therapy (ESWT)

ESWT is used by some clinicians for the treatment of SSL desmitis. Conflicting results still exist in the literature regarding its effect on healing tissues versus temporary post-treatment local analgesia of the area [66,67]. However, horses undergoing treatment of suspensory ligament desmitis had a better prognosis if ESWT was used, although this study did not include a control group [68].

Mesotherapy

This technique consists of multiple intra-dermal injections with a 5 mm needle of a mixture or a single drug or drugs (steroid, local anaesthetic and a muscle relaxant) in order to mediated the responses of pain fibers; although the author has no experience with such techniques, they have been suggested by others [19].

Prognosis

The prognosis for this condition has not been reported. The prognosis depends on the concomitant problems in the back and hindlimbs. Full resolution of clinical signs can often be achieved, but many chronic cases have a frustrating progress with recurrence of clinical signs when the horse returns to ridden work. It is not uncommon for behavioural problems to develop unrelated to pain. Identifying these cases following an injury can be challenging.

Dorsal Sacroiliac Ligament Pathology

Anatomy and Biomechanics

There are three pairs of sacroiliac ligaments: the dorsal, the ventral and the interosseous. The dorsal sacroiliac ligaments (DSIL) are divided into two parts, a dorsal (or short) and a lateral (or long) (Figure 13.11). The dorsal portion is a strong cord-like structure, which attaches on to the dorsocaudal aspect of the tuber sacrale and on the abaxial side of the sacral spinous processes (Chapter 10). Dorsally it is intimately associated with the caudal tendinous portion of the *longissimus dorsi* muscles (thoracolumbar facia), and these two structures fuse in their caudal portion before inserting on to the abaxial surface of the sacral spinous processes. The lateral portion of the ligament is a triangular thin sheet that covers the sacrocaudal muscles. The cranial side inserts on to the caudal margin of the proximal ilium and the ventral side on to the lateral sacral crest of the transverse processes of the sacrum and is contiguous with the sacrosciatic ligament.

The sacroiliac ligaments stabilize the connection between the spine and pelvis and therefore the sacroiliac joints (Chapter 2). The dorsal sacroiliac ligaments prevent dorsal rotation (counternutation) of the pelvis. Thus, injury to the DSIL can lead to sacroiliac joint instability.

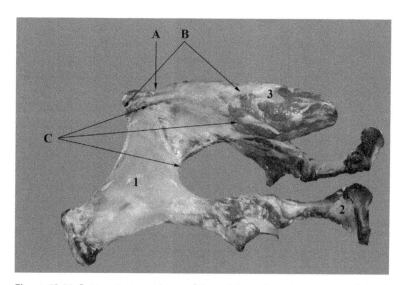

Figure 13.11 Postmortem specimen of the pelvis to show the anatomy of the dorsal sacroiliac ligament. Arrow A points to the insertion of the thoracolumbar fascia of the *longissimus dorsi* muscle. Arrow B points to the insertion sites of the dorsal sacroiliac ligament. Arrow C shows the triangular shape of the lateral sacroiliac ligament. 1: wing of the ilium; 2: ischium; 3: caudal sacrum.

Aetiology

Biomechanical injury to the DSIL occurs by excessive dorsal rotation of the sacrum about the pelvis. This can happen acutely following a traumatic injury like a fall or flipping over backwards [61]. Strains can also occur during exercise as the hindlimbs transmit their propulsive force through the spine mainly by the DSIL [58]. These forces are more dramatic during jumping activities and high-speed gaits [59].

As with other joints following injury to the stabilizing ligaments, osteoarthritis of the sacroiliac joint could occur following injury to the sacroiliac ligaments. This will aggravate the clinical signs and worsen the prognosis.

Pain or lameness originating from injury to the lateral portion of the DSIL has not yet been reported. This might reflect the difficulty in imaging this portion of the ligament. Biomechanically these two portions of the ligament come under tension with the same forces (counternutation) and such injuries may occur to both of them in the same traumatic event.

Clinical Signs

The severity of clinical signs depends on the amount of sacroiliac instability resulting from DSIL injury. As with other causes of back and pelvic pathology, the clinical signs of DSIL injury are variable and non-specific to the condition. Usually the presenting complaint is loss of performance or intermittent hindlimb lameness. On visual inspection, asymmetry of the *tubera sacralia* is a sensitive clinical sign. In one study, 33% (6/18) of horses with ultrasonographic abnormalities of the DSIL had a visible asymmetry [21]. If associated with acute ligament inflammation, pain on palpation is usually present. Manipulation of the pelvis to stress the DSIL can be done by placing dorso-ventral pressure on the caudal portion of the sacrum. Also, when lifting one hindlimb up in a similar way to a proximal limb flexion test, the horse might become uncomfortable on the weight-bearing leg and the lameness might deteriorate, as has

been described for sacroiliac dysfunction (Chapter 14).

The author performs relatively firm palpation on the abaxial side of each DSIL by reaching over from the opposite side of the horse, as part of a routine examination of lameness cases. Sensitivity to such palpation is common in horses with hindlimb gait abnormalities and is not per se indicative of DSIL pathology. No particular characteristic gait abnormality appears to be associated with horses with DSIL desmitis but a difficulty in maintaining a good-quality canter when lunged on a soft surface is a common feature. In some cases the tail may be 'clamped down' and the epaxial muscles may be very tense, suggesting a guarding of the lumbosacral region. Further deterioration in gait quality is expected when the horse is ridden. Ridden exercise should be performed by the owner and another experienced rider. Different saddles should be used if clinical signs are only obvious under ridden exercise.

Diagnosis

Ultrasonography

Diagnosis is based on ultrasonographic detection of ligament disruption. The ultrasonographic technique has been described in Chapter 10 and the ultrasonographic appearance of the DSIL has been elegantly described in three separate studies [69–71].

The dorsal portion of the sacroiliac ligament and the adjacent thoracolumbar fascia (Figure 13.12) can be followed caudally in transverse section from its attachment on to the corresponding *tuber sacrale* to its common attachment with the thoracolumbar facia on to the apices of the sacral spinous processes [69]. In its cranial portion the ligament is intimately associated with the caudal tendinous portion of the *longissimus dorsi* insertion, making them difficult to distinguish ultrasonographically. They gradually fuse to form one structure as they course caudally. The caudal insertion is on to the abaxial surface of the sacral dorsal spinous processes.

The cross-sectional shape of the dorsal portion of the DSIL changes as it courses

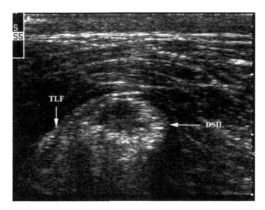

Figure 13.12 A transverse ultrasonogram of the dorsal sacroiliac ligament (DSIL). The DSIL is seen as a rounded structure (DSIL) and the thoracolumbar fascia is seen on the medial aspect of the DSIL (TLF). Note the central hypoechogeneic lesion (black) within the DSIL.

Table 13.3 Thickness at insertion and cross-sectional area of the dorsal sacroiliac ligament in different studies.

Thickness at insertion	Crosssectional area	Study
0.4 cm (02–1.9 cm)	1.9 cm^2 (1.1–2.4 cm^2)	[16]
1.09 cm (±0.07 cm)	1.1 cm^2 (0.89–1.59 cm^2)	[21]
0.6–1.0 cm		[2]
0.08–0.41 cm		[17]

caudally. At its cranial insertion it is a thin crescent-shaped hyperechoic structure underlying the subcutaneous tissue and the medial portion of the *gluteus medius* muscle. It then becomes round and close to the caudal insertion it becomes flattened and the lateromedially detail is lost. The echogenicity is homogeneous throughout the ligament, although a small hypoechoic area in the central portion of the ligament is a normal finding in some horses and should not be mistaken for a core lesion within the ligament. This presumably occurs as the thoracolumbar fascia and the DSIL are fused in that region.

Values for the thickness of the DSIL have been published in different studies (Table 13.3). The variation is proportional to the size of the animal. Measurement of the cross-sectional area of the fused dorsal portion of the dorsal sacroiliac ligament and the thoracolumbar fascia is subjective because of the difficulties in delineating all the borders of the medial extension of the thoracolumbar fascia on a single ultrasonographic image [69].

Pathology of the DSIL

Both an increase and a decrease in the size of the DSIL have been associated with desmitis, with the latter associated with chronic cases.

In longitudinal section the normal fibre pattern is seen to be disrupted (Figure 13.13).

The fibre alignment should also be evaluated in longitudinal images. It should be homogeneous throughout the ligament and quantitative methods of assessing fibre pattern can be used to evaluate damage and healing (Chapter 10).

At its insertion the ligament and bone interface should be carefully evaluated for signs of entheseopathy. An irregular shape of the *tuber sacrale* with or without avulsed osseous fragments as well as disruption in the fibre pattern can be seen in this form of pathology.

Due to the symmetry between the left and right ligaments, the normal variation of the ultrasonographic appearance of the DSIL and the low incidence of bilateral desmitis, a practical way of imaging the DSIL is by comparing left and right ligaments sliding the probe across each other at the same level.

Lateral (Long) Portion of the DSIL

The lateral portion of the dorsal sacroiliac ligament is visible as a thin hypoechoic line connecting the lateral portion of the sacral spinous processes and the lateral sacral crest ventrally. The lateral portion has been reported to be 4 mm thick [69]. Like the dorsal portion the size of the ligament is related to the size of the horse. Integrity of the ligament should be evaluated by continuity of the hyperechoic line. Although some fibre pattern

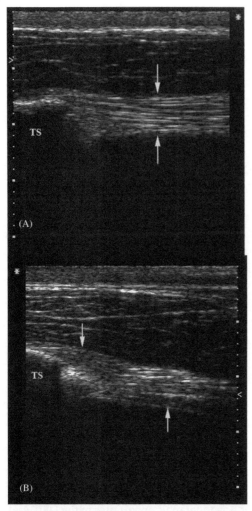

Figure 13.13 Longitudinal ultrasonograms of the dorsal sacroiliac ligament (DSIL). (A) Normal DSIL, margins delimitated by white arrows. TS: *tuber sacrale*. (B) Pathology within the DSIL. There is disruption of the fibre pattern and swelling close to the insertion of the DSIL (↓ arrow) and an area of fibre disruption in the body of the DSIL (↑ arrow).

is visible it is difficult to evaluate small areas of fibre disruption.

Radiography

Radiography of the *tuber sacrale* for diagnosis of enteseopathies is unrewarding because of the superimposition of both structures on lateral radiographs and difficulty in obtaining good-quality images due to the film-focal distance.

Thermography

Thermographic imaging of the DSIL can be a useful diagnostic technique (Chapter 11). One report found that 20/20 horses with ultrasonographic changes in the DSIL had thermographic abnormalities in the region [72], but no indication of its specificity was given. In the author's experience, thermographic imaging of the pelvic region must be carried out with care and over-interpretation avoided. An increase in surface temperature is expected in the acute stage of injury. The best way to detect this is to narrow the temperature range and compare the left and right regions for differences in temperature, rather than compare temperature differences to the more lateral portions of the gluteal region, which are normally at a lower temperature.

Nuclear Scintigraphy

Nuclear scintigraphic evaluation of the equine pelvis (Chapter 9), although extremely useful, can be misleading due the amount of soft tissue coverage of some areas [73]. Areas of increased radiopharmaceutical uptake over one *tubera sacralia* or any portion of the sacrum warrant ultrasonographic examination of the DSIL. Dorsal views, with the gamma camera parallel to the dorsal pelvic midline and centered over the sacrum, and with the camera parallel to the ground and centered over the *tubera sacralia*, are the most useful.

Local Analgesia

Local analgesia of the DSIL has not been reported. It is unlikely due to the size and thickness of and of the ligament that this may not be possible. Local infiltration may be attempted but a negative result should not rule out a diagnosis of desmitis. Local analgesia of the sacroiliac joints, however, is justified if ultrasonographic abnormalities of the DSILs are detected and sacroiliac joint laxity and dysfunction are suspected (Chapter 14).

Management

Acute Injuries

Management and treatment of DSIL ligament injuries in the post-traumatic period is based on rest and anti-inflammatory therapy. Strict box rest with regular hand walking for 10–20 min twice a day should be continued for two to three weeks. NSAIDs (e.g. phenylbutazone 2.2 mg/kg) should be administered for five to ten days. Topical NSAID (e.g. ibuprofen, diclofenac) can also be used during this stage. The horse should remain rugged in cold weather to improve blood flow to superficial structures like the DSIL. A few days after injury hot therapy may be started over the area.

Long-Term Management

The long-term management should include physiotherapy aimed at strengthening the muscles of the back, pelvis and thighs. This can be achieved by walking on sand surfaces, uphill work and swimming (Chapter 17). Ridden exercise should be delayed beyond resolution of clinical signs to avoid recurrence. The total recovery period can vary from three to six months and prognosis is likely to depend on secondary changes in the sacroiliac joint due to temporary instability.

References

1 Stover, S.M., Johnson, B.J., Daft, B.M. et al. An association between complete and incomplete stress fractures of the humerus in racehorses. *Equine Veterinary Journal* 1992; **24**:260–263.

2 Raidal, S.L., Love, D. and Bailey, G.D. Inflammation and increased numbers of bacteria in the lower respiratory tract of horses within 6–12 hours of confinement with the head elevated. *Australian Veterinary Journal* 1995; **72**:45–47.

3 Williams, J. and Dyson, S.J. Management of a recumbent horse. In: *A Guide to the Management of Emergencies at Equine Competitions.* Newmarket, Suffolk: EVJ Ltd, 1996, pp. 58–63.

4 Dyson, S.J. Pelvic injuries in the non-racehorse. In: Ross, M.W. and Dyson, S.J. (eds), *Diagnosis and Management of Lameness in the Horse.* St Louis, MO: Saunders, 2003, pp. 491–501.

5 Pilsworth, R.C. Diagnosis and management of pelvic fractures in the thoroughbred racehorse. In: Ross, M.W. and Dyson, S.J. (eds), *Diagnosis and Management of Lameness in the Horse.* St Louis, MO: Saunders, 2003, pp. 484–490.

6 Reef, V.B. (ed.) Musculoskeletal ultrasonography. In: *Equine Diagnostic Ultrasound.* Philadelphia, PA: W.B. Saunders Co., 1998, pp. 149–150.

7 Shepherd, M.C. and Pilsworth, R.C. The use of ultrasound in the diagnosis of pelvic fractures. *Equine Veterinary Education* 1994; **6**:23–27.

8 Barrett, E.L., Talbot, A.M., Driver, A.J., Barr, F.J. and Barr, A.R.S. A technique for pelvic radiography in the standing horse. *Equine Veterinary Journal* 2006; **38**:266–270.

9 Almanza, A. and Whitcombe, M.B. Ultrasonographic diagnosis of pelvic fractures in 28 horses. In: Proceedings of the 49th American Association of Equine Practitioners. New Orleans, LA: AAEP, 2003, pp. 50–54.

10 Collatos, C., Allen, D., Chamber, J. and Henry, M. Surgical treatment of sacral fracture in a horse. *Journal of the American Veterinary Medicine Association* 1991; **198**:877–879.

11 MacKay, R.J. The cauda equina syndrome. In: Robinson, N.E. (ed.), *Current Therapy in Equine Medicine 4.* Philadelphia, PA: W.B. Saunders, 1997, pp. 311–314.

12 Klide, A.M. Overriding dorsal spinous processes in the extinct horse *Equus occidentalis. American Journal*

of Veterinary Research 1989; **50**:592–593.

13 Jeffcott, L.B. Disorders of the thoracolumbar spine of the horse – A survey of 443 cases. *Equine Veterinary Journal* 1980; **12**:197–210.

14 Haussler, K.K. Osseous spinal pathology. *Veterinary Clinics of North America: Equine Practice* 1999; **15**(1):103–111.

15 Townsend, H.G.G., Leach, D.H., Doige, C.E. and Kirkaldy-Willis, W.H. Relationship between spinal biomechanics and pathological changes in the equine thoracolumbar spine. *Equine Veterinary Journal* 1986; **18**:107–112.

16 Jeffcott, L.B. Radiographic examination of the equine vertebral column. *Veterinary Radiology* 1979; **20**:135–139.

17 Walmsley, J.P., Pettersson, H., Winberg, F. and McEvoy, F. Impingement of the dorsal spinous processes in two hundred and fifteen horses: Case selection, surgical technique and results. *Equine Veterinary Journal* 2002; **34**:23–28.

18 Erichsen, C., Eksell, P., Holm, K.R., Lord, P. and Johnston, C. Relationship between scintigraphic and radiographic evaluations of spinous processes in the thoracolumbar spine in riding horses without clinical signs of back problems. *Equine Veterinary Journal* 2004; **36**:458–465.

19 Denoix, J.-M. and Dyson, S.J. Thoracolumbar spine. In: Ross, M.W. and Dyson, S.J. (eds), *Diagnosis and Management of Lameness in the Horse.* Philadelphia, PA: Saunders, 2003, 509–521.

20 Erichsen, C., Eksell, P., Widstrom, C. et al. Scintigraphy of the sacroiliac joint region in asymptomatic riding horses: Scintigraphic appearance and evaluation of method. *Veterinary Radiology and Ultrasound* 2003; **44**:699–706.

21 Pettersson, H., Stromberg, B. and Myrin, I. Das thorkolumbe, interspinale Syndrom (TLI) des Reitpferdes – Retriospektiver Vergleich konservativ und chirurgisch behandelter Falle. *Pferdeheilkunde* 1987; **3**:313–319.

22 Roberts, E.J. Resection of thoracic or lumbar spinous processes for the relief of pain responsible for lameness and some other locomotor disorders of horses. *Proceedings of the American Association of Equine Practitioners* 1968; **14**:13–30.

23 Comber, R.I., McKane, S.A., Smith, N. and Vanderweerd J.M. A controlled study evaluating a novel surgical treatment for kissing spines in standing sedated horses. *Veterinary Surgery* 2012; **41**:890–897.

24 Desbrosse, F.G., Perrin, R., Launois, T., Vanderweerd, J.-M.E. and Clegg, P.D. Endoscopic resection of dorsal spinous processes and interspinous ligaments in ten horses. *Veterinary Surgery* 2007; **36**:149–155.

25 Perkins, J.D., Schumacher, J., Kelly, G., Pollock, P. and Harty, M. Subtotal ostectomy of dorsal spinous processes performed in nine standing horses. *Veterinary Surgery* 2005; **34**:625–629.

26 Brink, P. Subtotal osteoctomy of impinging dorsal spinous processes in 23 standing horses. *Veterinary Surgery* 2014; **43**:95–98.

27 Jacklin, B.D., Minshall, G.J. and Wright, I.M. A new technique for subtotal (cranial wedge) ostectomy in the treatment of impinging/overriding spinal processes: Description of technique and outcome of 25 cases. *Equine Veterinary Journal* 2014; **46**:339–344.

28 Lauk, H.D. and Kreling, I. Surgical treatment of kissing spines syndrome – 50 cases. II. Results. *Pferdeheilkunde* 1998; **14**:123–130.

29 Rooney, J.R. Congenital equine scoliosis and lordosis. *Clinical Orthopaedics and Related Research* 1969; **62**:25–30.

30 Cook, D., Gallagher, P.C. and Bailey, E. Genetics of swayback in American Saddlebred horses. *Animal Genetics* 2010; Supplement 2: 64–71.

31 Gallagher, P.C., Morrison, S., Bernoco, D. and Bailey, E. Measurement of back curvature in American Saddlebred horses: Structural and genetic basis for early-onset

lordosis. *Journal of Equine Veterinary Science* 2003; **23**:71–76.

32 Kirberger, R.M. and Gottschalk, R.D. Developmental kyphoscoliosis in a foal. *Journal of the South African Veterinary Association* 1989; **60**:146–148.

33 Lerner, D.J. and Riley, G. Congenital kyphoscoliosis in a foal. *Journal of the American Veterinary Medical Association* 1978; **172**:274–276.

34 Wong, D.M., Scarratt, W.K. and Rohleder, J. Hindlimb paresis associated with kyphosis, hemivertebrae and multiple thoracic vertebral malformations in a Quarter Horse gelding. *Equine Veterinary Education* 2005; **17**:187–194.

35 Kothstein, T., Rashmir-Raven, A.M., Thomas, M.W. and Brashier, M.K. Radiographic diagnosis: Thoracic spinal fracture resulting in kyphosis in a horse. *Veterinary Radiology and Ultrasound* 2000; **41**:44–45.

36 Wong, D., Miles, K. and Sponseller, B. Congenital scoliosis in a Quarter Horse filly. *Veterinary Radiology and Ultrasound* 2006; **47**:279–282.

37 Faber, M., Van Weeren, P.R., Scheepers, M. and Barneveld, A. Long-term follow-up of manipulative treatment in a horse with back problems. *Journal of Veterinary Medicine Series A* 2003; **50**:241–245.

38 Girodroux, M., Dyson, S. and Murray, R. Osteoarthritis of the thoracolumbar synovial intervertebral articulations: clinical and radiographic features in 77 horses with poor performance and back pain. *Equine Veterinary Journal* 2009; **41**:130–138.

39 Cousty, M., Retureau, C., Tricaud, C., Geffroy, O. and Caure S. Location of radiological lesions of the thoracolumbar column in French trotters with and without signs of back pain. *Veterinary Record* 2010; **166**:41–45.

40 Jeffcott, L.B. The horse's back – soft tissue and skeletal problems – their diagnosis and management. Presented at the Dubai International Equine Symposium, Dubai, 1996.

41 Haussler, K.K., Stover, S.M. and Willits, N.H. Pathology of the lumbosacral spine and pelvis in Thoroughbred racehorses. *American Journal of Veterinary Research* 1999; **60**:143–153.

42 Denoix, J.M. Lesions of the vertebral column in poor performance horses. Presented at the World Equine Veterinary Association Symposium, Paris, 1999.

43 Vandeweerd, J.M., Desbrosse, F., Clegg, P. et al. Innervation and nerve injections of the lumbar spine of the horse: a cadaveric study. *Equine Veterinary Journal* 2007; **39**:59–63.

44 Manchikanti, L., Pampati, V., Bakhit, C.E. et al. Effectiveness of lumbar facet joint nerve blocks in chronic low back pain: a randomised clinical trial. *Pain and the Physician* 2001; **4**:101–117.

45 Coudry, V., Thibaud, D. and Riccio, B. Efficacy of tiludronate in the treatment of horses with signs of pain associated with osteoarthritic lesions of the thoracolumbar vertebral column. *American Journal of Veterinary Research* 2007; **68**:329–337.

46 Meehan, L., Dyson, S. and Murray, R. Radiographic and scintigraphic evaluation of spondylosis in the equine thoracolumbar spine: A retrospective study. *Equine Veterinary Journal* 2009; **41**:800–807.

47 Townsend H. and Leach D. Relationship between intervertebral joint morphology and mobility in the equine thoracolumbar spine. *Equine Veterinary Journal* 1986; **16**:461–465.

48 Haussler, K. Anatomy of the thoracolumbar vertebral region. *Veterinary Clinics of North America: Equine Practice* 1999; **15**:13–26.

49 Clark-Price, S.C., Rush, B.R., Gaughan, E.M. and Cox, J.H. Osteomyelitis of the pelvis caused by *Rhodococcus equi* in a 2 year old horse. *Journal of the American Veterinary Medical Association* 2003; **222**:269–272.

50 Sweers, L. and Carsten, A. Imaging features of discospondylitis in two horses. *Veterinary Radiology and Ultrasound* 2006; **47**:159–164.

51 Furr, M.O., Anver, M. and Wise, M. Intervertebral disc prolapse and discospondylitis in a horse. *Journal of the American Veterinary Medical Association* 1991; **198**:2095–2096.

52 Hillyer, M.H., Innes, J.F., Patteson, M.W. et al. Discospondylitis in an adult horse. *Veterinary Record* 1996; **139**:519–521.

53 Gaughan, E.M., Fubrini, S.L. and Patterson, M.W. Fistulous withers in horses: 14 cases (1978–1987). *Journal of the American Veterinary Medical Association* 1988; **201**:121–124.

54 Cohen, N.D., Carter, G.K. and McMullan, W. Fistulous withers: The diagnosis and treatment of open and closed lesion. *Veterinary Medicine* 1991; **86**:416–418.

55 Verheyen, K.L.P. and Wood, J.L.N. Descriptive epidemiology of fractures occurring in British Thoroughbred racehorses in training. *Equine Veterinary Journal* 2004; **36**:167–173.

56 Haussler, K.K. and Stover, S.M. Stress fractures of the vertebral lamina and pelvis in Thoroughbred racehorses. *Equine Veterinary Journal* 1998; **30**:374–381.

57 Collar, E.M., Zavodovskaya, R., Spriet, M. et al. Caudal lumbar vertebral fractures in California Quarter Horse and Thoroughbred racehorses. *Equine Veterinary Journal* 2015; **47**:573–579.

58 Denoix, J.M. Ligament injuries of the axial skeleton in the horse: Supraspinal and sacroiliac desmopathies. In: Rantanen, N.W. (ed.), *Dubai International Equine Symposium*, 1996, pp. 273–286.

59 Jeffcott, L.B. and Haussler, K.K. Back and pelvis, In: Hinchcliff, K.W., Kaneps, A.J. and Geor, R.J. (eds), *Equine Sports Medicine and Surgery*, 1st edn, Vol. 1Philadelphia, PA: W.B. Saunders, 2004, pp. 433–474.

60 Gillis, C. Spinal ligament pathology. *Veterinary Clinics in North America: Equine Practice* 1999; **15**(1):97–101.

61 Denoix, J.M. Ultrasonographic evaluation of back lesions. In: Haussler, K.K. (ed.), *Veterinary Clinics of North America:*

Equine Practice. Philadelphia, PA: Saunders, 1999, pp. 131–139.

62 Henson, F.M.D., Lamas, L., Knezevic, S. and Jeffcott, L.B. Ultrasonographic evaluation of the supraspinous ligament in a series of ridden and unridden horses and horses with unrelated back pathology. *BMC Veterinary Research* 2007; **3**:3.

63 Tunley, B.V. and Henson, F.M. Reliability and repeatability of thermographic examination and the normal thermographic image of the thoracolumbar region in the horse. *Equine Veterinay Journal* 2004; **36**(4):306–312.

64 Anderson, D., Kollias-Barker, C., Colahan, P. et al. Urinary and serum concentrations of diclofenac after topical application to horses. *Vet Theapeutics* 2005; **6**(1):57–66.

65 Stubbs, N.C., Kalser, L.J., Hauptman, J. and Clayton, H.M. Dynamic mobilisation exercises increase cross sectional area of musculus multifidus. *Equine Veterinary Journal* 2011; **43**(5):522–529.

66 Mcclure, S.R. VanSicle, D., Evans, R., Reinsertson, E.L. and Moran, L. The effects of extracorporeal shock-wave therapy on the ultrasonographic and histologic appearance of collagenase-induced equine forelimb suspensory ligament desmitis. *Ultrasound Medicine and Biology* 2004; **30**(4):461–467.

67 Bolt, D.M., Burba, D.J., Hubert, J.D. et al. Determination of functional and morphologic changes in palmar digital nerves after nonfocused extracorporeal shock wave treatment in horses. *American Journal of Veterinary Research* 2004; **65**(12):1714–1718.

68 Crowe, O.M., Dyson, S.J., Wright, I.M., Schramme, M.C. and Smith, R.K. Treatment of chronic or recurrent proximal suspensory desmitis using radial pressure wave therapy in the horse. *Equine Veterinary Journal* 2004; **36**(4):313–316.

69 Engelli, E., Yeager, A.E., Erb, H.N. and Haussler, K.K. Ultrasonographic technique and normal anatomic features of the

sacroiliac region in horses. *Veterinary Radiology and Ultrasound* 2006; **47**(4):391–403.

70 Kersten, A.A. and Edinger, J. Ultrasonographic examination of the equine sacroiliac region. *Equine Veterinary Journal* 2004; **36**(7):602–608.

71 Tomlinson, J.E., Sage, A.M. and Turner, T.A. Ultrasonographic abnormalities detected in the sacroiliac area in twenty cases of upper hindlimb lameness. *Equine Veterinary Journal* 2003; **35**(1):48–54.

72 Tomlinson, J.E., Sage, A.M., Turner, T.A. and Freeman, D.A. Detailed ultrasonographic mapping of the pelvis in clinically normal horses and ponies. *American Journal of Veterinary Research* 2001; **62**(11):1768–1775.

73 Erichsen, C., Eksell, P., Widstrom, C. et al. Scintigraphy of the sacroiliac joint region in erinaryasymptomatic riding horses: scintigraphic appearance and evaluation of method. *Veterinary Radiology and Ultrasound* 2003; **44**(6):699–706.

14

Sacroiliac Dysfunction

Leo B. Jeffcott

Introduction

Sacroiliac dysfunction (SID) is a relatively poorly understood condition in the horse. Historically it has been suggested that a diagnosis of SID was a 'dustbin' diagnosis – only made when no other condition could be found to explain the clinical signs of poor performance, lack of impulsion and mild hindlimb lameness exhibited by the horse (Box 14.1). However, studies have demonstrated a high incidence of pathological lesions within the sacroiliac region postmortem, which have made significant advances in our ability to establish a more definitive diagnosis of SID. A major obstacle to successful diagnosis has been the dearth of information on the biomechanics of the joint. The sacroiliac joint (SIJ) is particularly inaccessible due to its depth within the pelvis and the surrounding musculature, making it impossible to palpate the joint externally. Little is known about the three-dimensional movement of the SIJ in horses, and this has prevented the establishment of an effective model with which to study the biomechanics of this complex joint [1]. SID is most commonly seen in athletic horses. Affected horses are often older animals and it has been suggested that larger horses are more often affected. One study demonstrated that, in the UK, horses used for dressage and show-jumping are more prone to be affected with SID than general purpose or other athletic animals [2]. In addition, warmblood horses are more likely to be affected [3,4], although this may purely reflect the work done by warmblood horses in the UK. There is no reported sex predilection.

Anatomy

As described in Chapter 2, the vertebral column articulates with the pelvis at the sacroiliac joints (Figure 14.1A and B). The SIJ is a highly specialised point of contact between the two flat bony surfaces of the sacrum and the ilium. The point of contact is a synovial joint with some unusual histological characteristics. The majority of synovial joints in the body are formed between two hyaline cartilage surfaces; in the sacroiliac region the joint is formed between a hyaline cartilage surface (sacral side) and a fibrocartilaginous one (iliac side) [5].

Unlike other important synovial joints in the body, the SIJ does not have the advantage of osseous contouring to aid the maintenance of joint integrity, as is found, for example, in ball-and-socket joints. The morphology of the joint indicates that it is designed for gliding movements. This is based on suggestions that the sacroiliac articular cartilage may never be subject to full weight bearing like most joints. It is subject to shearing rather than orthogonally directed compressive forces [5,6]. The role of the SIJ is to transfer these forces from the horse's hindlimb to the thoracolumbar vertebral column [7]. To provide biomechanical stability

Equine Neck and Back Pathology: Diagnosis and Treatment, Second Edition. Edited by Frances M.D. Henson.
© 2018 John Wiley & Sons, Ltd. Published 2018 by John Wiley & Sons, Ltd.

Box 14.1 List of conditions that possibly show signs attributable to sacroiliac disease in the horse

'Jumper's or hunter's bump'
Thoracolumbar pathology (i.e. back problem)
Wing of ilium stress fracture (± sacroiliac pathology)
Other sites of pelvic fracture (tubera coxae, ischii, sacrale)
Fracture of wing of sacrum
Dorsal sacroiliac ligament desmitis
Sacrolumbar disc injury
Distal hindlimb lameness
Acute sacroiliac injury ± subluxation
Chronic sacroiliac dysfunction (SID)

---

to the meeting of two flat surfaces, the horse uses three strong sacroiliac ligaments (SILs): the dorsal sacroiliac ligaments (DSILs), the ventral sacroiliac ligaments (VSILs) and the interosseous sacroiliac ligaments (ISILs). These ligaments are discussed in detail in Chapter 2.

Incidence

Postmortem studies on horses have shown a high incidence (up to 100% in one study) of pathological lesions within the SIJ itself, most of which were degenerative [8]. Such a high incidence of lesions indicates that degeneration at this site is likely to be a significant clinical problem, although, at the current time, the exact progression from joint changes to pain and clinical signs is not known. Pain arising from the SIJ has long been considered to be associated with chronic mild instability of the joint, and this certainly fits with the other signs of poor hindlimb impulsion at slow paces. The pathology findings described at the SIJ [7] include enlargement of the joint surfaces, osteophyte formation, lipping of the edge of the joint and cortical buttressing. In some cases cartilage erosion is also noted, although loss of the joint space and ankylosis has not been recorded (in contrast to the situation in other low motion, high load joints, e.g. the tarsometatarsal joints). These changes have also been associated with the over-riding of the thoracolumbar DSPs and the lumbar

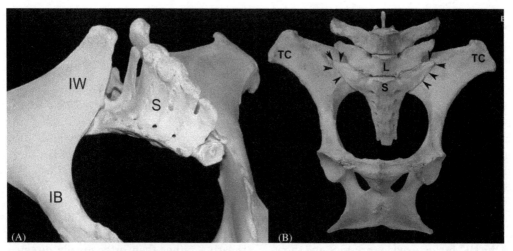

Figure 14.1 Postmortem specimens to show the anatomical position of the sacrum and ilium. (A) Caudolateral view of an anatomical specimen of the pelvis and the sacrum (S) illustrating the position of the sacrum within the pelvis, ventral to the iliac wing (IW) and medial to the iliac body (IB). (B) Ventral view of an anatomical specimen of the ventral pelvis, sacrum, sacroiliac and last two lumbar vertebrae (L) regions. The sacrum is positioned medially within the pelvis and articulates with the iliac wing. TC = tuber coxae. The position of the sacroiliac joint is outlined by the black arrowheads. *Source:* Courtesy of M.D. Whitcomb.

transverse processes, as well as with osteo-arthritis of the articular facets of the thoraco-lumbar spine, suggesting that alterations within the thoracolumbar area may cause compensatory SIJ lesions or vice versa.

Clinical Signs

Horses with SID can present as either acute or chronic cases, although chronic problems are far more common. Acute sacroiliac injury is usually the result of a serious traumatic injury, e.g. falling or sustaining impact. The clinical signs of acute sacroiliac injury include notice-able lameness and localised sensitivity to pal-pation of the soft tissues or tuber sacrale [9].

The clinical signs of chronic SID are much more vague and non-specific, and it appears that there can be two clinical presentations. These two variations of SID may, of course, simply be different ends of a single continuum, depending on the degree of bony change that has occurred. The first occurs principally in performance horses, still in work, where the main clinical findings are pain and poor performance, with the signs usually responsive to regional analge-sia [10,11]. The underlying pathology of these cases has not been established, but it is likely that they are associated with pain in periarticular structures rather than chronic bony changes of the SIJ. This may explain why there may be no significant asymmetry of the pelvis and the gait changes are variable.

The other, more debilitating, form of SID, resulting in poor performance and more marked gait changes with asymmetry of asso-ciated muscles and/or bone, has been reported to be associated with chronic pathological joint changes [5]. The clinical signs (Box 14.2) include poor performance, thoracolumbar pain [9], a failure to engage the hindlimbs, poor hindlimb action and lameness (either unilateral or bilateral), and the clinical signs are often worse when ridden, characterised by stiffness of the back and lack of hindlimb impulsion. A recent study has highlighted that the canter quality is worse than trot and horses often kick out or bunny hop in canter [3].

> **Box 14.2 The clinical signs reported to occur in horses with sacroiliac dysfunction**
>
> Reduced hindlimb impulsion
> Hindlimb lameness
> Stiff back
> Close behind
> Wide behind
> Plaiting
> Rolling hindlimb gait
> Reduced hindlimb engagement
> Poor-quality canter/breaks in canter
> Reluctance to work and/or work on the bit
> Resistant behaviour
> Poor quality lateral work
> Worsening of the clinical signs when ridden

In addition, the signs often worsen after a period of prolonged rest. Pelvic asymmetry, in particular tuber sacrale asymmetry, has long been reported to be significantly associated with SID [7]. Similarly, a close hindlimb action and dragging of the hind toes has been com-monly associated with this form of SID.

This lack of consistency in what constitutes the specific clinical signs of SID underlines the difficulties associated with making a definitive diagnosis. In relation to pelvic asymmetry the following guidelines may be helpful:

- Unilateral muscle wastage from one quarter without pelvic bone malalignment: *suspect hindlimb lameness (hock or stifle) or ace-tabular damage.*
- Elevation of one tuber sacrale ± gluteal muscle wastage: *suspect thickening and dam-age to DSIL* or *stress fracture of wing of ilium on opposite side (i.e. lowered quarter).*
- Lowering of tuber sacrale associated with muscle wastage and lowering of tuber coxae on same side: *suspect chronic sacroiliac disease.*
- Lowering of tuber coxae without lowering of tuber sacrale or ischii: *suspect fracture of tuber coxae.*
- Lowering of tuber ischii without deviation of tuber sacrale or coxae: *suspect fracture of tuber ischii.*

Table 14.1 The components of the SID scoring system DSIL – dorsal sacroiliac ligament.

Clinical sign	Grade
Pelvic shear	0-1
Close hindlimb action/plaiting	0-3
Muscle atrophy	0-3
Tuber coxae asymmetry	0-3
Tuber sacrale asymmetry	0-3
Left DSIL pain	0-3
Right DSIL pain	0-3
Left gluteal pain	0-3
Right gluteal pain	0-3

Of these clinical signs a number have been reported to occur with more consistency in horses with SID diagnosed postmortem, and have been used, with anatomical features, to assign an 'SID score' to horses (Table 14.1). The clinical signs that have been used as part of the SID score are close movement of HL/plaiting of the hindlimbs, pelvic bony asymmetry (of both tubera coxae and sacrale), gluteal muscle atrophy and a positive pelvic shear.

SIJ Provocation Tests

A number of specific tests to identify pain in the sacroiliac region and SIJ provocation tests have been described [9,12]. However, although these tests may well indicate that there is pain in the region of the SIJ in the horse, they are not specific for SID because other conditions, such as fractures (i.e. stress or traumatic) of the iliac wing, can also give a similar response. Tests to identify SIJ pain include the following.

Manual Compression of the Dorsal Aspects of the Tuber Sacrale

In this test the tubera sacrale are pushed together simultaneously. The aim is to bend the iliac wing and compress the sacroiliac articulation. Normal horses usually show no response, but SID horses show a pain response or even collapse.

'Sway Test'

In this test the horse has one hindlimb raised (i.e. like a flexion test). The horse is then gently rocked from side to side by the person holding the leg in order to produce movement in the contralateral SIJ. Normal horses tolerate this procedure well, but SID horses show a pain response or will refuse to pick up the leg on the normal side (in order to avoid shearing within the affected SIJ when the normal leg is raised).

Ventral Force

This test involves application of ventral force over the lumbosacral dorsal spinous processes (DSPs) in a rhythmic fashion. This test is considered to stress the ISIL. Normal horses should show no response and SID horses show a pain response. A modified version of this test is to apply the force focally over the DSPs of the sacrocaudal junction in order to specifically stress the dorsal portion of the DSIL.

Tuber Coxae Stress Test

This test involves application of rhythmic ventral force to the tuber coxae to induce general sacroiliac and lumbosacral joint motion. Normal horses respond with a smooth vertical motion of the lumbosacral region, while SID horses have a noticeable pain response and/or gluteal muscle spasm.

Application of Lateral Forces to the Pelvis

- Technique 1 requires that the ipsilateral tuber sacrale be pushed away from the veterinarian with one hand while the tail head is pulled towards the veterinarian with the other. This test is considered to compress the contralateral SIJ and distract the ipsilateral SIJ. Reversal of the movement distracts the contralateral SIJ and compresses the ipsilateral SIJ. Normal horses show no resentment to manipulation, but SID horses show a pain response. It has been proposed that pain on compression of the SIJ is more indicative of osteoarthritic changes, whereas pain on distraction of the joint is more indicative of ligamentous damage, although these associations have not been proved.

- Technique 2 requires that the tail head be pushed away from the operator while the contralateral tuber ischii is pulled towards the operator with the other hand, and then reversing the movement. This test is designed to stress the supporting ligaments of the SIJ. Normal horses show no resentment to manipulation.

Diagnosis of SID

The diagnosis of SID relies on a careful clinical evaluation and the exclusion of other conditions with similar clinical signs. However, diagnostic imaging modalities and local analgesic techniques do have an ever-increasing role, particularly with the improvements in technology and experience gained with their use.

Diagnostic Imaging of the SIJ Region

There is a range of imaging modalities available nowadays, although all have some limitations. Radiography and ultrasonography can certainly be of some benefit, but nuclear scintigraphy is considered the most useful aid to diagnosis.

Nuclear Scintigraphy

As discussed in Chapter 9, nuclear scintigraphy provides direct visualisation of the radionuclide uptake in the SIJ region relative to other areas of the pelvis, and allows an assessment of whether there is increased uptake at other sites in the back, pelvis or hindlimbs that may be causing the clinical signs noted in the horse. Both dorsoventral and oblique views of

the ilium are recommended in order to ascertain the positioning of areas of increased radionuclide uptake. The interpretation of scintigrams of the sacroiliac region is often not straightforward. The exact anatomical location of the SIJ on scintigrams has been described [13]. The joint itself covers a large area of the ilium, but due to soft tissue attenuation uptake in the more lateral part of the joint may be difficult to appreciate. An oblique view of the cranial pelvis may help in diagnosis and also allow better separation of any bladder shadow and genuine uptake within the SIJ itself. Analysis of scintigrams of the sacroiliac region is complicated by the finding of pathological changes in the sacroiliac region in normal horses [6] and the findings of significant overlap in the radionuclide uptake in the sacroiliac region in groups of normal horses [14] and horses with sacroiliac pain [2]. Also, it should be noted that there is an age-related change in the sacroiliac area [15].

Notwithstanding the problems of interpretation a number of attempts have been made to quantify uptake in the SIJ region using regions of interest and computer-generated profiles (Figure 14.2) to help with diagnosis. Although it is known that scintigrams of the sacroiliac region are bilaterally symmetrical and show little or no uptake in radionuclide uptake in normal horses, it is also known that there is significant overlap in nucleotide uptake ratios among horses affected with SID, normal horses and lame horses who do not have SID.

Ultrasonography

Ultrasonography of the SIJ region has been described by a number of authors [16] (Chapter 10). However, in the main, they have concentrated on the easily accessible DSIL rather than the more specific supporting ligaments of the SIL, and on the dorsal surface of the iliac wing to identify fractures of the dorsal cortices. The actual SIJ itself cannot be visualised by ultrasonography in its entirety, although transrectal ultrasonography has

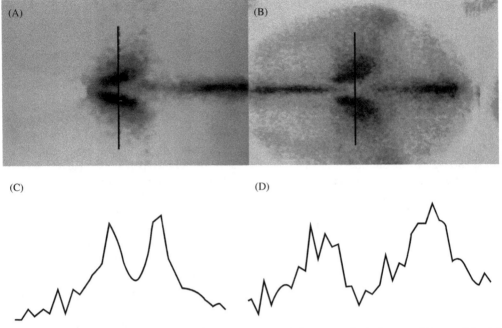

Figure 14.2 Nuclear scintigraphy of the sacroiliac region: (A, B) dorsoventral scintigrams of the cranial pelvis. (A) Normal horse: the paired tubera sacrale are seen as comma-shaped increases in radionuclide uptake either side of the midline. The black line through them is the reference line for generation of the profile of the region (C). (B) Horse with chronic bilateral sacroiliac dysfunction. In this case there is increased radionuclide uptake abaxial to the tuber sacrale at the site of the sacroiliac joint. The black line is the reference line for generation of the profile of the region (D). (C) Profile from (A): the normal profile is seen as a pair of peaks of radionuclide uptake. (D) Profile from (B): the abnormal profile is seen to have a wider peak of uptake associated with more radionuclide in the region of the sacroiliac joint.

been used to identify remodelling along the joint margins of the ventral border of the SIJ.

The ultrasonographic appearance of the VSIL has also been described using transrectal ultrasonography. In contrast there are no ultrasonographic descriptions of the ISILs. Unlike nuclear scintigraphy, ultrasonography is not a very useful imaging modality for the identification of SID.

Radiography

Radiography of the SIJ region is difficult, unrewarding and rarely diagnostic. A number of features conspire to make SIJ radiography difficult, including the depth of the joint within the body, the soft tissues overlying the joint, the artefacts caused by the viscera within the pelvis and the overlying bone of the iliac wing. Radiography of the SIJ is best

performed under general anaesthesia using ventrodorsal views. However, even when this is performed the resulting radiographs are frequently difficult to interpret in all except the smallest animals. A final complication of radiographic diagnosis of SID is that the radiographic features of chronic SID are non-specific and subtle, including non-specific increases in the joint space and enlargement of the caudomedial aspect of the joint. The use of linear tomography has been used with some success, but is really not a practical proposition nowadays because the equipment is no longer available [17].

Local Analgesic Techniques

The diagnosis of joint pain in lame horses usually relies on the response to intra-articular and perineural analgesia. However, until recently local analgesia of the SIJ was not performed due to its deep anatomical location and the difficulties in targeting the small, tightly bound joint capsule. In addition, the close proximity of the greater sciatic foramen with its neurovascular contents (including the sciatic nerve) and cranial gluteal nerve means that accurate placement of local anaesthetic solution into the SIJ is required. Inadvertent poor placement of local anaesthetic may lead to nerve damage, paresis and even marked lameness, and ataxia has been reported by a number of veterinarians.

A number of different approaches blocking the SIJ have been described, with and without the use of ultrasound guidance [2,9,18–20]. However, neither technique is 100% accurate in delivering local analgesia solutions to the SIJ – diffusion is seen within associated muscles and ligaments in experimental studies. Two techniques that have been reported are described below:

1) The dorsal approach: this approach aims to pass a needle down from the dorso-lateral surface of the pelvis, directly over the SIJ, to hit it just off the edge of the wing of the ilium. The technique involves the placement of a 20–25 cm spinal needle dorsally over the iliac wing ipsilateral to the SIJ that is being anaesthetised. The needle is directed ventrally and walked off the caudal border of the iliac wing in the region of the SIJ. A local anaesthetic solution is injected. This technique is easier to perform than technique 2, but is reported to be associated with a higher risk of significant ataxia/hindlimb paresis.
2) The medial approach: this approach aims to pass a needle down from just off the midline, between the divergent DSPs of L6 and S1, and into the space formed by the ventral aspect of the iliac wing and the dorsal part of the sacrum. This technique involves placement of a long (18–25 cm) spinal needle at the cranial margin of the tuber sacrale contralateral to the SIJ that is being anaesthetised. The needle is inserted along the cranial aspect of the tuber

sacrale, directed towards the greater trochanter of the femur of the opposite limb (at approximately 20° to the vertical). The needle is advanced along the medial aspect of the iliac wing (on the affected side) in a caudolateral direction until contact is made with bone. This should be near the SIJ margin. A local anaesthetic solution is then injected (20 ml). The response to the local analgesia is assessed at 15–20 minutes.

Management of SID

The treatment of SID remains largely empirical because of the lack of understanding of its primary pathogenesis.

Acute SID

In cases of acute SID the aim of treatment is to reduce inflammation at the damaged site and promote effective healing. It is recommended that the horse have a period of prolonged rest including a period of strict box rest for 4–6 weeks followed by hand walking. Restricted turnout is advised. During this initial period it is recommended that systemic non-steroidal anti-inflammatory drugs (NSAIDs) be given. There is no documented evidence for the efficacy of any other medical treatment of this condition.

Affected horses should be allowed 6–12 months to recover from acute injuries (analogous to the time required for healing in other ligaments and tendons in the body). The injection of anti-inflammatory medication, such as corticosteroids, into the joint (or at least around the joint) is also a logical option after the first repair phase has passed.

Chronic SID

Management of SID in horses should be based on clinical presentation, but includes use of rest, anti-inflammatory medication and exercise [9]. Reduction of pain associated with SID is important, but it should be noted that complete rest may be contraindicated due to the possible adverse effects of reduced pelvic and hindlimb muscle function and worsening functional instability of the SIJ [9]. NSAIDs can result in temporary improvement in performance [7,10]; however, it is ideal to rehabilitate the horse so improvement is consistent and lasting. A specific rehabilitation programme based on biomechanical findings may achieve this. Exercise to build up the muscles of the back and hindquarters [9] is more appropriately recommended. However, the use of exercise to manage SID has generally been non-specific, and there is a clear need for more specific muscle re-training to enhance functional stability of the region, and ultimately improve performance, in individual cases. An understanding of the biomechanics and neuromotor control of the equine SIJ region is needed to approach that of the human SIJ. This may lead to the development of manual mobilisation and/or manipulation techniques, which can be applied to the equine pelvis and SIJ, to improve joint kinematics.

In some cases, some veterinarians have described the injection of sclerosing agents at the site of the SIJ to aid management of the condition [1,15]. Chronic cases may well improve when the musculature around the SIJ strengthens.

Conclusion

Although sacroiliac dysfunction is still something of an anathema to equine veterinarians, many of the difficulties relating to diagnosis and management have greatly improved in recent years. Much progress has been made in research, and there is a better appreciation of the functional anatomy of the SIJ and the type of pathological lesions that can develop. This is complemented by the improvements in clinical evaluation, local analgesia and the use of modern diagnostic imaging modalities. The current thrust of research in biomechanics, kinesiology and various forms of physiotherapy bode well for the future.

References

1 Goff, L.M., Jeffcott, L.B., Jasiewicz, J. and McGowan, C.M. Structural and biomechanical aspects of equine sacroiliac joint function and their relationship to clinical disease. *Veterinary Journal* 2008; **176**:281–293.

2 Dyson, S., Murray, R., Branch, M. and Harding, E. The sacroiliac joints: Evaluation using nuclear scintigraphy. Part 2: Lame horses. *Equine Veterinary Journal* 2003; **35**:233–239.

3 Dyson, S. and Murray, R. Pain associated with the sacro-iliac joint region: A clinical study of 74 horses. *Equine Veterinary Journal* 2003; **35**:240–245.

4 Barstow, A. and Dyson, S. Clinical features and diagnosis of sacroiliac joint region pain in 296 horses: 2004–2014. *Equine Veterinary Education* 2015; **27**:637–647.

5 Dalin, G. and Jeffcott, L.B. Sacroiliac joint of the horse. 1. Gross morphology. *Anatomia, Histologia et Embryologia* 1986; **15**:80–94.

6 Dalin, G. and Jeffcott, L.B. Sacroiliac joint of the horse. 2. Morphometric features. *Anatomia, Histologia et Embryologia* 1986; **15**:97–107.

7 Jeffcott, L.B., Dalin, G., Ekman, S. and Olsson, S.-E. Sacroiliac lesions as a cause of poor performance in competitive horses. *Equine Veterinary Journal* 1985; **17**:111–118.

8 Haussler, K.K., Stover, S.M. and Willits, N.H. Pathology of the lumbosacral spine and pelvis in Thoroughbred racehorses. *American Journal of Veterinary Research* 1999; **60**:143–153.

9 Haussler, K.K. Diagnosis and management of sacroiliac joint injuries. In: Ross, M. and

Dyson, S. (eds), *Diagnosis and Management of Lameness in the Horse.* St Louis, MO: Saunders, 2003, pp. 501–508.

10 Dyson, S. and Murray, R. Pain associated with the sacroiliac joint region: A clinical study of 74 horses. *Equine Veterinary Journal* 2003; **35**:240–245.

11 Zimmerman, M., Dyson, S. and Murray, R. Close, impinging and overriding spinous processes in the thoracolumbar spine: The relationship between radiological and scintigraphic findings and clinical signs. *Equine Veterinary Journal* 2012; **44**:178–184.

12 Goff, L.M., Jasiewicz, J., Jeffcott, L.B. et al. Movement between the equine ilium and sacrum – *in vivo* and *in vitro* studies. *Equine Veterinary Journal* 2006; **38**(Suppl. S36): 457–461.

13 Erichsen, C., Eksell, P. and Berger, M. The scintigraphic anatomy of the equine sacroiliac joint. *Veterinary Radiology and Ultrasound* 2002; **43**:287–292.

14 Dyson, S., Murray, R. and Branch, M. The sacroiliac joints: evaluation using nuclear scintigraphy. Part 1: The normal horse. *Equine Veterinary Journal* 2003; **35**:226–232.

15 Dyson, S.J. Pelvic injuries in the non-racehorse. In: Ross, M.W. and Dyson, S.J. (eds), *Diagnosis and Management of Lameness in the Horse.* St Louis, MO: Saunders, 2003, pp. 491–501.

16 Denoix, J.M. Ultrasonographic evaluation of back lesions. In: Haussler, K.K. (ed.), *Veterinary Clinics of North America Equine Practice.* Philadelphia, PA: Saunders, 1999, pp. 131–139.

17 Jeffcott, L.B. Radiographic appearance of equine lumbosacral and pelvic abnormalities by linear tomography. *Veterinary Radiology* 1983; **24**:204–213.

18 Denoix, J. and Jacquet, S. Ultrasound guided injections of the sacro-iliac area in horses. *Equine Veterinary Education* 2008; **20**:203–207.

19 Engeli, E. and Haussler, K.K. Review of sacro-iliac injection techniques. In: Proceedings of the American Association of Equine Practitioners, Denver, 2004.

20 Engeli, E., Haussler, K.K. and Erb, H.N. Development and validation of a periarticular injection technique of the sacroiliac joint in horses. *Equine Veterinary Journal* 2004; **36**:324–330.

15

Muscular Disorders

Richard J. Piercy and Renate Weller

Introduction

Muscle disorders that affect the equine back can be broadly divided into two categories, depending on whether the condition is generalised (for example an exertional myopathy) or localised (for example a muscle tear). The investigation of such cases will depend largely on the presenting clinical signs, but often it is difficult to determine whether the problem is localised to the back or whether, in fact, the signs are a manifestation of a generalised problem.

Difficulty in discriminating between generalised and localised conditions partly reflects the underlying pathology. In particular, the response shown by skeletal muscle is somewhat limited despite varied underlying causes. Disruption of muscle fibre homeostasis results in osmotic imbalance: normally the myoplasmic Ca^{2+} concentration is tightly regulated and maintained at a resting concentration that is 60–100 times lower than that of the extracellular fluid; however, damage or disease allows Ca^{2+} to enter the cytoplasm from the interstitial fluid or sarcoplasmic stores, thereby activating destructive cellular proteases and inhibiting mitochondrial respiration [1,2]. Cell death by necrosis is often associated with inflammatory responses that result in the chemotaxis of circulating neutrophils and macrophages, the removal of damaged tissue and collagen deposition, which, if extensive, can result in fibrosis. However, in many circumstances, there is

muscle disease without a marked inflammatory response [3].

The regenerative capacity of muscle is dependent on a population of normally quiescent, 'stem cell'-like cells, known as satellite cells, which occupy a position beneath the fibre's basement membrane but outside the fibre's sarcolemma. Fibre damage results in satellite cell activation, division and transformation into myoblasts – cells that eventually fuse to form immature myotubes and subsequently new myofibres [4]. This process can take several months; in the intervening period, histopathology reveals immature fibres of variable sizes with internally located nuclei (Figure 15.1) [5]. Regeneration is, however, limited by the extent to which reinnervation and revascularisation are possible when these modalities are compromised and the degree of damage to the fibres' basement membranes [6]. It is generally assumed that when the basement membrane is compromised, there is a greater propensity for fibrosis and scar formation [6].

Diagnostic Procedures

Clinical Exam

Clinical signs vary depending on the extent of the underlying disease. Localised tears or inflammation will be manifest as guarding or avoidance responses to deep palpation of the region, whereas horses with generalised myopathies might show more severe systemic

Equine Neck and Back Pathology: Diagnosis and Treatment, Second Edition. Edited by Frances M.D. Henson.
© 2018 John Wiley & Sons, Ltd. Published 2018 by John Wiley & Sons, Ltd.

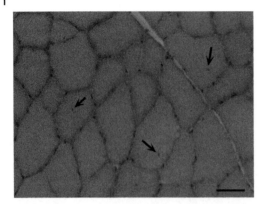

Figure 15.1 *Semimembranosus* muscle biopsy sample. 11-year-old TBx mare with a history of repeated episodes of exertional rhabdomyolysis. Note the internalised nuclei (arrows). Haematoxylin and eosin stain. Bar = 50 μm. (*For a colour version of this figure, see the colour plate section.*)

signs. Mild to moderately affected animals are tachycardic, with firm pelvic limb, epaxial and gluteal musculature that is painful when palpated and results in a stiff gait [7]. Pigmenturia might be evident in more severely affected animals: furthermore, these animals will often be severely painful, tachycardic and tachypnoeic. They often sweat profusely and are unwilling to move or they become recumbent [7].

Biochemistry

Many muscle strains and tears might not be detectable through routine biochemical assessment, but more generalised conditions (such as the exertional myopathies) or severe localised muscle damage are likely to be represented by elevations in the plasma of activities of the muscle-derived enzymes, creatine kinase (CK) and aspartate amino transferase (AST). CK remains the most convenient and specific marker of acute muscle damage, peaking at 4 to 6 hours following acute muscle damage [8]. AST activity usually peaks about 24 hours after an episode and can remain elevated for several days to weeks [9,10]. In some horses, provocative exercise testing (usually 20 minutes of lunged exercise at the trot) is informative, though individual clinicians vary in their methodology and interpretation of such testing. In general, plasma CK activity should not normally rise following moderate exercise of this type, provided the horse is fit (Piercy, personal observation), so a rise of more than 10–20% of the resting value, 4 hours postexercise, should be regarded as potentially relevant [11]. Note, however, that not all horses with underlying primary myopathies show a consistent positive response to such testing; indeed, it is highly likely that horses with different underlying primary conditions respond differently to this test. Further, different breeds with the same disease can respond differently [12,13]. There are many underlying primary myopathies in other species that are not reflected by elevated plasma CK activities, either resting or postexercise, likely because in these disorders the sarcolemmal membrane is not compromised. Despite this, such patients can have marked clinical signs (often paresis) and prominent underlying pathological changes [14].

DNA Testing

DNA testing for polysaccharide storage myopathy type 1 (PSSM1) is often indicated in horses of certain breeds that have an especially high prevalence of this genetic disorder, prior to, or concurrently with, muscle biopsy (see below), when horses present with back pain, paresis, gait abnormalities or a combination of these signs, and when conventional lameness evaluation has been uninformative. Elevations in plasma CK or AST activity (either resting or postexercise test) might be supportive, but can be absent in horses with PSSM1 [13]. A blood sample (in EDTA) or hair plucks (containing hair roots) should be submitted for genetic testing: the horse can be tested specifically for the R309H mutation in the equine glycogen synthase, the *GYS1* gene [15] responsible for PSSM1, and will be identified as either normal or a heterozygote or homozygote. Genetic testing is useful to help prompt management and treatment options and especially when the animal might be used for breeding. Since the test is inexpensive and minimally invasive, genetic testing is often sensible early during any investigation.

Biopsy

Muscle biopsy might be indicated in an animal that is presented because of suspected back pain, where no other credible cause has been identified and, in particular, when there are persistent elevations in serum muscle enzyme activities or when a horse has shown a significant rise in muscle-derived enzymes following an exercise test. Note, however, that less invasive diagnostics, in particular DNA testing, might be indicated prior to biopsy, or performed concurrently, when PSSM1 is suspected, especially when the breed in question is one of several with a high prevalence of the mutated allele (see the section on DNA testing above). Muscle biopsy might be sensible in horses with appropriate clinical signs, when DNA testing has returned negative for PSSM1.

The site of the biopsy should be based on results of the physical examination, but epaxial, gluteal and semimembranosus muscles are usually chosen [9,11]. A semimembranosus muscle biopsy is likely to result in fewer complications and is generally indicated in suspected exertional myopathies (Figure 15.2). Both open and needle biopsy techniques have been described and ideally both fresh and formalin-fixed samples should be submitted to a specialist laboratory. Open biopsy generally results in less artefact, especially when samples are shipped with a delay (e.g. overnight). Careful packaging, in particular keeping the sample cold (with icepacks) and avoiding wrapping the sample in saline-soaked gauzes will minimise artefact [16].

Ultrasonography

Ultrasonography is widely used for the evaluation of soft tissue structures in the horse.

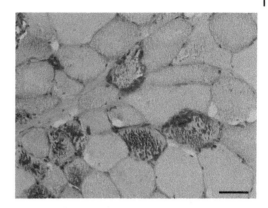

Figure 15.2 *Semimembranosus* muscle biopsy sample stained with periodic acid Schiff (PAS) following diastase digestion. 8-year-old Cob gelding with exertional rhabdomyolysis. Note the abundant dark staining inclusions in multiple fibres, consistent with abnormal polysaccharide and a diagnosis of polysaccharide storage myopathy. Bar = 50 μm. (*For a colour version of this figure, see the colour plate section.*)

Although it is mainly used for tendons, ligaments and joints, its use for the evaluation of equine muscle has been described [17,18].

Technique

For accurate and repeatable assessment, the skin over the area of interest has to be clipped and thoroughly cleansed. Owners are often reluctant to have their horses clipped over a wide area and in short-haired horses soaking the skin for a few minutes can result in images of diagnostic quality. An ultrasound machine used for the evaluation of the flexor tendons is suitable for the ultrasonographic examination of the epaxial muscles. The epaxial muscles vary in depth depending on the location and a 5–10 MHz transducer with a central frequency of 7.5 MHz will allow visualisation of the iliocostalis, the longissimus dorsi, the spinalis and the multifidi muscles. For the deeper laying multifidi muscle, a technique using a 5 MH curvilinear transducer has been described for the assessment of changes in cross-sectional area [19,20].

Muscle tissue appears less echogenic ultrasonographically than the connective tissue

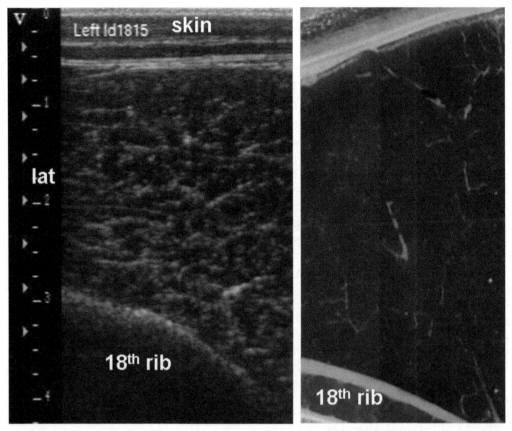

Figure 15.3 Transverse ultrasound scan of the *longissimus dorsi* at the level of the 18th thoracic rib and the corresponding dissection. Muscle tissue appears less echogenic than the connective tissue enveloping the muscle fascicles, resulting in a speckled appearance. (*For a colour version of this figure, see the colour plate section.*)

enveloping the muscle fascicles. This results in a speckled or marbled appearance of muscle on transverse scans (Figure 15.3) and multiple, parallel, linear lines on longitudinal scans (Figure 15.4). Aponeurotic sheets appear as hyperechogenic lines within muscles or separating muscle bellies (Figure 15.4). Each muscle has a characteristic ultrasonographic appearance that is dependent on its architecture and by its contraction status: care should be taken to standardise the ultrasonographic examination by ensuring that the horse is positioned on a level surface, equally weight bearing on all four limbs with the head and neck positioned in line with the back. As with any ultrasound examination, a thorough knowledge of the anatomy is prerequisite: the gross architecture of some of the

perivertebral muscles has been described in detail [21].

Indication for Muscle Ultrasonography

Ultrasonography has been used to diagnose muscle tears, myositis, haemorrhage, foreign bodies and abscesses [18], though this has not been described for these lesions in equine back muscles. In some horses with suspected muscle strain based on a localised increase in uptake of radiopharmaceutical over the thoracolumbar region, an increase in echogenicity with changes in pennation angle has been found on ultrasound.

Ultrasonography can also be used to evaluate muscle architecture as an indicator of muscle fitness, to monitor training and to

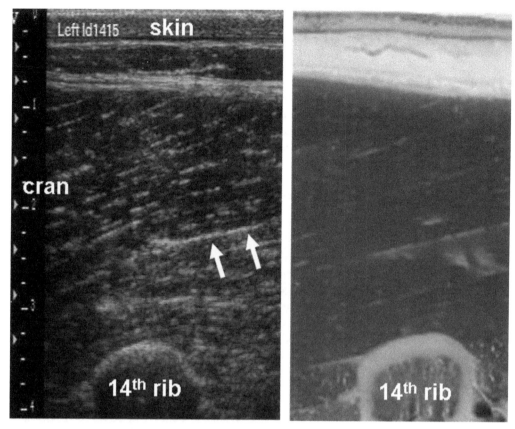

Figure 15.4 Longitudinal ultrasound scan of the *longissimus dorsi* at the level of the 14th thoracic rib, 15 cm ventral to the midline and the corresponding dissection. Muscle is less echogenic compared to the connective tissue, the muscle fascicles appear as multiple, parallel, linear lines and aponeurotic sheets appear as distinct hyperechonic lines within muscles (arrows) and separating muscle bellies. (*For a colour version of this figure, see the colour plate section.*)

assess horses with suspected back pain with a view to determining efficacy of interventional treatments. Muscle architecture including volume, fibre length and pennation angle greatly influences muscle function [22]. These architectural parameters are used to calculate the physiological cross-sectional area of a muscle (which is proportional to the force potential of the muscle) [23]. The amount of fibrous tissue within a muscle also determines its passive force–length properties. Active and passive properties of the muscle are important in back function, since back muscles do not only contribute to spinal movement but are crucial in spinal stabilization [24,25]. Muscle responds to its usage: atrophy or hypertrophy occurs with decreased

and increased use (training) respectively, which in humans can be assessed ultrasonographically as a decrease or increase in muscle volume and pennation angle [26,27]. The same effect has been observed in a cohort of six untrained ponies undergoing a 12-week low-intensity training program (Weller et al., unpublished data), and an increase in cross-section area of the multifidi muscles as an effect of dynamic mobilisation exercises has been described [20].

It is well documented in humans that back pain is associated with changes in the volume of back muscles [28]. Affected muscle groups undergo hypertrophy in the acute stage and atrophy with an increase of connective tissue in chronic cases. This has been illustrated in denervated laryngeal muscle in horses [29]. This seems to hold true for the *longissimus dorsi* in the horse: preliminary data from horses with chronic back disorders show an increased fibrous:muscle tissue ratio, a decrease in muscle depth and a change in pennation angle in the *longissimus dorsi* muscle (Weller, unpublished data). These measurements should be considered in the context of the overall muscular condition of the horse to differentiate between generally unfit animals and horses with impaired back muscle function. Note that the pennation angle decreases from cranial to caudal and from dorsal to ventral, ranging from 30 to 45° [30]; hence standardisation of location is important. There is a correlation between osseous spinal pathology and epaxial muscle ultrasonography in Thoroughbred racehorses, with horses showing asymmetrical multifidi cross-section at or close to the site of pathology and relating to severity of the pathology [19]. This further illustrates the relationship between back function, muscle development and pathology.

Scintigraphy

Scintigraphic evaluation follows a standard procedure for musculoskeletal examination in the horse (Chapter 9).

Generalised radiopharmaceutical uptake over the back muscles has been described in racehorses following an episode of exertional rhabdomyolysis. This has been reported 24 hours after treadmill exercise [31] and also up to 10 days after training [32]. These findings have been observed in the bone phase rather than the soft tissue phase of the scintigraphic examination. Not all horses with evidence of exertional rhabdomyolysis, however, show abnormal findings on scintigraphy. Figure 15.5 shows the scintigraphic findings in a horse with acute rhabdomyolysis. The image shows linear areas of increased radiopharmaceutical uptake 3 hours after injection of 1GBq Tc^{99m}-methylendiphosponate. Radiopharmaceutical uptake over

specific portions of the epaxial muscle has also been identified in sport horses with concurrent ipsilateral pelvic limb lameness, possibly due to muscle strains or tears [32]. This can be associated with an increase in echogenicity and changes in pennation angle on ultrasound (see above). Mineralising lesions, for example calcifying melanomas, can show a diffuse increase in radiopharmaceutical uptake and this might guide further imaging procedures, especially ultrasonography.

Electromyography

An electromyographic (EMG) signal can be collected using surface or fine-wire needle electrodes and provides information on the timing and amplitude of muscle activity and also clinical information regarding the state of innervation and pathology within the muscle.

Surface EMG

EMG using surface electrodes has been used to relate muscle activity to changes in gait characteristics in normal horses in different gaits and under different conditions [25,33,34]. It has also been used to assess the efficacy of physiotherapeutic intervention in horses [35] and the effect of training aids (Wakeling, personal communication). The signal and its interpretation is very sensitive to the position and placement of the electrode over the muscle of interest and great variability can exist between signals collected from the same and between different animals. Electrodes are placed over the mid-belly region of the muscle of interest; hence surface EMG is restricted to evaluation of superficial muscles.

To ensure a good quality signal, the area on which the surface electrode will be placed should be clipped and shaved. The skin should be wiped clean to remove any remaining dust and grease. The surface electrodes, which are usually self-adhesive, should then be placed on to the skin and held in place with suitable

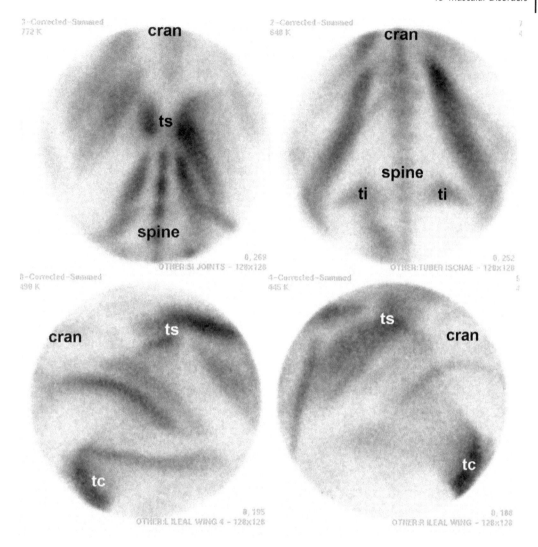

Figure 15.5 Scintigraphic images of a horse with acute rhabdomyolysis three hours after injection of Tc^{99m}-methylendiphosphonate. The top two images show two dorsal views of the pelvis region, the two bottom images show a left lateral oblique and a right lateral oblique image (tc = *tuber coxae*, ts = *tuber sacrale*, ti = *tuber ischii*). Note the striped/linear increase in radiopharmceutical uptake over the musculature typical for this condition. (*For a colour version of this figure, see the colour plate section.*)

tape to help prevent movement and introduction of low-frequency noise artefact. The dimensions of the electrodes (size and inter-electrode distance) should be known and reported, as these factors influence the signal components. Several manufacturers offer complete EMG systems with varying numbers of channels and sampling frequencies to suit different needs.

Needle EMG

A needle EMG requires specialist equipment and expertise and is sometimes helpful in cases where the clinician suspects neurogenic or primary myopathic disease. Unlike surface EMG, with needle EMG the clinician can evaluate very specific regions and the electrical activity of individual groups of muscle fibres. Normal muscle at rest is electrically inactive; hence following a brief period of activity caused by the placement of the needle disrupting muscle fibres (insertional activity), a resting muscle should quickly fall silent (unless the needle is close to a neuromuscular junction). Prolonged insertional activity is considered abnormal.

Electrical activity within the muscle after needle insertion can be either normal or pathological. Normal activity occurs when the muscle contracts or is held contracted, making assessment in standing, conscious horses sometimes difficult to interpret (the latter is aided by a quiet environment, stocks and a sedated animal). Pathological findings include fibrillation potentials and positive sharp waves, which are often encountered with denervation. The reader is referred to additional sources for further information [36]. Generally, conventional needle EMG is best interpreted in an anaesthetised horse if practicalities allow, although specialist testing for the morphology and duration of the compound motor unit action potential has been used to assess normal electrical activity in equine muscles [37].

Disorders: Aetiopathogenesis and Treatment

Muscle Strains, Bruises and Tears

Although there may be a history of trauma, frequently muscle tears and strains at first go unnoticed because the condition only becomes painful after several hours. Generally, these injuries occur during exercise or while at pasture and in some circumstances injuries can result from inexperienced riding or poorly fitting saddles. Show jumpers and eventers are particularly prone to lumbar and gluteal strain, which may be reflected as unwillingness to jump or turn sharply [38]; however, often horses exhibit only mild to moderate lameness or stiffness. The propensity for muscle injury to result in chronic back pain, and in particular myofascial trigger points, is an active area of investigation. These points are regarded as the sites of painful nodules, located within taut bands of skeletal muscle [39,40].

Adequate rest followed by a gradual return to exercise forms the mainstay of treatment in horses with these kinds of injuries. Non-steroidal anti-inflammatory drugs (NSAID) (e.g. phenylbutazone 4.4 mg/kg IV or PO BID for one day followed by 2.2 mg/kg PO BID for several days, or flunixin meglumine 0.5–1.1 mg/kg IV or PO BID or SID) provide analgesia and might help limit the fibrotic response. Various forms of physiotherapy, such as massage, electrical stimulation and swimming exercise might aid healing and speed recovery.

Exertional Myopathies

Exertional myopathies have received considerable attention in recent years, as investigators have recognised that specific entities exist within this multifactorial syndrome. Horses with exertional myopathies usually have generalised disease, of which back stiffness, soreness and pelvic limb lameness may be part. There is convincing evidence that both acquired and genetic causes contribute to the clinical scenario: within the former group, overexertion, electrolyte imbalance, hormonal influence and infectious disease have all been proposed as potential causes [41], but supportive evidence is sometimes scant. Note, however, that some of these factors may be the precipitating cause of disease in a genetically susceptible animal or they are detected concurrently in such a patient and might not be the underlying primary cause.

Injury resulting from overexertion is likely to have several components and depends on the nature of the exercise. For instance, eccentric muscle contraction (contraction that occurs during muscle lengthening), as might occur as strain is taken in contracted back muscles on landing from a jump, results in more severe muscle damage than other types of contraction and, in particular, in sarcomeric disruption and damage to the excitation-contraction coupling mechanism and the sarcolemma [42]. The result is a local inflammatory response accompanied by oedema and the sensitisation of nociceptors [43].

Other factors that contribute to overexertion-induced myopathy include metabolic exhaustion (for example in endurance animals) and antioxidant status. For the latter, evidence suggests that production of reactive oxygen species (such as free radicals) correlates with energy expenditure [44] and that oxidative stress occurs in horses, especially when ambient humidity and temperature are high [45]. Causal links with myopathies and oxidative stress are hard to prove; however, though antioxidant supplementation does not attenuate exercise-induced elevations in muscle enzymes in horses [46–48] the link between vitamin E and/or selenium deficiency in foals with nutritional myodegeneration [49] suggests that antioxidants play an important role. Animals with antioxidant deficiencies might be especially prone to damage or disease of other underlying causes.

There are two well-characterised forms of exercise-related myopathy in horses with known or suspected underlying genetic causes. These include a condition examined extensively in a group of Thoroughbreds in the US that has been termed 'recurrent exertional rhabdomyolysis' (RER) [50,51] and another condition, termed (equine) polysaccharide storage myopathy (PSSM or EPSM) [52–54]. These conditions have clinical and clinicopathological similarities and are managed similarly, though they have different aetiologies, other key differences and different breed susceptibilities [55]. The word 'recurrent' in Thoroughbreds with exercise-related myopathy has been used variably to describe certain Thoroughbreds with apparent abnormalities in muscle calcium regulation [50,51], a wider group of Thoroughbreds with a possible inherited form of exertional rhabdomyolysis [55–57] and all Thoroughbreds with a susceptibility to the syndrome. In humans there are many genetic causes of rhabdomyolysis (e.g. mutations in genes encoding enzymes involved in cellular metabolism or

structural proteins); it is currently unknown how many different forms of rhabdomyolysis affect horses. Active investigation of horses with use of genetic testing, muscle biopsy, immunohistochemistry and advanced genomic techniques will very likely help identify additional causes [58,59].

Recurrent Exertional Rhabdomyolysis (RER)

Estimates of prevalence or incidence of exercise-associated rhabdomyolysis in Thoroughbreds suggests that 5–7% of Thoroughbreds worldwide are affected, although it remains unknown whether all these animals have the same disorder. Pedigree analysis of some lines of Thoroughbreds in the US supports autosomal dominant inheritance of the trait [56,60], but a multigenic disorder is now considered likely based on large-scale genetic studies [61,62]. Given that acquired forms of rhabdomyolysis are common in humans and other species it seems possible, or likely, that some Thoroughbreds develop acquired forms of the syndrome as a result of triggering environmental or management factors [63]. Despite this, a common underlying genetic predisposition within the breed remains a distinct possibility. Furthermore, it is possible that exertional myopathies in other breeds (such as Standardbreds) may have an identical underlying cause or share genetic risk factors [64].

The abnormality in muscle calcium regulation identified in some Thoroughbreds shares certain experimental similarities to a condition recognised in humans and other species, known as malignant hyperthermia (MH). In particular, muscle from horses with RER and other species with MH is hypersensitive to agents (such as caffeine and halothane) that stimulate release of calcium from the muscle calcium store (sarcoplasmic reticulum) through a calcium release channel known as the ryanodine receptor (RYR1) [50,51]. However, though MH has been reported in some horses following halothane anaesthesia and, indeed, though an RYR1 receptor, mutation has been identified in MH-susceptible Quarter Horses [65]. Thoroughbreds with abnormal calcium regulation do not share the same mutation and there is evidence suggesting that the RYR1 receptor is not mutated in Thoroughbred RER [66]. Given that inhalational anaesthesia is common in equine veterinary work, but MH-like episodes are extremely rare, this seems unsurprising. Despite this, the basic research similarities between RER and MH do still suggest the involvement of another protein or proteins that influence intracellular calcium regulation in muscle. Indeed mutations in other proteins are known to cause or are implicated in human MH [67]. Alternatively, formerly detected defects in calcium homeostasis in equine muscle samples [50] (but notably not sarcoplasmic reticulum derived vesicles [51]) might be due to a secondary rather than primary defects.

Currently it is not easy to document calcium regulation abnormalities in horses with suspected RER because the techniques involved are invasive, technically challenging and unavailable in the clinical setting, although experimental techniques based on cultured cells are now available in the research setting [68]. Furthermore, muscle biopsy and histopathology, though confirming myopathy and providing information regarding severity, is not specific for this form of the disease (see Figure 15.1). As such, many of these cases are treated or managed without establishing the definitive diagnosis and remain in the idiopathic category.

Polysaccharide Storage Myopathy

Polysaccharide storage myopathy (PSSM or EPSM) is currently definitively diagnosed by muscle biopsy. Pathognomonic changes include diastase-resistant inclusions detected by periodic acid Schiff staining [52]. Some, but not all horses with this disorder are hypersensitive to insulin [69]. This disease was first reported in detail in Quarter Horses with exertional rhabdomyolysis in the US [52]. Since then, a disease with the same

histopathological features has been reported in a variety of other breeds, in particular certain European continental Draught horses [53,54,70]. Although there are sometimes clinical differences in the presentations of this disease (rhabdomyolysis in athletic animals and weakness or muscle atrophy in the draught horses), these diseases share the same underlying genetic cause (genotype). The disease is inherited as an autosomal dominant trait and a single, gain of function mutation, associated with a missense DNA base change in a gene integrally involved in glycogen metabolism, glycogen synthase (*GYS1*), is present in many breeds [15,70]. Evidence suggests that in Quarter Horses the prevalence is between 6 and 12% [15] but prevalence in some European draught breeds can approach 50% [13]. Many horses have only sub-clinical involvement, or only vague signs, but homozygotes have more extensive pathological changes than heterozygotes [13]. The glycogen storage disorder associated with the *GYS1* founder mutation are defined as having type 1 PSSM (PSSM1).

In comparison with genetic testing, muscle biopsy diagnosis of PSSM1 lacks sensitivity and specificity [71] and some horses have clinical signs and histopathological features suggestive of PSSM, but they lack the specific *GYS1* R309H mutation in genetic testing [70,71]. In these horses, alternative glycogen storage disease(s) is/are a possibility. Furthermore, identification of amylase-resistant polysaccharide inclusions seems to be associated with secondary myopathic features in mammals [72]. The group of horses that have histopathological features of PSSM, but that lack the GYS1 mutation, are currently diagnosed with type 2 PSSM (PSSM2); however, note that it remains unclear whether these horses have a single or various different disorders and, further, that the optimal management and treatment of these animals is unknown.

Treatment of Exertional Myopathies

The management and treatment of exertional rhabdomyolysis in Thoroughbreds depends on whether the horse is seen in the acute setting or between intermittent episodes [11]. The treatment of acute exertional rhabdomyolysis depends on the severity. Mildly affected horses (the majority) can often be managed conservatively, through controlled exercise with or without non-steroidal anti-inflammatory medication, whereas severely affected animals require hospitalisation, analgesics, intravenous fluids and sometimes diuresis (the latter to diminish the possibility of myoglobin-induced nephrotoxicity). Various other drugs, such as acepromazine and corticosteroids, are sometimes administered, but largely with unproven efficacy [11].

Prophylaxis is important for horses that appear predisposed to repeated episodes of exertional rhabdomyolysis. There is currently widespread use of oral dantrolene in Thoroughbred racehorses. The rationale is based on two published reports that suggest some efficacy, either in Thoroughbreds where calcium regulation abnormalities have been documented or in a group of uncharacterised racehorses [73,74]. Dantrolene is an RYR1 receptor antagonist (though it has other less specific effects in muscle cells); as such, its main effect is probably to reduce the release of calcium from the sarcoplasmic reticulum that is required for muscle contraction. Further, the drug lowers resting sarcoplasmic calcium concentration in cultured equine muscle cells [68], which might reduce the propensity towards activation of destructive cellular proteases. Effects of the drug on performance are currently unknown, though it has been associated with weakness in some experimental horses at high doses [75]. Early evidence that suggested that gastrointestinal absorption is poor without feed withdrawal [74] is not supported by more recent data; indeed, the opposite seems to be the case [76]. Various other treatments (such as phenytoin) and vitamin, mineral, electrolyte and hormonal supplements are administered to horses prone to repeated episodes of exertional rhabdomyolysis, but most have unproven efficacy [41].

There is, however, good evidence that episodes of exertional rhabdomyolysis in some susceptible Thoroughbreds can be reduced in severity or frequency through manipulation of the diet, in particular, by increasing the proportion of dietary energy derived from fat and decreasing the proportion derived from carbohydrate [77]. Similar dietary alterations are recommended for the management of PSSM1 [78,79], but it remains unclear why such management results in a beneficial response in these two separate disorders. Regular and consistent exercise in both groups also appears to be important.

Muscle Atrophy

Atrophy of the back musculature usually falls into one of two categories: (1) generalised and symmetrical atrophy and (2) localised and asymmetric atrophy. In the former cases, close attention should be given to the nutritional status (and dentition) and systemic disease in animals that may have generalised weight loss. In addition, disuse atrophy (perhaps manifest as increased prominence of the tuber sacrale) can occur in horses that are rested, in older horses or in animals that have another source of lameness. If these are ruled out, then other rarer causes, for example equine motor neuron disease (EMND) and chronic grass sickness (in affected countries), should be considered. Both these latter conditions can usually be distinguished by other characteristic clinical signs that accompany the diseases and the reader is referred to general medicine and neurology texts for more detailed descriptions. Equine motor neuron disease can often be confirmed through muscle biopsy of the sacrocaudalis dorsalis medialis muscle (Figure 15.6).

In horses with localised and asymmetric muscle atrophy, a neurogenic cause or primary muscle disease should be considered. Neurogenic muscle atrophy of the back musculature can result from damage or pressure to spinal nerve roots, caused by vertebral osteoarthritis, vertebral injury or a space-occupying lesion, or to localised grey matter

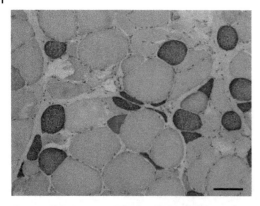

Figure 15.6 *Sacrocaudalis dorsalis medialis* muscle biopsy specimen. 2-year-old filly with marked muscle atrophy and weakness, labelled (immuno-peroxidase) with an antibody to slow myosin heavy chain. Note the angular atrophy of particularly the darker, type I fibres, characteristic of equine motor neurone disease. Bar = 100 μm. (*For a colour version of this figure, see the colour plate section.*)

disease (for example with equine protozoal myelitis). With spinal cord lesions, additional involvement of white matter tracts can result in other clinical signs (such as asymmetric pelvic limb ataxia or paresis). Neurogenic causes of muscle atrophy result in characteristic changes identifiable by needle electromyography (see above); however, definitive diagnosis is achieved with the aid of muscle biopsy.

A primary (and presumed immune mediated) myositis has been identified in horses with severe muscle atrophy of the dorsal musculature (and elsewhere) [80]. This can be either symmetrical or asymmetrical. Recent exposure to *Streptococcus equi equi* appears to be a risk factor and, given this organism's propensity to cause purpura, the causative agent of equine strangles may be a primary cause of many horses with immune mediated myositis, though a breed predisposition (Quarter Horses) might also exist [78]. Diagnosis in these cases is based on identification of a lymphocytic myositis by muscle biopsy and many affected horses respond to rest, combined with corticosteroid administration [78].

References

1 Belcastro, A.N., Shewchuk, L.D. and Raj, D.A. Exercise-induced muscle injury: a calpain hypothesis. *Molecular and Cellular Biochemistry* 1998; **179**(1–2):135–145.

2 Gissel, H. and Clausen, T. Excitation-induced Ca^{2+} influx and skeletal muscle cell damage. *Acta Physiologica Scandinavia* 2001; **171**(3):327–334.

3 Sandri, M. and Carraro, U. Apoptosis of skeletal muscles during development and disease. *International Journal of Biochemistry and Cell Biology* 1999; **31**(12):1373–1390.

4 Zammit, P. and Beauchamp, J. The skeletal muscle satellite cell: Stem cell or son of stem cell? *Differentiation* 2001; **68**(4–5):193–204.

5 Dubowitz, V. and Sewry, C. Changes in sarcolemmal nuclei. In: *Muscle Biopsy: A Practical Approach*. Philadelphia, PA: Saunders and Elsevier, 2007, pp. 92–94.

6 Kaariainen, M., Jarvinen, T., Jarvinen, M., Rantanen, J. and Kalimo, H. Relation between myofibers and connective tissue during muscle injury repair. *Scandinavian Journal of Medicine and Scence in Sports* 2000; **10**(6):332–337.

7 McEwen, S.A. and Hulland, T.J. Histochemical and morphometric evaluation of skeletal muscle from horses with exertional rhabdomyolysis (tying-up). *Veterinary Pathology* 1986; **23**(4):400–410.

8 Toutain, P.L., Lassourd, V., Costes, G. et al. A non-invasive and quantitative method for the study of tissue injury caused by intramuscular injection of drugs in horses. *Journal of Veterinary Pharmacology and Therapeutics* 1995; **18**(3):226–235.

9 Snow, D. and Valberg, S. *Muscle Anatomy, Physiology, and Adaptions to Exercise and Training*. Philadelphia, PA: W.B. Saunders Company, 1994.

10 Harris, P.A., Marlin, D.J. and Gray, J. Plasma aspartate aminotransferase and creatine kinase activities in thoroughbred racehorses in relation to age, sex, exercise and training. *Veterinary Journal* 1998; **155**(3):295–304.

11 Piercy, R. and Lopez-Rivero, J. (2014). Muscle disorders of equine athletes. In: Hinchcliff, K., Kaneps, A. and Geor, R. (eds), *Equine Sports Medicine and Surgery*. London, Saunders, 2014, pp. 109–143.

12 Schwarz, B., Ertl, R., Zimmer, S. et al. Estimated prevalence of the GYS-1 mutation in healthy Austrian Haflingers. *Veterinary Record* 2011; **169**(22):583.

13 Naylor, R.J., Livesey, L., Schumacher, J. et al. Allele copy number and underlying pathology are associated with subclinical severity in equine type 1 polysaccharide storage myopathy (PSSM1). *PLoS One* 2012; 7(7):e42317.

14 Bohm, J., Vasli, N., Maurer, M. et al. Altered splicing of the BIN1 muscle-specific exon in humans and dogs with highly progressive centronuclear myopathy. *PLoS Genetics* 2013; **9**(6): e1003430.

15 McCue, M.E. and Valberg, S.J. (2007). Estimated prevalence of polysaccharide storage myopathy among overtly healthy Quarter Horses in the United States. *Journal of American Veterinary Medical Assocation* 2007; **231**(5):746–750.

16 Stanley, R.L., Maile, C. and Piercy, R.J. Storage-associated artefact in equine muscle biopsy samples. *Equine Veterinary Journal* 2009; **41**(1):82–86.

17 Leveille, R. and Biller, D. Muscle evaluation, foreign bodies and miscellaneous swelling. In: Rantanen, N. and McKinnon, A. (eds), *Equine Diagnostic Ultrasonography*. Baltimore, MD: Williams and Wilkins, 1998.

18 Reef, V. Musculoskeletal ultrasonography. In: Reef, V. (ed.), *Equine Diagnostic Ultrasound. V*. Philadelphia, PA: Saunders, 1998.

19 Stubbs, N.C., Kaiser, L.J., Hauptman, J. and Clayton, H.M. Dynamic mobilisation exercises increase cross sectional area of musculus multifidus. *Equine Veterinary Journal* 2011; **43**(5):522–529.

20 Stubbs, N.C., Riggs, C.M., Hodges, P.W. et al. Osseous spinal pathology and epaxial muscle ultrasonography in Thoroughbred racehorses. *Equine Veterinary Journal* 2010, November; Suppl. 38:654–661.

21 Rombach, N., Stubbs, N.C. and Clayton, H.M. Gross anatomy of the deep perivertebral musculature in horses. *American Journal of Veterinary Research* 2014; **75**(5):433–440.

22 Lieber, R.L. and Friden, J. Functional and clinical significance of skeletal muscle architecture. *Muscle Nerve* 2000; **23**(11):1647–1666.

23 Epstein, M. and Herzog, W. *Theoretical Models of Skeletal Muscle: Biological and Mathematical Considerations*. New York: John Wiley & Sons Inc., 1998.

24 Robert, C., Audigie, F., Valette, J.P., Pourcelot, P. and Denoix, J.M. Effects of treadmill speed on the mechanics of the back in the trotting saddlehorse. *Equine Veterinary Journal* 2001; Suppl. 33:154–159.

25 Licka, T.F., Peham, C. and Frey, A. Electromyographic activity of the longissimus dorsi muscles in horses during trotting on a treadmill. *American Journal of Veterinary Research* 2004; **65** (2):155–158.

26 Kawakami, Y., Abe, T. and Fukunaga, T. Muscle-fiber pennation angles are greater in hypertrophied than in normal muscles. *Journal of Applied Physiology* 1993; **74**(6):2740–2744.

27 Kawakami, Y., Muraoka, Y., Kubo, K., Suzuki, Y. and Fukunaga, T. Changes in muscle size and architecture following 20 days of bed rest. *Journal of Gravitational Physiology* 2000; 7(3):53–59.

28 Hides, J.A., Stokes, M.J., Saide, M., Jull, G.A. and Cooper, D.H. Evidence of lumbar multifidus muscle wasting ipsilateral to symptoms in patients with acute/subacute low back pain. *Spine* 1994; **19**(2):165–172.

29 Chalmers, H.J., Caswell, J., Perkins, J. et al. Ultrasonography detects early laryngeal

muscle atrophy in an equine neurectomy model. *Muscle Nerve* 2015, July 30. doi: 10.1002/mus.24785.

30 Ritruechai, P., Weller, R. and Wakeling, J.M. Regionalisation of the muscle fascicle architecture in the equine longissimus dorsi muscle. *Equine Veterinary Journal* 2008; **40**(3):246–251.

31 Morris, E., Seeherman, H.J., O'Callaghan, M.W. et al. Scintigraphic identification of skeletal muscle damage in horses 24 hours after strenuous exercise. *Equine Veterinary Journal* 1991; **23**(5):347–352.

32 Ross, M. and Stacey, V. Nuclear medicine. In: Ross, M. and Dyson, S. (eds), *Diagnosis and Management of Lameness in the Horse*. Philadelphia, PA: Saunders, 2003.

33 Robert, C., Valette, J.P. and Denoix, J.M. The effects of treadmill inclination and speed on the activity of three trunk muscles in the trotting horse. *Equine Veterinary Journal* 2001; **33**(5):466–472.

34 Robert, C., Valette, J.P. Pourcelot, P., Audigie, F. and Denoix, J.M. Effects of trotting speed on muscle activity and kinematics in saddlehorses. *Equine Veterinary Journal* 2002; Suppl. 34:295–301.

35 Wakeling, J., Barnett, K., Price, S. and Nankervis, K. Effects of manipulative therapy on the longissimus dorsi in the equine back. *Equine and Comparative Exercise Physiology* 2006; **10**:1–8.

36 Andrews, F. Electrodiagnostic aids and selected neurological diseases. In: Reed, S., Bayley, W. and Sellon, D. (eds), *Equine Internal Medicine*. Philadelphia, PA: Saunders, 2004, pp. 546–560.

37 Wijnberg, I.D. and Franssen, H. The potential and limitations of quantitative electromyography in equine medicine. *Veterinary Journal* 2016; **209**:23–31.

38 Rivero, J. and Letelier, A. Skeletal muscle profile of show jumpers: physiological and pathological considerations. In: *Equine Sports Medicine and Science*. Dortmund: Gestalt Manufaktur, GmbH, 2000.

39 Gerwin, R.D. Myofascial pain syndromes in the upper extremity. *Journal of Hand Therapy* 1997; **10**(2):130–136.

40 Gerwin, R.D. and Duranleau, D. Ultrasound identification of the myofacial trigger point. *Muscle and Nerve* 1997; **20**(6):767–768.

41 Beech, J. Chronic exertional rhabdomyolysis. *Veterinary Clinics in North America: Equine Practice* 1997; **13**(1):145–168.

42 Proske, U. and Morgan, D.L. Muscle damage from eccentric exercise: Mechanism, mechanical signs, adaptation and clinical applications. *Journal of Physiology* 2001; **537**(2):333–345.

43 MacIntyre, D.L., Reid, W.D. and McKenzie, D.C. Delayed muscle soreness. The inflammatory response to muscle injury and its clinical implications. *Sports Medicine* 1995; **20**(1):24–40.

44 Ji, L. and Leichtweis, S. Exercise and oxidative stress: Sources of free radicals and their impact on anti-oxidant systems. *Age* 1997; **20**:91–106.

45 Mills, P.C., Smith, N.C., Casas, I. et al. Effects of exercise intensity and environmental stress on indices of oxidative stress and iron homeostasis during exercise in the horse. *European Journal of Applied Physiology and Occupational Physiology* 1996; **74**(1–2):60–66.

46 Brady, P.S., Ku, P.K. and Ullrey, D.E. Lack of effect of selenium supplementation on the response of the equine erythrocyte glutathione system and plasma enzymes to exercise. *Journal of Animal Science* 1978; **47**(2):492–496.

47 Siciliano, P.D., Parker, A.L. and Lawrence, L.M. Effect of dietary vitamin E supplementation on the integrity of skeletal muscle in exercised horses. *Journal of Animal Science* 1997; **75**(6):1553–1560.

48 White, A., Estrada, M., Walker, K. et al. Role of exercise and ascorbate on plasma antioxidant capacity in thoroughbred race horses. *Comparative Biochemistry Physiology Part A: Molecular and Integrative Physiology* 2001; **128**(1):99–104.

49 Lofstedt, J. White muscle disease of foals. *Veterinary Clinics of North America: Equine Practice* 1997; **13**(1):169–185.

50 Lentz, L.-R., Valberg, S.J., Balog, E.M., Mickelson, J.R. and Gallant, E.M. Abnormal regulation of muscle contraction in horses with recurrent exertional rhabdomyolysis. *American Journal of Veterinary Research* 1999; **60**(8):992–999.

51 Lentz, L.R., Valberg, S.J., Herold, L.V. et al. Myoplasmic calcium regulation in myotubes from horses with recurrent exertional rhabdomyolysis. *American Journal of Veterinary Research* 2002; **63**(12):1724–1731.

52 Valberg, S.J., Cardinet, 3rd, G.H., Carlson, G.P. and DiMauro, S. Polysaccharide storage myopathy associated with recurrent exertional rhabdomyolysis in horses. *Neuromuscular Disorders* 1992; **2**(5–6):351–359.

53 Valentine, B.A., Credille, K.M., Lavoie, J.P. et al. Severe polysaccharide storage myopathy in Belgian and Percheron draught horses. *Equine Veterinary Journal* 1997; **29**(3):220–225.

54 Valentine, B.A., Habecker, P.L., Patterson, J.S. et al. Incidence of polysaccharide storage myopathy in draft horse-related breeds: a necropsy study of 37 horses and a mule. *Journal of Veterinary Diagnostic Investigation* 2001; **13**(1):63–68.

55 Valberg, S.J., Mickelson, J.R., Gallant, E.M. et al. Exertional rhabdomyolysis in quarter horses and thoroughbreds: one syndrome, multiple aetiologies. *Equine Veterinary Journal* 1999; Suppl. 30:533–538.

56 MacLeay, J.M., Valberg, S.J., Sorum, S.A. et al. Heritability of recurrent exertional rhabdomyolysis in Thoroughbred racehorses. *American Journal of Veterinary Research* 1999; **60**(2):250–256.

57 MacLeay, J.M., Valberg, S.J., Pagan, J.D. et al. Effect of ration and exercise on plasma creatine kinase activity and lactate concentration in Thoroughbred horses with recurrent exertional rhabdomyolysis. *American Journal of Veterinary Research* 2000; **61**(11):1390–1395.

58 Massey, C.A., Walmsley, G.L., Gliddon, T.P. and Piercy, R.J. Vacuolar myopathy in an adult Warmblood horse. *Neuromuscular Disordorders* 2013; **23**(6):473–477.

59 Valberg, S.J., McKenzie, E.C. Eyrich, L.V. et al. Suspected myofibrillar myopathy in Arabian horses with a history of exertional rhabdomyolysis. *Equine Veterinary Journal* 2015, August 1. doi: 10.1111/evj.12493.

60 Dranchak, P.K., Valberg, S.J., Onan, G.W. et al. Inheritance of recurrent exertional rhabdomyolysis in thoroughbreds. *Journal of American Veterinary Medical Association* 2005; **227**(5):762–767.

61 Tozaki, T., Hirota, K., Sugita, S. et al. A genome-wide scan for tying-up syndrome in Japanese Thoroughbreds. *Animal Genetics* 2010; **41**(2):80–86.

62 Fritz, K.L., McCue, M.E., Valberg, S.J., Rendahl, A.K. and Mickelson, J.R. Genetic mapping of recurrent exertional rhabdomyolysis in a population of North American Thoroughbreds. *Animal Genetics* 2012; **43**(6):730–738.

63 MacLeay, J.M., Sorum, S.A., Valberg, S.J., Marsh, W.E. and Sorum, M.D. Epidemiologic analysis of factors influencing exertional rhabdomyolysis in Thoroughbreds. *American Journal of Veterinary Research* 1999; **6560**(12): 1562–1566.

64 Isgren, C.M., Upjohn, M.M. Fernandez-Fuente, M. et al. Epidemiology of exertional rhabdomyolysis susceptibility in standardbred horses reveals associated risk factors and underlying enhanced performance. *PLoS One* 2010; **5**(7):e11594.

65 Aleman, M., Riehl, J. Aldridge, B.M. et al. Association of a mutation in the ryanodine receptor 1 gene with equine malignant hyperthermia. *Muscle Nerve* 2004; **30**(3): 356–365.

66 Dranchak, P.K., Valberg, S.J., Onan, G.W. et al. Exclusion of linkage of the RYR1, CACNA1S, and ATP2A1 genes to recurrent exertional rhabdomyolysis in Thoroughbreds. *American Journal of Veterinary Research* 2006; **67**(8): 1395–1400.

67 Jurkat-Rott, K., McCarthy, T. and Lehmann-Horn, F. Genetics and

pathogenesis of malignant hyperthermia. *Muscle Nerve* 2000; **23**(1):4–17.

68 Fernandez-Fuente, M., Terracciano, C.M., Martin-Duque, P. et al. Calcium homeostasis in myogenic differentiation factor 1 (MyoD)-transformed, virally-transduced, skin-derived equine myotubes. *PLoS One* 2014; **9**(8):e105971.

69 Firshman, A.M., Valberg, S.J., Baird, J.D., Hunt, L. and DiMauro, S. Insulin sensitivity in Belgian horses with polysaccharide storage myopathy. *American Journal of Veterinary Research* 2008; **69**(6):818–823.

70 Stanley, R.L., McCue, M.E., Valberg, S.J. et al. A glycogen synthase 1 mutation associated with equine polysaccharide storage myopathy and exertional rhabdomyolysis occurs in a variety of UK breeds. *Equine Veterinary Journal* 2009; **41**(6):597–601.

71 McCue, M.E., Armien, A.G., Lucio, M., Mickelson, J.R. and Valberg, S.J. Comparative skeletal muscle histopathologic and ultrastructural features in two forms of polysaccharide storage myopathy in horses. *Veterinary Pathology* 2009; **46**(6):1281–1291.

72 Sierra, E., Fernandez, A., Espinosa de Los Monteros, A. et al. Complex polysaccharide inclusions in the skeletal muscle of stranded cetaceans. *Veterinary Journal* 2012; **193**(1):152–156.

73 Edwards, J.G., Newtont, J.R., Ramzan, P.H., Pilsworth, R.C. and Shepherd, M.C. The efficacy of dantrolene sodium in controlling exertional rhabdomyolysis in the Thoroughbred racehorse. *Equine Veterinary Journal* 2003; **35**(7):707–711.

74 McKenzie, E.C., Valberg, S.J., Godden, S.M., Finno, C.J. and Murphy, M.J. Effect of oral administration of dantrolene

sodium on serum creatine kinase activity after exercise in horses with recurrent exertional rhabdomyolysis. *American Journal of Veterinary Research* 2004; **65**(1):74–79.

75 Court, M.H., Engelking, L.R., Dodman, N.H. et al. Pharmacokinetics of dantrolene sodium in horses. *Journal of Veterinary Pharmacology and Therapeutics* 1987; **10**(3):218–226.

76 McKenzie, E.C., Garrett, R.L., Payton, M.E. et al. Effect of feed restriction on plasma dantrolene concentrations in horses. *Equine Veterinary Journal* 2010; Suppl. 38: 613–617.

77 McKenzie, E.C., Valberg, S.J., Godden, S.M. et al. Effect of dietary starch, fat, and bicarbonate content on exercise responses and serum creatine kinase activity in equine recurrent exertional rhabdomyolysis. *Journal of Veterinary Internal Medicine* 2003; **17**(5):693–701.

78 Firshman, A.M., Valberg, S.J., Bender, J.B. and Finno, C.J. Epidemiologic characteristics and management of polysaccharide storage myopathy in Quarter Horses. *American Journal of Veterinary Research* 2003; **64**(10): 1319–1327.

79 Ribeiro, W.P., Valberg, S.J., Pagan, J.D. and Gustavsson, B.E. The effect of varying dietary starch and fat content on serum creatine kinase activity and substrate availability in equine polysaccharide storage myopathy. *Journal of Veterinary Internal Medicine* 2004; **18**(6): 887–894.

80 Lewis, S.S., Valberg, S.J. and Nielsen, I.L. Suspected immune-mediated myositis in horses. *Journal of Veterinary Internal Medicine* 2007; **21**(3):495–503.

16

Integrative and Physical Therapies

Joyce Harman and Mimi Porter

16.1 Integrative Therapies

Joyce Harman

Introduction

Back pain is an important cause of loss of performance and economic loss in the horse industry. Conventional medicine may help treat back pain, but integrative medicine, also known as complementary and alternative medicine, can offer, in the author's opinion, many more solutions. The successful treatment of back pain requires multiple modalities, time and patience to achieve the best results. In most cases a return to the previous level of comfort and performance can be achieved. In many cases the level of comfort exceeds expectations with the horse better able to perform than before when sidelined due to back pain.

The major integrative modalities used in the treatment of back pain include acupuncture, spinal manipulation (chiropractic, osteopathy), massage and the physical therapies (e.g. heat, cold, laser, ultrasound and electrical stimulation discussed later in this chapter). Herbal and homeopathic medicines are also used as adjunctive therapies. It is critical to check saddle fit and important to use various rehabilitation exercises.

The successful treatment of back pain, whether done with conventional or integrative therapy, requires a combination of treatment modalities and management changes. Management practices that directly influence back pain are saddle fit, feet, teeth, bitting, training styles, training aids and, of course, the rider's influence on the horse. When all aspects related to the back are corrected, the horse often returns to a higher level of performance than before it was diagnosed with a back problem.

Integrative Approach to Diagnosis of Back Pain

As discussed in Chapter 6, the symptoms of back pain can range from mild to intolerable and some symptoms are not as specific for back pain as others. In the author's opinion sinking down as the rider mounts is likely to be a symptom of back pain, while refusing a jump could be due to back or orthopaedic pain, as well as rider interference or just that the horse hates to jump. However, many of the persistent difficulties encountered in training horses can be traced to back pain or back and neck pain.

The integrative practitioner uses similar techniques to those used by the veterinarian to make a diagnosis of back pain. However, the emphasis of the clinical examination is slightly different with closer attention paid to the way of moving and muscular function and will be discussed in full. As with a veterinary examination, a complete history needs to be taken, followed by observation of the horse at rest

Equine Neck and Back Pathology: Diagnosis and Treatment, Second Edition. Edited by Frances M.D. Henson.
© 2018 John Wiley & Sons, Ltd. Published 2018 by John Wiley & Sons, Ltd.

and in motion, with and without tack. The muscles and joints are palpated thoroughly. Standard diagnostic procedures such as nerve blocks and diagnostic imaging can be used. Therapies mentioned in this section, such as acupuncture and chiropractic, will be discussed in more detail later in the text.

History of the Horse with Back Pain

Pertinent history questions to focus on are:

- What is the primary complaint?
- When does the problem show up?
- What makes the problem better?
- What makes the problem worse?

Many riders want to blame their problems on the horse's attitude rather than back pain. Tables 16.1 and 16.2 summarize common behavioural and performance-related symptoms of back pain in horses that are presented to the author.

Observation of the Horse

Observe the shape of the back for muscle development or atrophy. Also note if there are any visible physical signs of trauma from the saddle. Trauma from an ill-fitting saddle almost invariable leaves some degree of back

Table 16.1 A summary of behavioral problems related to back pain.

Objects to being saddled
Hypersensitive to brushing
Exhibits a 'bad attitude'
Difficult to shoe
Bucks or rolls excessively
Rearranges the stall bedding constantly
Displays repetitive behaviours
Piles up bedding in stall to stand on or leans on the wall

Table 16.2 A summary of performance problems that may indicate back pain.

'Cold-backed' during mounting
Slow to warm up or relax
Resists work
Reluctant to stride out
Hock, stifle and obscure hindlimb lameness
Front leg lameness, stumbling and tripping
Excessive shying, lack of concentration on rider and aids
Rushes downhill or pulls uphill with the front end (exhibits improper use of back or hindquarters)
Demonstrates an inability to travel straight
Is unwilling or unable to round the back or neck
Displays difficulty maintaining good stride
Falters or resists when making a transition
Bucks or rears regularly

pain, even if the problem occurred with the previous owner (Table 16.3).

The horse should be observed standing at rest with no saddlery on. Note the natural stance of the horse, as many horses develop a compensatory positioning of the legs at rest when there is pain present. Some horses stand stretched out or 'parked out' to rest their back, while others stand with their limbs underneath their bodies. Look at the shoeing, as unbalanced feet lead to alterations in stance, movement [1] and to upper body pain. Does the horse always rest one foot or place one foot in a certain position? Can the horse stand square if asked?

Table 16.3 Physical evidence of poor saddle fit.

Obvious sores
White hairs
Temporary swellings after removing the saddle
Scars or hard spots in the muscle or skin
Muscle atrophy on the sides of the withers
Friction rubs in the hair

Look at the horse from all angles for symmetry and asymmetry. Many horses' shoulders are uneven. Stand the horse squarely on level ground and look at the points of the shoulders, the carpi and slope of the distal metacarpals, as well as the shape of the feet. Stand directly behind the horse, noting asymmetries in the pelvic structure, muscle mass over the hindquarters and in the gaskins, and the shapes of the feet. Make note of the differences.

Place a stool behind the horse and stand above the horse's back, looking down. Be sure the horse is standing square, though it may be impossible to be square in front and behind at the same time due to discomfort. The shoulders often appear asymmetrical from differences in muscle tension. This can lead to saddle-fitting problems, stiffness and imbalances in movement. Observe the entire spine up into the neck for asymmetries.

Observe the horse walking and trotting/jogging in hand, while being lunged and with a rider mounted. Many horses move freely on the lunge line, but with a rider the horse loses its free movement or adversely changes its movement, a strong indication of back pain.

Biomechanically, the head, neck, back and hindquarters are connected and move together, so if a horse carries its neck in a raised 'upside-down' (dorsi-flexed), hollow position, the back is also going to be hollow. The hollow position of the back will alter the position of the pelvis, making it impossible to engage the hindquarters correctly underneath its body. To allow the horse to use its back properly the *rectus abdominus* muscles, *ileopsoas*, *tensor fasci latae* and the quadriceps (all protractor muscles of the hindlimbs) must contract.

As the horse's back becomes hollow or stiff, the hind legs cannot engage properly and the front feet tend to hit the ground hard. Common incorrect back movement leads to horses with an attractive headset, a motionless back and relaxed abdominal muscles.

The rider may feel that the horse is 'off' or just not quite right on a particular limb. To the observer, the main sign is often stiffness or resistance in one direction or another, but the horse is not lame enough to warrant the use of local analgesic techniques to localize pain in the suspect limb. In some horses, multiple limbs may be involved, which may well manifest as a general stiffness. A stiff spine means that the horse is not moving correctly and the muscles of the back are painful or in spasm. In other cases it is clear that the horse is protecting a painful part of the body, often the back. As the horse moves stiffly and incorrectly, over time the distal limbs may become affected secondarily, slowly resulting in overt lameness. In the author's opinion, correct treatment during the back pain stage may prevent distal limb lameness.

Palpation of the Back

Palpation skills are enhanced by learning acupuncture and chiropractic approaches for treating horses. The information gathered by specific palpation allows the practitioner to make a complete diagnosis and treatment plan.

The first palpation is a gentle passing of the practitioner's hands over the entire neck, back and thorax looking for muscle tension, sensitivity, flinching or discomfort. A light touch often reveals more than a heavy touch and much practice is needed to develop the light touch.

Acupuncture Palpation and Diagnosis

The next stage in the examination is the acupuncture palpation and diagnosis. This involves palpation of the acupuncture meridians looking for pain or tension. The most common meridian to palpate for back pain is the *bladder meridian*. The section of the bladder meridian used is about 10 cm lateral to the midline of the spine in an average-sized horse, beginning in the pocket just behind the shoulder blade and ending near the tail. This meridian is one of the most important pathways in the body and is easily affected by ill-fitting saddles.

As the practitioner's fingers gain experience palpating for acupuncture points, subtle changes can be found. Any sensitivity found along the back will cause the horse to alter its gait. Pain in the back and neck acupuncture points may, in the author's opinion, be the origin of distal limb problems.

Chiropractic Examination

The chiropractic examination is the next stage. All joints in the body including the spine should move smoothly through their entire range of motion. Many horses have lost normal motion throughout their spine, resulting in stiffness and pain. To examine the range of motion, the practitioner gently moves the spine through its normal range, looking and feeling for stiffness. A carrot can be held by the horse's hip, stifle and down between the front limbs to check neck mobility (the 'carrot stretch'), then the back can be raised (ventroflexion) by pressing on the ventral midline to contract the *rectus abdominus* ('sit-ups' for horses).

A normal horse can reach its hip and close to its stifle, as well as reach down well between its forelimbs. The back should be able to rise up easily, resulting in the horse extending and lowering its neck. A horse can become very upset if raising its back is painful. If the horse cannot raise its back while standing still, it will not be able to raise its back with a rider in place, which is the goal in many sports. Loss of normal motion at the junction of the ribs and the sternum or loss of motion through the withers, midthorax or the thoracolumbar area usually produces pain when raising the back.

The practitioner then does a specific motion palpation of the individual joints of the spine and extremities, looking for restrictions. Healthy joints move freely and have spring to them, while problem joints often feel stiff.

Muscle palpation is also important, starting with a light touch and moving deeper to assess muscle quality. A healthy muscle will feel soft and springy; the horse will not object in any way to the palpation. A muscle under tension will feel tight and hard, and will have little spring. A muscle in spasm will be more likely to become injured and will take a long time to warm up, as there is less blood flow through the spasm. Sometimes a horse will 'splint' its back or hold it rigidly in place while being examined to avoid moving it. This reflects pain.

As the palpation is being done, if signs of saddle-induced injuries are found, they indicate that there has been a problem with a saddle, either past or present (see Table 16.3. If a poorly fitted saddle has been used on a horse for any length of time, there will be residual back pain and probably loss of normal motion of the thoracic and lumbar vertebrae.

The Use of Diagnostic Imaging

When evaluating horses for back pain, diagnostic imaging of all types can be used to complete the picture. However, as noted in other chapters, it is common to have minimal or non-specific radiographic and scintigraphic changes. This is partly because considerable back pain in the horse and indeed other species is often due to soft tissue injury rather than the degenerative bone and joint disease that radiography and nuclear scintigraphy provide information about. A diagnostic imaging modality that can provide information on soft tissue inflammation is thermography (Chapter 11). Thermography detects areas of increased and decreased blood flow and in horses that have inflammatory processes causing pain, an increase in body surface temperature may be detected. In contrast, chronic pain, in many cases, shows up as decreased blood flow and cool areas in the muscle [2]. Anti-inflammatory therapy will not affect the cool areas; manual therapies such as acupuncture, chiropractic, osteopathy and massage will increase blood flow and reduce pain and may be useful in these cases.

Saddle Fit

Poor saddle fit is perhaps one of the primary contributors to back pain and must be addressed in an examination for back pain (Table 16.4). Saddle fit should be considered as important as, and similar to, shoe fit in a person.

Saddle Structure

Saddle structure is extremely important and the manufacture of saddles has seldom included quality control. Many new saddles are purchased with serious defects such as panels and flaps installed asymmetrically and/or twisted trees. The initial cost of the saddle seems to have no bearing on the number or severity of structural defects to be found. Examine the saddle carefully from all angles to check for balance and symmetry. Minor differences from one side to the other can be tolerated, but most differences that can be easily seen will create pain or cause the rider difficulty in finding the correct position in the saddle.

Saddle Position

Saddle position is the most critical aspect of saddle fit. Commonly, the saddle is placed too far forward. This position places the rigid tree over the top of the shoulder blade, which significantly restricts the movement of the front legs. If the saddle is moved back to the correct position the stride will generally lengthen immediately. When an English saddle is placed too far forward, the pommel is too high. This causes the seat to slope down towards the cantle and places the rider's legs too far forward in an unbalanced position. The rider then tries to level the seat with pads under the back of the saddle.

Western saddles, when too far forward, exert enormous pressure on the top of the scapula. Moving the saddle back to the correct position frees the scapula but can put the rider and the saddle too far back. Saddles with shorter bars, such as those used in barrel racing or for Arabians, can be easier to move back into the correct position due to the shorter bar. The shorter bar may still be too straight.

If the saddle, no matter what type it is, does not fit, no change in position will correct the problem.

Saddle Panels and Bars

The saddle must sit squarely down the middle of the back supported by the bars or panels sitting evenly over the longissimus dorsi. The dorsal spinous processes have no muscle covering; therefore, there is little soft tissue to protect them from saddle pressure.

A bar or panel should conform to the shape of the back. If it is too flat or long, a bridge will be created with pressure on the shoulders and

Table 16.4 Considerations when assessing saddle fit in a horse with suspected back pain.

The structure of the saddle
The position of the saddle on the back
The contact of the bars or panels against the horse's back; absence of bridging
Must have enough rocker and twist to the bars to conform to the horse's back (Western)
Whether the panels are wide enough for good support (English)
Whether the gullet is wide enough to clear the spine completely (2½ to 3 inches) (English)
Whether the gullet is the correct width and tall enough to clear the withers (Western)
The fit of the tree to the horse's back, especially across the withers
Whether the saddle sits squarely in the centre of the back
The levelness of the seat
The placement of the girth
How the rider fits in the saddle
Position of the stirrup bars or stirrup placement

the back of the saddle. The weight becomes distributed on four points, one on each side of the withers/shoulder blade and one on each side of the back at the rear of the saddle. Some flexible panelled endurance saddles cannot follow the contour, while a treeless saddle naturally follows the shape of the back.

English panels need to be wide enough to offer good support. The gullet needs to be wide enough (2½ to 3 inches) to allow the spine complete freedom from pressure and to allow the spine to bend slightly laterally during movement. The angle of the panels needs to follow the angle of the horse's back under the cantle. Saddles can have too acute an angle, putting pressure on the outer corner of the panel.

English saddles need to be reflocked (restuffed) every year or even more frequently. Finding a competent saddler to do this can be a challenge. Wool stuffing is very useful as it is resilient and offers a smooth surface to the horse's back. High-quality foam-stuffed panels can be excellent, while low-quality ones lose their resilience in a few years' time. Foam is hard to adjust and replace but does not need restuffing.

Western bars should only put pressure on the rib cage; any part of the saddle extending past the 18th rib should not put any pressure on the loins. Bars need to have enough rocker (curve to the bottom) and flair (curve at the ends) so the bar shape conforms to the shape of the horse's back. Very few trees have enough shape. Skirts need to be short and flared so they do not interfere with the shoulders or loins.

Saddle Trees

The tree must follow the contour of the withers without the use of pads. If the tree is too narrow for the withers, the front will sit up high, unbalancing the rider. If the rider then places pads under the back of the saddle to raise it, more pressure is placed on the withers. If a saddle is too wide across the withers the rider will be tipped forward and the saddle may make contact with the withers.

Unfortunately many saddles are poorly designed. Cheap Western saddles may have the bar grooved too deeply for the stirrup leathers, leaving what appears to be a bulge at the base of the fork. English close-contact jumping saddles may have an outward flare in the tree where the withers are flat in shape. Other saddles, especially dressage and a few Western/endurance saddles, have pressure points underneath the stirrup bars or attachments.

The Importance of a Level Seat

An important aid in determining saddle fit is that the seat must be level when viewed from the side and the rider must be placed in the centre of the seat. If the seat is not level or the lowest point is incorrectly placed, the rider will be out of balance, either tipped forward if the saddle is down at the front, or tipped back into a chair seat if the saddle is too high at the front. Roll a pill bottle on the seat to see where the lowest point is.

Position and Shape of the Girth

The girth will always finish the ride in the narrowest point of the rib cage. It must drop naturally perpendicularly into this space or the saddle will move either forward or back as the girth finds its natural spot. Some horses have girth spots close to the elbows, while others are one to two hand-breaths behind the elbow. An otherwise well-fitting saddle can become a poorly fitting saddle just by having the girth attached in the wrong place.

Short girths (both the Western girths and the short dressage girths) can cause discomfort. The correct length is to have the buckle or rigging D just below the saddle, out of the rider's way and away from the horse's elbow.

Rider Fit

If the saddle does not fit the rider, the rider becomes the saddle-fitting problem. The most common fault is having the seat too small for the rider, forcing them to sit at the back of the saddle.

The position of the stirrup attachment is critical to the comfort and balance of the rider. Stirrup leathers placed too far forward will cause the rider's legs to drift forward, leaving them in a chair-seat position.

On Western saddles particularly, the ground seat is made too wide for the rider's legs to drop comfortably down to the side. The wide seat pushes the thigh out to the side so the knees cannot lie against the horse's side. This rolls the pelvis back and prevents the correct use of the lower leg.

Locating Pressure Points

The most obvious way of ascertaining whether chronic pressure points have been experienced under a saddle is if white hairs appear under the saddle. If these white hairs appear there will be a pressure point above them. On a Western saddle the sheepskin covering of the panels will become worn down over the pressure points. One way to locate pressure points is to ride with a thin, clean, white saddle pad. Dark spots that appear after 15 or 20 minutes usually will be pressure points. Light areas or areas with no sweat are generally from a lack of pressure, but be careful, these can also be caused by excess pressure, which decreases the amount of sweat produced.

Measuring the Back for Saddle Fitting

To measure the horse's back for some assistance in fitting saddles a flexible ruler from an office supply store is a tool that is easy to use, and works well as a rough guide to the fit of the tree. Such a ruler can be moulded to the shape of the horse's withers; then a drawing can be made on cardboard and cut out. If this is done at four-inch intervals along the saddle area, a basic diagram of the horse's back can be constructed. By holding the cut-out shapes of the back inside a saddle, a very general idea of whether the saddle may fit can be obtained. Several new methods, including computerized pressure analysis and thermography, are available to help with fitting saddles.

Rider Variables

The rider, by virtue of the fact that he/she is sitting on top of the horse, has an enormous influence on the horse's back. Sally Swift and her concept of 'centered riding' [3] has demonstrated very clearly that if a part of the rider is stiff, that stiffness will be reflected in the horse directly. Most riders have some degree of back pain or other old injuries that create stiffness in their body; this is transferred directly to the horse.

As veterinarians, making suggestions about the rider is the most difficult aspect of the problem to solve, as most riders do not want to hear that they need to change; they have hired the veterinarian to 'fix' their horse. Riders must be handled carefully, because if they are offended they will look elsewhere for someone to 'fix' their horses.

The Use of Therapeutic Pads

Therapeutic pads are often used to try to solve saddle-fit problems. Much of the time the pads provide only temporary relief and may cause more problems than they solve in the long run. The addition of the pad to a saddle is similar to a person adding an extra sock to his shoe. If the tree of the saddle is wide enough the pad may help. If the tree is already too narrow, and this is the most common scenario, the addition of the pad causes more pressure on the withers, the pommel may sit higher in front which unbalances the rider, who then adds some more pads under the back of the saddle, raising the back of the saddle and driving more pressure on to the withers. Muscles will atrophy along each side of the withers from increased pressure.

The addition of a pad may cause a dramatic improvement in a horse's performance. This may last for a short time, but the same problems usually return, because the pad changes the fit of the saddle and moves the pressure points slightly but seldom eliminates them. Over time pressure points find their way through the pads.

A saddle properly fitted with a pad to act as an interface and shock absorber can be a big help. Many pads are useful; the secret is to select the pad with care and fit it with the saddle, just as you would fit a shoe with the type of sock it will be worn with. For long-distance horses it is especially important that the pads breathe due to the long hours in the saddle.

Shims are thin pads that can be placed under a part of the saddle to make a temporary change in fit. If shims are used carefully they can solve many problems. Be sure they do not interfere with saddle fit.

Teeth, Mouth Pain

Pain in the mouth, either from poorly cared for teeth or bit pain, can mimic or cause back pain. Mouth pain will cause a horse to travel with its head high and neck hollowed, which leads to a hollow or dropped down back. As the back hollows muscle tightness is created, altered gait patterns occur and back pain is the result. Mouth pain must be corrected, either with quality teeth care, a change in bits or an improvement in rider skill.

Additional Management Factors Influencing Back Pain

Many other management and training practices can, in the author's opinion, cause back pain.

- *Ponying racehorses* – torques the muscles and vertebrae in the neck and back, primarily done in America.
- *Lunging, round pen work*, especially for long periods of time, or at a fast pace as is done in round pen training with young horses.
- *Training aids* range from benign to abusive. These cause at least one joint to brace against the device. The best way to use them is to interval train for a few minutes, then release and reconnect after a few minutes of rest.
- *Mechanical hot-walkers* place the horse in a hollow position with the head and neck up in the air, causing the back to hollow also. Old-fashioned hand walking or caged hot-walkers are much better

- *Swimming* has an excellent place in the rehabilitation of lameness. However, the hollow position of the back tightens back muscles and can increase back pain.
- *Blankets* are an important source of back and wither pain. Blankets cut out over the withers cause a vice-like tightness between the caudal aspect of the withers and the points of the shoulders. The cranial thoracic vertebrae with their long dorsal processes often become subluxated, as do the attachments of the first few ribs to the sternum. The shoulder muscles become compressed and the stride shortens significantly. To compensate, the horse then tightens up the entire back and shortens the stride. Blankets should be selected to fit as loosely over the shoulder as possible so that, after the horse has been turned out all night, it should still be easy to open the buckles. The most effective shape is one that comes over the withers and up on to the neck. Use new lightweight and durable materials. An old blanket can be adapted by adding darts in the centre of the neck area; this pulls the blanket away from the shoulder [4].

Treatments for Back Pain

Acupuncture

In this author's practice, acupuncture is an extremely useful treatment for back pain. Approximately 85 to 90% of the horses treated return to their previous level of performance in one to four treatments given about one month apart. When clients are unwilling or unable to correct management issues or the horses are in hard work, the horse must be maintained with regular preventative treatments. Human athletes have discovered it is necessary to maintain some regular form of musculoskeletal therapy to keep maximum performance with minimum injury since continued athletic activity puts a certain degree of strain on the musculoskeletal system.

Acupuncture is best known for its treatment of back pain and arthritis. It is best performed by a veterinarian with advanced training in the technique. Practitioners who just pick a few standard points or follow a single formula will find that their results are inconsistent. A significant improvement with one to three or four treatments is considered a normal response. If a significant positive response (not necessarily a cure, but a definite improvement) is not achieved in horses after four treatments, either the diagnosis was wrong, the pathology is too far advanced or the treatment is incorrect. Maintenance treatments can often slow the progression of degeneration and give pain relief even if no cure is possible.

Acupuncture operates on the concept that there is another system in the body in addition to the cardiovascular and neurological systems [5]. Similar to vessels in the cardiovascular system and the nerves in the nervous system, there are pathways along the body through which there is a flow of energy, or as the Chinese call it – 'Chi' or 'Qi'. Along these pathways, called meridians, are acupuncture points. Acupuncture points are real structures with arterioles, venules, fine nerve endings and mast cells [6]. The points have a lower electrical resistance than the rest of the body so it is possible to measure the points with a modified ohm meter [7].

It is easiest to understand the acupuncture system if it is compared to an electrical system. The points are like dimmer switches in that if the flow of Qi becomes blocked, it is similar in concept to turning the dimmer switch down and not allowing much electricity through. If a point is treated with acupuncture, it is like turning the dimmer switch back on and allowing Qi to flow again. Sometimes Qi gets backed up behind the blockage or the dimmer switch, and treating the point allows a more even flow of energy.

Acupuncture points can be stimulated in many ways, including by needles, electrical stimulation, Moxa (a herbal form of heat), injection of vitamin B12, cold laser stimulation and massage or acupressure. Horses are generally very receptive to the treatment. Several excellent textbooks are available on the subject [5,6] and courses are taught internationally (IVAS, Chi).

Chiropractic and Spinal Manipulation

Restricted motion in a joint may either be primarily due to osseous pathology or, conversely, in the author's opinion, lead to pain, reduced performance and osseous pathology. As described elsewhere in this book, significant spinal pathology is well recognised in the horse. Restoration of normal spinal movement is the goal of spinal manipulation [8]. Full range of motion in all joints allows the horse to perform comfortably and with flexibility in his back [9,10].

During motion palpation of the back the chiropractic practitioner locates joints with restricted motion and aims to restore motion to that segment of the spine.

Spinal manipulation of horses is usually performed using chiropractic or osteopathy. These are different modalities though their goal is to restore function to the spinal cord and nerve supply. Training is critical before a practitioner is qualified to work on a horse and cannot be accomplished in a weekend or through a correspondence course. Courses are available worldwide and only qualified practitioners should be referred to.

Chiropractic is often misunderstood partly due to the use of the word 'subluxation'. The traditional medical definition of a subluxation is a partial dislocation. Modern chiropractic terminology uses the vertebral subluxation complex (VSC) to describe all the manifestations of the biomechanical and neurological components of the alteration of normal dynamics, anatomic or physiological relationships of contiguous articular surfaces in the spine – the term does not necessarily refer to a partial dislocation. The research behind chiropractic techniques is extensive, though only a few studies have been done directly within the equine field [11,12].

The physiological stages of the VSC show that symptoms (pain) do not begin to manifest until kinesiopathy, myopathy, neuropathy, vascular abnormalities, connective tissue disorders and inflammation have all begun. Once signs of pain are present the next stage is degeneration of the joints [8]. Consequently, the reason for regular chiropractic adjustments is to prevent getting to the stage of pain.

A chiropractic adjustment is a short-lever, high-velocity, controlled thrust, by hand or instrument, directed at a specific articulation in a single motor unit (two vertebrae and the associated nerves, tendons, ligaments and soft tissue) [8]. Chiropractic adjustments do not require great strength, just skill in making the short, sharp thrust, and knowledge of how to direct that thrust. This author adjusts all sizes of horses from ponies to draft horses with her hands with no difficulty.

A manipulation, as is frequently done in the name of chiropractic or osteopathy, is a non-specific, forceful passive movement of a joint beyond its active range of motion, generally done with a long lever by jerking a leg or twisting the entire neck. Manipulations can result in damage to the joint capsules and to the joints themselves. Initially improvement in flexibility and performance is often seen, so these practitioners stay in business, but the long-term joint damage starts immediately. The effects of manipulations may not show up for several years. This style is most common with lay practitioners, but is unfortunately seen with trained veterinarians, chiropractors and osteopaths who should know better.

Untrained practitioners can use some simple exercises, such as the carrot stretches and belly lifts described below, and can find restricted or abnormal areas of motion and begin to restore that motion to the spine; owners can continue those exercises.

Stretching

Stretching is one of the simplest, most effective ways to enhance back pain treatment, aid in rehabilitation after injury or to help locate areas that may be of concern. Stretching can be performed by the owner on a regular basis or by the veterinarian as part of an examination and treatment. In this author's experience horses who are stretched on a regular basis (daily or at least 2–4 times a week) are generally more flexible through their back and stay sounder than horses who are not stretched.

Stretching must be done correctly and carefully to avoid injury. The use of force can damage muscles and joints. Any joint can be stretched safely to restore its full range of motion if the handler holds the leg in position and waits for the horse to release and relax the muscles. The stretch can be taken farther as the horse continues to release muscle tension. A horse is always stronger than its handler, so if force is applied and the horse pulls back it will only tighten the very muscle the handler is trying to loosen.

- *Carrot stretch.* The horse is asked with a carrot or other treat to reach to the *tuber coxae* and down between the front legs. A horse with normal flexibility can reach its *tuber coxae* by moving its head and neck directly around without twisting it down. This stretch restores flexibility to the neck, withers and thoracic area, with some muscle stretching as far as the lumbar area. Often a horse has restricted motion in its neck and cannot complete the stretch. Some horses may need spinal manipulation to restore complete motion.
- *Belly lifts.* These stretches (regular and lateral) restore dorsoventral and lateral motion through the thorax and are perhaps the most important stretches for the back. Many horses are incapable of performing all or parts of this stretch without significant pain and will kick or bite, so caution must be used. Perform this stretch very gently and carefully, to try to keep the horse comfortable and relaxed so the muscles stretch rather than contract.
  - Dorsoventral belly lift. The handler places fingertips on the midline of the sternum behind the elbows and presses upwards. The fingers can be moved along the midline to the centre of the

abdomen to raise and stretch different parts of the back. Start with a light touch and increase pressure until the back rises. In some cases a blunt plastic tool such as a needle cap or plastic writing pen may be needed to raise the back.

- Lateral belly lift. Stand on one side of the horse and reach across the midline up into the girth area behind the elbows on the opposite side. Pull the rib cage diagonally upwards towards the withers on the side the handler is standing (towards the handler's head). When belly lifts are comfortable for the horse, the abdominal muscles should contract, the longissimus muscles should fill out and relax, the withers should rise and then the head and neck should stretch forward and down. With the lateral belly lifts the rib cage should move easily laterally, the same on both sides. The withers on the side the handler is standing should fill with relaxed muscle, while the opposite side should form an even concave bend. The head and neck should stretch down and forward curved slightly away from the handler. When there is pain and tension, parts of the longissimus group of muscles will contract. This can be seen by depressed areas or muscle spasms in the muscle as the back is raised. Pain may be from muscle tension or as a result of the loss of motion or arthritis that may be present throughout the spine and may require chiropractic care to restore. When back pain is present the head and neck usually rise up during this stretch.

- *Wither stretch.* This can relieve tension and pain through the cranial thorax. The handler places his hands over the withers and leans back, gently pulling on the withers. Start at the cranial edge (T3–T4) and move towards the caudal part (T9–T11). When the stretch is ended, the handler should release the withers slowly. If there is little pain and the horse is enjoying the stretch, it will pull against the handler and relax into the stretch. If there is significant pain,

muscle fasiculations and spasms may be felt under the handler's hands and the horse will not pull into the stretch. Proceed gently if this reaction should occur and hold the stretch until the muscles relax. This stretch is especially useful for horses wearing tight blankets.

- *Psoas stretch.* This is one of the most important stretches for the back and it can be combined with a stretch for the semimembranosis and tendonosis (hamstring). When the psoas muscle is tight it prevents the caudal stretch of the hind leg.
  - This stretch is performed by holding the leg either caudal (psoas) or cranial (hamstring) to the vertical at the limit of the range of motion, and then waiting for the horse to release the leg a bit. As the muscle relaxes, the stretch can go farther until the leg reaches the back of the knee (hamstring stretch) or can touch the ground behind the vertical (psoas). If force is used, the horse will pull back and tighten the muscle. If the horse is comfortable with the stretch, it will release the leg quickly: if uncomfortable, it may only release small amounts at a time.

- *Psoas release.* An excellent therapeutic release for the psoas, sacroiliac and lumbar muscles can be performed.
  - The leg is held up a few inches off the ground in a comfortable position for the horse; gentle movements are made in a circular fashion for a minute. Then, for the next two minutes, the leg is brought progressively higher until it is flexed, much as the leg would be for a regular flexion test. The gentle movement is kept, and if the horse needs to put the leg down, set it gently on the ground vertical or forward of vertical, not in a caudal position. This is not a daily stretch as much as it is used as therapy for the caudal part of the back. The activity is performed daily for about a week, then two to three times a day for another week or two, to be repeated if necessary.

Massage

Massage therapy consists of manipulation of the muscle using a variety of techniques depending on the problem and the background of the practitioner. Massage can be very specific to treat a small area such as trigger point therapy (also known as myotherapy or neuromuscular therapy) where the practitioner applies concentrated finger pressure to 'trigger points' (painful irritated areas in muscles) to break cycles of spasm and pain. Trigger points commonly can occur in any muscle, but are common in the gluteal muscles and *longissimus dorsi* over the last few ribs and lumbar muscles.

Massage techniques can be used to treat specific muscle injuries, for prevention of injuries, for pre-event preparation and post-event recovery. Damaged, contracted muscle has less blood flow through the capillaries than healthy muscle. If an injury to a muscle is recent, massage techniques are used to enhance the clearing of lymphatic fluid and blood from the area of damage and to reduce swelling. Once the injury is older and has become chronic, massage is used to restore circulation and flexibility. Massage is currently routinely used on many human athletic teams to prevent and treat muscle injuries and should be used more routinely with equine athletes.

Massage is performed, in most cases, by lay people, many of whom have little training other than a one-week course. At the present time, the best way to find a qualified person is to locate someone who has completed a full 500-hour human massage course and who has then taken one of the more extensive equine courses offered. Veterinarians would be well advised to locate a few top-quality massage therapists for client referrals so that effective therapy is performed.

Homeopathic Treatment of Back Pain

Homeopathy is a branch of complementary medicine [13] that is perhaps least well understood of the modalities, yet it is useful in the treatment of back pain, especially that due to injury. Homeopathic remedies can be used in conjunction with any conventional treatments, though, as a practitioner becomes more comfortable with this type of therapy, faster results can be achieved by using the remedies alone, along with any required supportive care.

Homeopathic medicine approaches disease in a different manner than allopathic (conventional) medicine. Conventional thinking considers each disease to have a consistent, recognizable set of signs and symptoms that should then be treated with a specific drug or therapy. In homeopathic medicine symptoms are regarded as an expression of an imbalance present in the body, which can be from internal weakness or an external force that disturbs the workings of the body. The symptoms are the result of the body trying to correct the imbalance.

Allopathic treatment of a disease such as arthritis asks questions about how much pain the patient has and whether the current treatment is helping. Treatment usually includes one of a variety of similar-acting anti-inflammatories or a COX-2 inhibitor type of drug. As the disease progresses, the drug dosage is usually increased in order to counteract the symptoms.

Homeopathic treatment of the same disease examines the patient from a broader perspective and asks questions about the type of pain (sharp, dull, stiff) and the modalities – what makes the pain better, worse (weather, season of the year, motion or lack of motion) and whether there are visible changes to the shape of the joints. The treatment is tailored to the individual, with a different remedy for each presenting set of symptoms. This variability in treatment plan depending on the individual's response to a disease is what makes it difficult to perform traditional double-blind research studies [14].

Homeopathic remedies are usually supplied in small tablets or sand-sized granules listed with a potency (strength) of 6X, 12X, 12C, 30X, 30C or 200C. The standard dose for an adult horse is six to eight tablets, or one-half teaspoon granules, three to five for a pony or foal. The remedies can be given once or twice a day (for the 200C), or two to three times a day for the 30X or 30C potency and can be fed with small quantities of food or placed directly in the mouth.

Homeopathic remedies are prepared by diluting the original substance; therefore they will not test positive in a drug test during competition in the strengths described here. They are prepared according to exacting standards and are regulated by the Food and Drug Administration in the United States (Homeopathic Pharmacopoeia). Several remedies are particularly useful in treating back pain.

Arnica montana is a homeopathic remedy used by this author very successfully to decrease the pain, swelling, stiffness and healing time in many traumatic injuries of the back. Arnica, in this author's experience, is useful in helping chronic or long-standing back pain. The remedy can be given one to three times daily, with the more frequent dosing used when the injury is more severe. Arnica can be administered at any point in the healing process to improve the healing; however, if it is started at the time of the injury, the results are quicker than if started later [15].

Ruta graveolens (Ruta grav) is a remedy that has particular affinity for injuries to the periosteum, tendons and ligaments. The back contains many small joints and associated structures. In cases of chronic back pain, Ruta grav can be given two to three times a week for several weeks, followed by the next remedy (Rhus tox).

Rhus toxicodendron (Rhus tox) is indicated when an injury to muscle, tendon, ligament or joint has healed to the point where the horse is stiff when starting out, but warms up and moves much better. Rhus tox can be given for two to five days in a row, then may be given one to three times a week for a few weeks. Rhus tox is also commonly used for arthritic conditions of any joint, since the most common complaint is that the condition is better after being warmed up.

Ledum Palustra (Marsh Tea)

Ledum is a remedy that is well-indicated for arthritic pains of the small joints including those in the back, with or without inflammation and worse with motion. The pains associated with Ledum may move from place to place, as is often the case in Lyme's disease. Pain is better with cold hosing, but can be worse after bandaging.

Traumeel

Traumeel is a combination of many homeopathic remedies, used in low potencies. It is available as a topical, internal, and an injectable format in most countries. Clinical studies in Germany have shown Traumeel to be useful in treating muscle pain. Clinically this author has found Traumeel to be a helpful adjunct in treating back pain.

Herbal Therapy for Back Pain

Herbs have been used for centuries to treat various injuries and in China, the martial arts practitioners used herbal preparations to strengthen tendons and also ligaments. Herbs can be used internally (as powders or teas) as well as externally as an ointment, liniment or poultice. Herbs contain active ingredients and certain herbs can cause a positive in blood tests for drugs, mainly when ingested. Practitioners should become aware of herbs that may test positive (yucca, white willow bark, for example) and use caution when prescribing.

Arnica montana can be used as a poultice, ointment, body wash or liniment, as a topical treatment for bruising, or muscle, tendon and ligament injuries as well as overworked and tired muscles. Arnica should never be used on broken skin as it is irritating. Its primary action is anti-inflammatory, but it is not powerful enough to mask pain as a non-steroidal anti-inflammatory would.

Internally, dried herbs or liquid extracts of *devil's claw, meadowsweet, white willow bark and yucca* are all known for their anti-inflammatory action. In general, herbs such as these take several days of feeding or longer for the effects to be seen, so they are usually more effective when given for chronic problems rather than acute ones. Products containing anti-inflammatory herbs can be used in acute situations. However, for more immediate results, the practitioner may wish to try the homeopathics listed above. Please note that some 'herbal' supplements may contain additives that are not permitted by the Governing Council under which the horse competes and the veterinarian must consider this before recommending a remedy.

16.2   Physical Therapies

Mimi Porter

The Role of the Equine Physical Therapist

There is considerable evidence that pre-emptive pain management can be effective in decreasing the development of chronic pain states and is beneficial to the health, recovery and quality of life of horses. The role of the equine therapist is to identify the site/area of the pain and to apply the appropriate therapy. There are a number of different therapies available to the equine physical therapist. The following are, in the author's opinion, the most useful in the treatment of the equine athlete.

Therapies

Ice

A simple and effective intervention in the pain–spasm–pain cycle is the use of ice massage directly on the area of inflammation. To create a handy tool for ice massage, fill a Styrofoam cup with water and freeze it. Remove the lip of the cup to expose half of the ice block, keeping the rest of the cup intact to insulate your fingers from the ice. Massage the affected area for 5–10 minutes, depending on the depth of the involved tissue. The area

should feel quite cold to the touch. This will interrupt the pain–spasm cycle and cause local capillary constriction, reducing the leakage of fluid and blood from the damaged capillaries, and reduce the release of harmful chemicals involved in prolonged inflammation. Ice massage and a reduction in training intensity can provide effective therapy in the acute phase of injury development.

Therapeutic Ultrasound

Therapeutic ultrasound makes use of the kinetic energy of particle vibration within the high-frequency sound wave. Absorption of this energy takes place at the molecular level with protein in the tissue acting as the absorbing agent. Therapeutic ultrasound is delivered as either a thermal (continuous wave train) or a non-thermal (pulsed or intermittent wave train) application, generally at frequencies of 1 MHz or 3 MHz. A topical transmission gel must be applied to the hair coat to eliminate air, which is a deterrent to ultrasound transmission. Determination of frequency, duration and whether to use pulsed or continuous application depends on the nature of the injury, its acuteness or chronicity, and the depth of the injured tissue. Ultrasound delivered at 1 MHz will penetrate to deeper-lying soft tissue and bone, whereas 3 MHz ultrasound is absorbed superficially. It is the sound wave frequency that determines the depth of ultrasound energy penetration, not output intensity. Increasing the intensity setting when delivering ultrasound at 3 MHz could cause overheating of the superficial tissues and will not drive the sound wave deeper. Continuous wave ultrasonography of over $1.5 \, \text{W/cm}^2$ can cause a significant rise in tissue temperature, even beyond the therapeutic range. Used correctly this modality can benefit the horse through:

- Increased elasticity of collagen in tendons, joint capsules and scar tissue.
- Increased motor and sensory nerve conduction velocities, which assist in reducing pain.

- Altered contractile activity to skeletal muscle, which reduces muscle spasm.
- Diminished muscle spindle activity, another factor in muscle spasm reduction.
- Increased blood flow.

Therapeutic Laser

Therapeutic laser, also known as phototherapy, was introduced to the arena of equine health care in the 1980s. At that point collimated, monochromatic light devices did not have approval from the US Food and Drug Administration (FDA) for use on humans, so these devices were marketed to the horse industry. As the devices commonly used in the horse industry are not true lasers, the name phototherapy is a more accurate identifier. Many phototherapy devices in use today use a combination of light-emitting diodes and infrared-emitting diodes.

Research on the effects of phototherapy has shown that it stimulates cell growth, increases cell metabolism, improves cell regeneration, induces an anti-inflammatory response, reduces oedema, fibrous tissue formation and levels of substance P, stimulates production of nitric oxide, decreases the formation of bradykinin, histamine and acetylcholine, and stimulates the production of endorphins.

Phototherapy must be applied in contact and perpendicular to the skin surface. The horse's hair coat can absorb and scatter the energy, so diodes that protrude from the pad are better suited to contact the skin surface. The number of sessions required varies according to disorder, length of time that the disorder has been present and its severity.

Electrical Stimulation – The Longitudinal Muscle Channel System

Electrical stimulation is a tool available to the equine therapist for many purposes, such as tissue repair, reduction of swelling and mental relaxation, as well as for pain relief. A treatment strategy that the author has found to be particularly successful involves the use of the traditional Chinese medicine concept of the longitudinal muscle channel system combined with the Western approach of the use of dermatome patterns.

Dermatomes are areas of skin that are innervated, essentially, by one spinal nerve. Sensory fibres and nociceptors from the skin, muscles, joints and viscera enter a specific spinal cord segment via the dorsal nerve root. These dermatomal patterns correspond loosely with the longitudinal muscle channels, as described in traditional Chinese medicine.

The longitudinal muscle channel system is an adaptation of the more familiar meridian system of acupuncture. Similar to the acupuncture meridians, each of the muscle channels has its own pathway, which generally follows the acupuncture meridian pathway but is much wider, covering larger areas of the body. All muscle channels start in the extremities and go to the trunk or head. Dermatome pathways begin in the extremities and go to the spine.

Electrical stimulation, using four electrodes, provides a convenient agent for applying this system of pain control for the horse. The equine therapist begins by identifying the dermatome and spinal segment involved. An electrode is then placed on the lesion site or on a distal area of the dermatome. A second electrode is placed on the related spinal segment.

The next step is to determine the muscle channel involved and to place an electrode on a significant point along the muscle channel. This trigger point may be a muscle–tendon junction or a point that is significant acupuncturally. A fourth electrode is placed on the association point of the channel; these association points are found along a line running parallel to the spinal cord on the horse's back.

The electrical stimulation protocol is supported by a generally accepted model of pain control mechanisms, i.e. large sensory fibres in the area of pain are stimulated to block nociceptor transmission in ascending pathways in the spinal cord – a modified Wall's gate control theory. In contrast, another commonly used therapy available to the equine therapist, acupuncture, relies on the stimulation of peripheral sites in the body to activate descending influences on pain transmission. The stimulation of acupuncture sites enhances the release of endogenous opiates for prolonged pain relief.

Twelve muscle channels are described in traditional Chinese medicine, each covering a specific area of the body. By incorporating these transmission pathways into an electrical stimulation treatment protocol, the equine therapist has the opportunity to combine a traditional Western therapeutic approach with an Eastern therapeutic paradigm that has stood the test of time.

Pulse Signal Therapy

The label 'kissing spine' syndrome or ORDSPs is often given to any pain in the lumbar area of both humans and horses, although it is likely that much of the pathology comes from osteoarthritis and soft tissue damage in the region. Pulsed signal therapy (PST), a device that has been developed over the last 20 years, has been tested in double-blind clinical trials and has shown effectiveness and safety in horse and human patients suffering from osteoarthritis of the cervical and lumbar spine. Data were collected over a 10-year period in the US, Canada, France, Italy and Germany, at major medical centres. The PST device produces a pulsed magnetic wave, which induces a weak electrical signal that mimics the physiological signalling normally occurring in healthy tissue. PST has been shown to restore normal cell differentiation and stimulate joint cartilage maturation by means of passively generating streaming potentials that emulate chondrocyte activity in the healthy joint under load [16]. This device is easy to use because it requires only proper placement of the magnetic coil pads and activation of the unit. This device is relatively new to the equine world, but shows promise of efficacy in the treatment of osteoarthritis.

Therapeutic Exercise

The equine therapist's model of rehabilitation is based on that of the human athletic trainer. The therapeutic aspect is aggressive in terms of symptom relief and exercise plays an equally important role. Ground exercises improve musculoskeletal flexibility and increase the horse's kinaesthetic awareness, a factor in prevention of re-injury. Experimental and clinical studies demonstrate that early, controlled movement is superior to immobilisation for treatment of acute musculoskeletal soft tissue injuries and postoperative management. There are many books and videos that provide examples of ground exercises for the horse. Rehabilitation is dealt with in detail in Chapter 17, but three ground exercises that are of particular value to the horse with a stiff and painful back are described here.

Lateral Flexion–Extension Exercise

Begin with the horse moving around the handler on a long rope, at least 8 feet (2.5 m) long. If the horse is moving in a clockwise direction the rope is in the handler's right hand. The handler reaches with the left hand to grasp the rope and direct the horse to bend its torso to the left and change directions on the circle. The handler must not step back to offer the horse a bigger space in which to turn. The horse must demonstrate lateral flexion–extension of the thoracolumbar spine to complete the movement. This exercise could be called 'the waltz' because, when it is done correctly and repeatedly going from one direction to the other, it should be fluid and smooth like a dance.

Hip Disengagement Exercise

Using the long rope, bring it from the head down the right side of the body around the horse's hips to its other side. Gently pull the rope to direct the horse's head to the right until the rear legs move in an abduction–adduction motion. Continue until the horse faces the handles. This creates lateral flexion and extension throughout the entire spine, strengthens the adductor/abductor muscles in the hips and gives the equine therapist clues to the functionality of the rear hip joints.

Dorsiflexion–Extension Exercise

Downward fingertip pressure on the horse's back alternates with upward pressure from the fingertips on the belly. A clinical manifestation of back pain results in diminished flexion–extension movement at or near the thoracic lumbar junction. Carrying out this exercise with several repetitions daily will enhance spinal mobility over time.

Conclusion

Treatment of back pain requires a whole-horse approach to be consistently successful. The rewards are great as performance often improves to better than the previous level. There are many causes of back pain that need to be identified, followed by an individually tailored program to best aid in the recovery.

References

1 Chateau, H. et al. Normal three-dimensional behaviour of the metacarpophalangeal joint and the effect of uneven foot bearing. *Equine Veterinary Journal* 2001; **33**:84–88.

2 von Schweinitz, D.G. Thermographic diagnostics. In: Haussler, K.K. (ed.), *Veterinary Clinics of North America: Back Pain*, Philadelphia, PA: W.B. Saunders, 1999, pp. 161–170.

3 Swift, S. http://www.centeredriding.org/sallyswift.asp.

4 Harman, J.C. Does your blanket fit? In: *Practical Horseman*. AIMmedia, 1996.

5 Xie, H., Colahan, P. and Ott, E.A. Evaluation of electroacupuncture treatment of horses with signs of chronic thoracolumbar pain. *Journal of the American Veterinary Medicine Association* 2005; **227**:281–286.

6 Schoen, A. *Veterinary Acupuncture, From Ancient Art to Modern Medicine*, 2nd edn. St Louis, MO: Mosby Publications, 2001.

7 Steiss, J.E. Neurophysiological basis of acupuncture. In: Schoen, A.M. (ed.), *Veterinary Acupuncture: Ancient Art to Modern Medicine*, St Louis, MO: Mosby Publications, 2001.

8 Haussler, K.K. Chiropractic evaluation and management. In: Haussler, K.K. (ed.), *Veterinary Clinics of North America: Back Problems*. Philadelphia, PA: W.B. Saunders Company, 1999, pp. 195–209.

9 Denoix, J.M. and Audigié, F. The neck and back. In *Veterinary Clinics of North America Equine Practice: Equine Locomotion*. Philadelphia, PA: W.B. Saunders Company, 2000, pp. 167–192.

10 Denoix, J.M., Audigié, F., Robert, C. and Pourcelot, P. Alteration of locomotion in horses with vertebral lesions. In: Conference in Equine Sports Medicine Science, Taormina, Italy, 2000.

11 Haussler, K.K., Bertram, J.E.A., Gellman, K. and Hermanson, J.W. Dynamic analysis of *in vivo* segmental spinal motion: An instrumentation strategy. *Veterinary and Comparative Orthopaedics and Traumatology*. 2000; **13**:9–17.

12 Haussler, K.K., Bertram, J.E.A., Gellman, K. and Hermanson, J.W. Segmental *in-vivo* vertebral kinematics at the walk, trot and canter: A preliminary study. *Equine Veterinary Journal* 2001; Suppl., **33**:160–164.

13 Kleijnen, J., Knipschild, P. and ter Riet, G. Clinical trials of homeopathy. *British Medical Journal* 1991; **302**:316.

14 Birnesser, H., Klein, P. and Weiser, M.A. A modern homeopathic medication works as well as COX 2 inhibitors for treating osteoarthritis of the knee. *Der Allgemeinarzt*. 2003; **25**:261.

15 Macedo, S.B., Ferreira, L.R., Perazzo, F.F. and Carvalho, J.C. Anti-inflammatory activity of *Arnica montana* 6cH: Preclinical study in animals. *Homeopathy* 2004; **93**:84–87.

16 Markoll, R., Da Silva Ferreira, D. and Toohill, T. PST: An overview. *Journal of Rheumatology* 2003; **6**:89–100.

17

Rehabilitation

Mary Bromiley

Introduction

The processes of physiotherapy and rehabilitation should complement each other. In terms of personnel, in some cases the physiotherapist undertakes both, but rehabilitation is very time-consuming and a specialist trainer – the rehabilitation trainer (RT) – is the best person to effect rehabilitation. The RT should work together with the physiotherapist and any other involved professional, e.g. the vet, osteopath, chiropractor, acupuncturist or masseur.

At the outset of rehabilitation there are some important factors to be recognised. Following a diagnosis of the cause of the symptoms displayed by the horse the resultant musculoskeletal problems should never be addressed as a single entity as it is widely acknowledged that disruption of normal function in one area leads to a cascade of interrelated problems. When considering pain arising within the vertebral column, the core of the axial skeleton, associated primary limb dysfunction is a common finding. Unfortunately, the secondary complications are often those targeted by the owner or untutored RT.

One major problem when initiating back rehabilitation is to identify which of the epaxial muscle groups is affected. Until recently visualisation has been the only method to assess muscular integrity. Significant atrophy of superficial muscles is usually obvious, seen as increased prominence of the dorsal spinous

processes (DSPs), either in localised sites or throughout the thoracic and/or lumbar areas. Unfortunately, atrophy of deep-sited muscles, like the scalene group (leading to instability at the cervicothoracic junction), is not usually visually obvious in the early stages. However, the ability to diagnose muscle problems at this site is very important because loss of stability at C7–T1 leads to impaired neck function and this area is, probably after L6–S1, the most important junction within the vertebral complex.

In addition to the problems of assessing muscular atrophy or loss of function, ligaments are very important as loss of nuchal ligament support affects the entire back, leading to secondary loss of traction throughout the supraspinous ligament with consequent vertebral instability.

Ultrasound is the best imaging modality to diagnose muscle and ligament damage (Chapter 10). In addition to providing primary information on the presence of pathology, the technique is useful for rehabilitation as it enables determination of the relative size of the epaxial groups before and after rehabilitation. In addition a quantitative comparison of response to treatment might allow a more selective use of appropriate techniques.

The Back

Anatomically the vertebral column is described with each section presented individually rather

Equine Neck and Back Pathology: Diagnosis and Treatment, Second Edition. Edited by Frances M.D. Henson.
© 2018 John Wiley & Sons, Ltd. Published 2018 by John Wiley & Sons, Ltd.

than the structure being considered as a whole. In most descriptive literature the term 'back' is generalised, and then discussed as though it comprises only the section from the withers to the lumbosacral junction with no reference to the importance of the cervical spine.

When undertaking rehabilitation, it is essential, for a successful outcome, to consider the vertebral column as a whole; stability and normal function throughout the complete structure determine efficient locomotion of the entire body mass. The RT needs to appreciate that the skeletal and soft tissue components of all sections (cervical, thoracic, lumbar, sacral and pelvic) form an interdependent, interreliant mechanism. In addition it must be appreciated that the function of the appendicular skeleton relies on stability of the axial skeleton. To deliver effective rehabilitation for the equine back it is therefore necessary to consider not just the section from the withers to the loins, but also the cervical, sacral and pelvic areas. In rehabilitation the cause of the malfunction must be addressed as there is little or no benefit gained in removing back discomfort, and restoring mobility and stability, if the primary cause has not been addressed. One of the complicating functional consequences of the intercommunication and interdependence between all body parts is that disuse muscle atrophy (secondary to loss of proprioception) occurs after all traumatic incidents, be they as a result of accident, direct injury, a musculoskeletal condition or any form of disease.

When examining the horse, a broad approach should be adopted, with significant attention being paid to the skeletal and soft tissue components of the body. In addition the following all require consideration before designing an appropriate rehabilitation programme in order to achieve a successful outcome and restoration of preinjury function: neural and circulatory supply; the feet; teeth and general health of the horse, including nutrition; the age of the horse; the breed; the discipline and eventual level of activity required by the rider.

Anatomy

To achieve acceptable results an understanding of the interaction of the varied tissues and a detailed knowledge of the anatomy and physiology of the components involved in locomotion are required, in addition to an appreciation of the function of proprioceptors (the receptors that provide information on where the body is in space and relative to the ground; this information is used to adjust and correct imbalance).

Anatomical understanding should include:

- Skeletal components
- Ligaments
- Individual muscles, origin and insertion, and the functional nerve supply
- The neural supply of dermatomes
- The range of movement expected under normal circumstances, within and appropriate to the area targeted.

It should be appreciated that the anticipated range of movement will also, to a degree, be governed by age, conformation, muscle tone and any residual underlying bone or joint pathology.

Vertebral Ligaments

Back rehabilitation necessitates an understanding of the ligament support structure of the back and the ligament/muscular interactions that occur in the back, in particular the specialist activity of the nuchal and all associated ligaments. From a functional perspective, when considering the back, the vertebral ligaments can be imaged as two interacting chains influencing the dorsal and ventral sections of the whole.

Ligaments Influencing the Dorsal Section of the Body

Of great importance dorsally are the nuchal ligament and its direct continuation, the supraspinous ligament (SSL, see Chapter 10). In situations in which the nuchal ligament is affected, for example following wither injury, if the musculature of the neck (intimately connected to the nuchal ligament) is compromised, or if there is pain in the mouth or at the poll that affects the correct positioning of head and neck, nuchal ligament tension will be affected. Alterations in nuchal ligament tension lead, in turn, to SSL dysfunction with consequent minute changes in vertebral positioning. The interspinous ligaments and the ventral ligament of the spinal column work as stabilisers and are closely associated with the multifidus muscles, the deep muscles sited on the dorsal aspect of the entire vertebral column.

Muscles Influencing the Dorsal and Ventral Sections of the Body

Just as with the ligament chain, the dorsal (epaxial and hypaxial muscles, see Chapter 2) and ventral muscle chains contribute to the positioning of the back, and their functional development influences the 'top line' and 'bottom line', terms adopted by the riding fraternity.

Dorsal Section

The dorsal section is comprised primarily of the longissimus dorsi system, which functions to extend the vertebral column. The system extends from the pelvis to the cervical spine. Thus, an unidentified problem in the cervical segment of the muscle can affect other areas; conversely, problems in the lumber segment of the muscle will affect the cervical area.

The muscles that make up the *longissimus dorsi* system and the effects of loss of function of these dorsal muscles are shown in Table 17.1.

Ventral Section

The 'bottom line' comprises the cervical ventral muscles and continues, extending from sternum to pelvis, via the abdominal musculature. Without synergistic interaction of the dorsal and ventral musculature, the vertebral column is compromised with subsequent malfunction, so rehabilitation must also be targeted to involve the muscular chains.

In the lumber region, the ventral placement of iliopsoas creates an important bridge assisting the ventral ligament. The abdominal muscles complete the muscular part of the chain.

Table 17.1 The muscles that make up the *longissimus dorsi* system and the effects of loss of function of these muscles.

Muscle	Effects of pathology	Notes
Iliocostalis cervicis and thoracis	Reduction in stability of the lumbar spine	
Longissimus, lumborum, thoracis, cervicis, capitis et atlantis	Reduction of vertebral stability	
Spinalis, thoracis, cervicis	Reduction of stability of the cranial thoracic and caudal cervical areas	
Multifidus muscle system, lumborum, thoracis, cervicis	Reduces vertebral stability	Deep muscles. Span up to six vertebrae in lumbar area. Lumbar atrophy manifests in a roach back appearance, often unilateral, associated with atrophy of contralateral gluteus muscles

Table 17.2 The muscles that make up the ventral muscle system and the effects of loss of function of these muscles.

Muscle	Effects of pathology
Abdominal muscles	Reduces vertebral stability
Iliopsoas	Reduces stability of the lumbar spine and sacroiliac joint

The muscles that make up the ventral muscle system and the effects of loss of function of these muscles are shown in Table 17.2.

Back Pain

Pain actually *originating* in the back appears, from field experience, to be less common than is generally supposed by the lay public. True primary back pain is usually associated with a known incident: the horse getting a cast, a travel accident, a fall or identified pathology. In the author's experience back pain, disuse, muscle atrophy and skeletal changes are often secondary to a seemingly often remote, primary cause.

Possible Causes Associated with Back Discomfort

As discussed in Chapter 6, there are many possible causes of back discomfort including the following:

- *Inappropriate training/preparation*: this can be considered a 'chain malfunction'. When evaluating the effects of inappropriate training, consider the breed characteristics of the horse as well as the muscle characteristics of the breed.
- *Limb dysfunction* resulting in abnormal vertebral stresses: consider foot balance, conformation, adductor muscles.
- *Interrupted neural supply*: consider dermatome responses to identify the nerve involved, and so identify muscles compromised.
- *Muscle imbalance* within the ring of muscle groups supporting the axial skeleton:

consider the abdominals, neck and hindquarter musculature; test for possible power asymmetry, agonist/antagonistic balance.
- *Mouth discomfort* with associated incorrect head carriage: consider teeth, bit position, type and size.
- *Poll discomfort*: often associated with a history of the horse pulling back when tied or rearing and falling over backwards. Test movement of the atlanto-occipital and atlantoaxial joints.
- *Restricted respiratory function*: this can cause, in the author's opinion, a reluctance to flex at the poll or break overcorrectly; consider narrow jaw angle, oedema of parotid glands.
- *Metabolic malfunction*: consider diet, to include water, inappropriate protein levels, azoturia, gastric ulceration. Does the horse lack the necessary dietary balance to maintain a competent musculature?
- *Mares*: although not generally accepted, ovarian cysts or uterine discomfort can, in the author's experience, give rise to back discomfort.
- *Saddle fit*: the greater the area of back covered by the under panel, the more evenly distributed is rider weight; many modern saddles create a fulcrum at approximately T12, T13, T14, causing a seesaw motion at trot with consequent local bruising (Chapter 16). Note that the purchase of a new expensive saddle, endless pads or reflocking to suit the shape of the back is often the unsuccessful route chosen by the rider to alleviate back pain.
- *Rider position*: consider disparity of leg length, a common cause of rider imbalance necessitating adaptive repositioning of the vertebral column of the horse to counteract asymmetrical weight distribution.

Rehabilitation Programmes

The aims of a rehabilitation programme are first to restore muscle competence in affected groups and then to re-train normal movements. However, the RT must be aware that it should never be assumed that the normal, pre-injury pattern of movement will be automatically restored after muscle recovery.

In the human model, electromyography (EMG) has determined the role and level of activity of muscles during selected movement patterns, including athletic tasks. It is also possible, in the human model, to isolate an individual or number of individual muscles by incorporating apparatus to fix body parts. After isolation and EMG identification, experimentation has resulted in appropriate choice of activities in order to recruit and so influence selected muscles.

When trying to determine appropriate activities in order to rebuild the musculature in specific areas of the horse, and although currently work to determine muscle recruitment is ongoing, with some undertaken having been published, it should be remembered that the work is far from complete and unfortunately somewhat inadequate, particularly as experimentation is generally undertaken utilising a treadmill.

Movement isolation in the horse is not possible as it is in the human model, so general activity must form the basis of rehabilitation; however, by careful positioning of the head and neck, the choice of appropriate movement patterns and creating situations to increase load, at the same time influencing and targeting normal limb activity, it is possible to partially localise muscle recruitment.

Only with underpinning knowledge of the functional role of individual muscles, insofar as is currently known, and utilising group muscle activity can the RT select appropriate exercises and activities to ensure that the muscles that need to be influenced are exercised effectively, both to recover their pre-injury tensile strength and to ensure restoration of their pre-injury capability.

After re-establishment of muscle competence, it is necessary to select appropriate activities to re-establish the cortical pattern of natural balanced movements.

Rebuilding Muscle

A programme incorporating progressive resistance is considered to be the most efficient means of improving muscle but consideration of fibre type is also necessary. From the human model it has been demonstrated that type I fibres (slow twitch) respond to exercises incorporating slow repetition against a load, whereas type II fibres (fast twitch) respond to exercises involving rapid repetitions against a lesser load. It has also been established in the human model that fibre type can, to a small degree, be changed; this change is influenced by the type of muscle activity demanded.

Each breed of horse, before cross-breeding was introduced, retained its own specific characteristics, including that of muscle fibre type; this made the choice of an exercise regime relatively simple; e.g. the Arabian, with muscles predominantly endurance-type fibre, responds best to slow work against a load.

The crossing of a warmblood (slow twitch/endurance) to a thoroughbred (fast twitch/speed) can result in a thoroughbred-type frame and appearance but with predominantly warmblood-type muscle. Many problems arise from a lack of appreciation of this fact, with inappropriate muscle training often resulting in poorly prepared muscles leading, among other problems, to back pain.

The body musculature needs to be considered as consisting of stabilising or postural muscles, which function to stabilise the axial skeleton; the latter achieve movement and are concerned in the main with the appendicular skeleton.

Postural muscles are considered to consist, predominantly, of endurance (slow-twitch)-type fibres. The deep postural muscles, adjacent to the vertebral column, are linked functionally, as previously described, to the supporting ligaments; these and the joint capsules are all richly enervated. The role of the postural muscles throughout the vertebral column is to ensure correct positioning of individual vertebrae; their rich innervation also contributes to balance and to stability throughout the entire axial skeleton.

Stability is the essence of recovery, so early work in any rehabilitation programme should be aimed at rebuilding the stabilising musculature of the back. This is achieved through the use of long reins, and necessitates slow work with the back unencumbered by rider weight. With experience, it is possible to observe restoration of muscle activity. The musculature appears to 'ripple' as the horse is worked from the ground.

The basic exercises of the classical school were designed to 'strengthen' a horse before the introduction of ridden work, although it is unlikely that the exponents of these basic schooling activities appreciated that they were achieving axial stability.

The RT should incorporate such exercises in the daily routine, because, when the horse subconsciously appreciates that it possesses a stable frame, it will automatically begin to increase the range of appendicular movement.

A recent, much discussed schooling position, 'rolkur', undoubtedly focuses, by subtle positioning of head and neck, on activating and so strengthening the 'bridge' of muscles spanning the important junction of the base of the neck to the thorax. Stability of the cranial portion of the thoracic cage is achieved, which allows exaggerated forelimb extension, the horse instinctively realising that the forelimbs are attached to a firm underlying frame.

When the horse can work in long reins at both walk and trot, a gradual introduction of appropriate loading is required. Loading is achieved by the use of a weight boot, heavy shoe, suitably arranged poles in the arena, blocks, varied surfaces and, later, slopes.

If available, the walker, water treadmill or water walker can be incorporated to vary activity. Only when back stability has been restored, a process that often takes up to 6 weeks, should the programme be advanced to include ridden work.

When riding is introduced, working diagonally across a slope, wading in the sea and working in sand all achieve muscle loading.

Throughout the programme the discipline of the horse must be considered. Although the thoroughbred requires, in the early stages, exercises involving slow work to influence postural recovery, as rehabilitation progresses the speed and type of activity should be varied, to ensure fibre-type recruitment that is appropriate to discipline. Little benefit is gained if the rehabilitation programme produces endurance muscle in a horse that requires only speed.

Long Reins

Tack required for successful work in long reins:

- Snaffle bridle
- Cavesson
- Roller with at least three sets of side rings
- Pair of side reins with a rubber couple adjustable at both ends
- Pair of long reins, medium weight.

Horses take 2–3 days to become accustomed to being driven.

The side reins are used when the horse is first introduced to long reins; acting as an essential control aid, they run from cavesson to roller, not bit to roller. The side reins can also be utilised, for very short periods, to position the head and neck in order to influence body position and so influence muscle recruitment.

Why Rehabilitate in Long Reins Rather than Lunge?

The horse's back was designed to suspend the weight of the abdominal contents and resist gravity, not to carry weight. To achieve muscle recovery it is sensible to exercise the horse by working it as nature intended, riderless. Down the ages, and until quite recently, horses 'broken' in the old-fashioned manner in long reins were subjected, probably without the nagsman appreciating the fact, to the basic exercises of the classical school, involving as they do movement in both longitudinal and lateral directions.

Longitudinal exercises 'unite' the horse: they develop connection; as muscles strengthen in response to load, the frame stabilises.

Secondary to this stability is an improvement in the ability to shift the centre of gravity.

Lateral exercises result in improved flexibility. The effect of the exercises is to target and so strengthen muscles with a normal function, i.e. in general, to work, not in an active but in a static/stabilising mode.

Following sufficient lateral work, horses are considered to have become supple, or to move easier, with increased range. This improved range is possible because their joints are ably supported due to the improved condition of the muscle groups targeted by lateral work, and known collectively as adductor and abductor muscles. Lateral exercises can also be used to influence one-sidedness and/or to build one side of the back.

Early Rehabilitation

The horse should be worked in straight lines when active rehabilitation commences: work off a straight line gradually introduced, first by incorporating serpentines, then lateral work and finally circles. *Long reins* are preferable to the *lunge* due to the ability to control the hindquarters, in particular the outside hindleg, when work off a straight line is introduced.

A horse does not, as a natural activity, perform circles. To execute a 10-m circle, in perfect balance and perfect cadence, is probably one of the most difficult coordinations demanded and circle work should be avoided in early rehabilitation. Indeed, horses working in small circles often have areas of skeletal stress (Figure 17.1).

There is an apparent lack of understanding about the direct effects of individual exercises. Those described in texts state 'X exercise improves X movement' or that the activities described 'improve performance'. Unfortunately these statements do not identify the muscles affected by the particular exercise, explain the requirement for joint stability in order to improve general suppleness or describe the linkage between the influence of muscles on activity, stability and/or movement range. Understanding the effects of exercises, in particular *serpentines*, *lateral work* and *transitions down*, enables appropriate selection.

Why Classical Exercises?

The exercises of the classical school were designed to recruit differing muscle

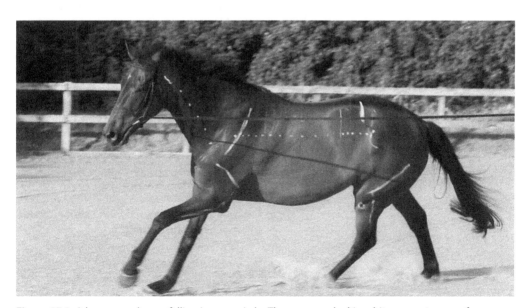

Figure 17.1 A horse on a lunge, falling in, on a circle. The areas marked in white suggest areas of skeletal stress.

combinations, in order to stabilise the axial skeleton, so enabling a safe change of gravitational position; this was necessary, before the introduction of the difficult movements demanded by Haute Ecole (all human dancers start their training using the basics of classical ballet!).

The use of an arena, equipped with poles and cavalletti, enables the RT to vary the limb action of the horse, not only changing the work of active muscles, from outer to middle range, but also as a result of the change of head and neck position influencing the position of the centre of gravity.

Muscle Loading

Added to an understanding of the effects of the basic classical exercises is the appreciation that increased resistance or loading is necessary for muscle recovery and appropriate loading is the only way to address unilateral muscle atrophy. Weight, either by the use of a heavy shoe or boot, increases the load of the selected limbs, with a secondary requirement for the stabilising musculature to also work against an increased load.

In addition to the addition of weights directly to the limb, the introduction of water and slopes can be employed to provide a variety of resistance. Increased loading is used for both muscle recovery and movement re-education because proprioceptive stimulation is affected by unnatural weight. Proprioceptive stimulus can also be enhanced by varying both terrain and footing.

There is no programme formula appropriate for all cases, even when considering a single body area. Each case requires an individual, specific programme. This programme should be appropriate for:

- The type of injury
- The primary site of damage
- Location of pain
- Muscles involved
- Eventual requirement.

The RT should remember that he or she is dealing with a recovery situation and that the speed of recovery will vary with each case, as will the ability to restore muscle competence.

Lateral Work

The muscle masses of the hindquarters may be considered as two pistons, each of which should produce equal power; to achieve this, the hindlimb thrust must be even, and the horse moves forward as design intended, with the vertebral column straight. If one hindlimb produces less thrust, the vertebral column will be subjected to a torque-type stress and the horse, as it moves forward, will not move truly straight.

With the *left hindquarter* affected the gluteal tongue and the deep musculature of the *right loins* (the antagonistic stabilisers) *atrophy*). If the problem in the hindquarter is not addressed or noticed, the horse rapidly becomes a "back pain" case, because, due to muscular imbalance, vertebral stress has occurred. The horse has become one sided, displaying back discomfort/pain, usually at the thoracolumbar junction, the range of vertebral movement is compromised and the horse's performance suffers. To counteract this situation, it is necessary to create an activity that loads the weaker hindquarter and works the back musculature unilaterally. To achieve this, the horse must be made to move off a straight line. By moving diagonally forward, one hind leg will need to exert a greater force in order to project the body mass, laterally, over the underloaded, contralateral limb. The requirement for the horse to move laterally has increased the workload of one leg, the leg of thrust, powered by the musculature of the appropriate hindquarter. The antagonistic, stabilising muscles of the vertebral column, sited on the opposite side to the muscles of thrust, are activated, because they work to retain the vertebral column in its functional position, straight.

Thrust supplied by the *left hindlimb* will load the *left hindquarter* muscles, and the movement will automatically influence the muscles down the *right side* of the back. Thus, by working to the right, employing the classic half-pass, the desired result, that of strengthening the musculature of the left hindquarter and right loins, is achieved.

Serpentines

The natural horse relies, for survival, on flight, necessitating a straight rather than a curved alignment of the vertebrae. When the horse performs a series of curves or loops a slight curve/rotation is created in the vertebral column, secondary in part to the movement of the weight of the abdominal mass.

The vertebral column is naturally designed to remain straight. If subjected to forces that create a curve, the subconscious reflex muscular response is to remove the curve and straighten the vertebral column. Thus work necessitating a series of loops or curves achieves increased activity within the muscle groups lying on the created convexity. Where the RT is aiming to treat a situation of bilateral muscle atrophy, even curves are employed, i.e. true serpentines. In cases with unilateral atrophy, the convexity is created on the same side as the muscle atrophy; the horse is then driven straight for a few strides, before executing another identical curve.

Transitions Down (Deceleration)

Movement at the lumbosacral junction recruits, among other muscles, iliopsoas and the gluteal tongue. A downward transition requires movement at the lumbosacral joint and these muscles, as they work to control the force generated by deceleration, are strengthened.

When to Start Early Rehabilitation

This is best described as the period immediately following injury, surgery or during the acute phase of muscle disease. Movement will be affected as a result of inflammatory responses (i.e. pain, muscle spasm, oedema).

At this stage it is the physiotherapist who uses his or her skills to reduce pain, retain optimum mobility and prevent excessive muscle atrophy. Activity, in the acute phase, unless box rest has been ordered, should be curtailed to hand walking, and/or turn-out in a small paddock or cage, rather than an immediate gymnastic approach.

Why Is a Period of Rest Important in the Rehabilitation Programme?

Before initiating a carefully controlled exercise programme it is best to observe a period of rest. This is recommended because, although the horse is still painful (from surgery or injury), it may recruit muscles other than those normally used when asked to perform specific activities by the RT or rider. The adaptation of incorrect muscle recruitment leads to an incorrect, inefficient, movement pattern. The adaptation is subconscious and adopted to attempt to reduce the pain experienced during movement. *In the author's opinion, persuading a horse that has changed its way of going to readopt the appropriate economic biomechanical pattern is one of the most exacting and difficult tasks for the RT.*

Examples of Inefficient Patterns

Neck Discomfort

The horse balances using neck and head and is instinctively aware of the necessity to remain ready and fully functional for flight. Discomfort in the neck changes the entire biomechanical function as pain or lack of mobility results in a change in limb function with stride compromised to maintain balance.

Forelimb Pain

The horse with pain in a forelimb may shorten the length of normal forelimb protraction, and by so doing will reduce the weight-bearing period at each stride, but will create uneven vertebral stress in and just caudal to the withers. Standing base narrow and placing the forelimbs along a central line, rather than standing and moving four square, is another change observed; these horses often show as having a 'cold back' when mounted.

Hindlimb Pain

A horse with hindquarter discomfort may attempt to overcome a loss of hindquarter impulsion by recruiting forelimb musculature, e.g. the brachiocephalic muscle may be used to exert traction at the sternal origin and pull the thoracic cage forward. In such cases, over time, an upside-down neck develops creating incorrect neck positioning, compromising nuchal ligament function and leading to a hollow, painful back.

Incorrect patterns rapidly become established, in the cortex, as normal, *and will be retained*, even after the condition giving rise to the pain has subsided, and often after a rehabilitation programme has been initiated and delivered. This is not successful rehabilitation.

Introduction of Active Rehabilitation

It is important to ensure that the acute injury phase is subsiding before a programme of active rehabilitation, involving as it does specific movements to order, is initiated. The time involved in each stage of specific tissue healing must always be considered.

The aims at this stage are to design a programme of exercises incorporating, at the appropriate time, varied aids and activities to encompass the following:

- Prevent development of soft tissue contractures.
- Prevent adhesions.
- Minimise ongoing loss of muscle.
- Restore muscle competence in all groups following atrophy.
- Restore normal levels of mobility.
- Re-educate to restore normal movement.

Throughout the programme, it is important that the RT liaise with the veterinary surgeon, owner, trainer and/or rider to ensure that the anticipated outcome, and the time required to achieve this, are understood and agreed by all concerned.

Failure

The prime reason for an unsuccessful outcome is that the RT has failed to:

- Recognise incorrect movement patterns.
  - Identify and rebuild appropriate muscle groups.
  - Re-educate movement.
- Re-establish normal biomechanics.
- Mobilise the neck.

Another common mistake, if an incorrect movement pattern has been noticed, is to introduce 'training aids' when trying to re-educate a way of going, e.g. the Chambon, de Gogue or Abbot Davies. In a rehabilitation programme, horses rapidly learn to rely on these, using them as a balance aid, rather as a child uses stabilisers when learning to ride a bicycle. Remove the stabiliser and the programme falls apart *because static positioning does not build muscle.* In some cases:

- The pain of injury is still present, inhibiting movement.
- The primary cause of the pain has not been elicited and addressed.
- The condition causing the pain has been so long term that cortical adaptation may have become irreversible.

Diagnosis and prognosis should have indicated whether the condition will resolve or whether irreversible changes are present. In the latter case any rehabilitation programme should be tailored appropriately.

Slopes as a Rehabilitation Aid

Walking a horse across a slope, either led or in long reins, can be used to exercise, strengthen and restore function in the long back muscles. The slope needs to be sufficiently steep to cause the positioning of a pair of limbs to be below, or downhill to, the contralateral pair; the body weight will then exert a 'down-hill' pull, creating a mild lateral or convex curve in the thoracolumbar spine, with the convexity downhill. The cortical pattern automatically attempts to restore equilibrium and re-establish the normal, straight configuration of the vertebral column. This attempt is achieved by the muscles on the 'downhill' side of the column working to reduce the convexity and pull the column straight. The muscle activity is similar to that achieved by the use of serpentines – restoration of a straight column – but demand is increased. Due to the use of a slope, the body weight is shifted laterally and the length of time for holding the position can be manipulated by the distance travelled across the slope; both these factors increase muscle loading.

The activity has been used not only for rehabilitation after atrophy of the back musculature, but also by a number of international riders to strengthen their horse's loins. The specificity of this activity is not fully known; however, rectal examination suggests that iliopsoas is the prime muscle targeted. In addition, in cases of iliac wing fracture, repeated rectal examination has suggested that this activity reverses the atrophy that occurs after fracture.

Treadmill

A treadmill can provide a very useful method of controlled exercise during rehabilitation. In some cases, rehabilitation exercises in the arena using poles will restore a balanced cadence; however, some cases fail to respond and retain an unlevel gait sequence. One of the advantages of the treadmill is that the horse requires a more balanced stride sequence when on the treadmill, in order to remain upright, than it would on solid ground. A treadmill with an uphill slope, as found in most rehabilitation centres, necessitates a lift to advance each individual limb rather than the normal swing-through, making the limb and its muscles work harder than on a flat surface.

Balance becomes established after three to five 5-minute sessions at walk, and is normally retained when the horse is worked over ground.

Hydrotherapy – Water as a Rehabilitation Aid

As previously stated, to improve muscle efficiency work effort needs to be increased. The swimming pool, hydrospa, water treadmill and water walker all make use of the weight of water as an aid to recovery, i.e. to increase muscle efficiency. Before the invention/marketing of the above devices, rivers, lakes and the sea were incorporated by some RTs into their rehabilitation programmes. All rehabilitation programmes using water have been reported as being very effective, although unfortunately little or no scientific research has been published detailing their efficacy.

Cardiovascular and Muscular Effects of Water Therapy

Equine Pools

The shape of equine pools vary: some are round, some straight with a ramp for entry and exit at each end and some oval, but with a straight section that can be used either as a straight section on its own or incorporated into the oval. The straight section is useful when teaching horses to swim and is the preferred option for rehabilitation. The ease with which horses adapt to swimming varies from individual to individual. However, even in horses that do learn to swim, unfortunately not all horses follow the required limb pattern in order to swim with a straight spine; some swim using front legs only, others just kick from behind, trailing their front legs, or screw the hindquarters to one side and then kick both hind limbs simultaneously sideways.

Benefits of Swimming

The resistance supplied by water is even, but, when swimming is incorporated as a rehabilitation aid, it is suitable only for horses that adopt a one-, two-, three- or four-limb pattern, or four-limb sequence, similar to the walk. The horses should also swim in a manner that keeps their back just out of the water, with head and neck comfortably positioned. Swimming benefits include the following:

- The muscles of the shoulders and hindquarters, and to a degree those of the loins and possibly the abdominal tunic.
- Joints: human studies suggest that movement of joints in a non-weight-bearing situation is of value in rehabilitation. Thus, the equine knee and hock, subjected to considerable stress in all competition animals, and often the primary cause of vertebral stress, may well benefit.
- Swimming does not benefit the tendons of the distal limbs. Movement in the distal limbs is entirely reliant on tendon stretch and recoil, affected only by weight bearing and weight transference.

Cardiovascular Stress

Swimming has an effect on the cardiovascular system. It has been observed that a straight pool raises the heart rate to over 200 beats/min and that a circular/oval pool might further increase this cardiovascular stress. Thus the hydrotherapy pool does cause a marked cardiovascular effort; however, swimming should not replace ground-based exercise but should be considered useful as a cardiorespiratory adjunct to rehabilitation.

Side Effects of Swimming

It is possible that stress to the cervicothoracic and lumbosacral junctions can occur, particularly in bad or poor swimmers. It is also postulated that possible damage to the back may result, secondary to the loss of proprioceptive input and when a horse is tired. A tired horse usually begins to drop its back and becomes noisy as it gasps for air. Experienced swimming personnel should never allow a horse to reach this stage of exhaustion. Excessive chilling is also a theoretical problem to the equine swimmer, although this is a rarity. In an ideal situation, in cold weather, a horse

should be put on a walker or stood under heat lamps to be dried off.

The dense mineral water of the thermal spas of Europe is warm, so there is no danger of muscle damage due to chilling in midwinter.

Pools obviously have their place but it should be accepted that swimming does not activate all over ground muscles; the prime benefit of swimming must be considered to be a non-weight-bearing, cardiovascular activity.

Water Walking

To improve muscular efficiency it is necessary to increase the workload of the muscle. This can be done in a number of ways, as described above. Water walking achieves this by using the resistance of water to increase the work required by the muscle to move the limb. Walking in a stream provides some resistance; walking in the sea is harder work due to the density of the water. The depth of the water that is being walked through does affect the work done. Water that is only fetlock deep does not change the action of the limb, but it has been noted that the splashing created appears to stimulate abdominal sensors and achieve abdominal muscle contraction. Work in deeper water, e.g. mid-cannon, does change the action. Mid-cannon work requires recruitment of the musculature of the loins to help lift the hindlimb and also activates the musculature at the base of the neck. In contrast, observation of horses wading shoulder deep suggests that they utilise normal limb activity, albeit with a shortened stride. For horses that, despite extensive rehabilitation from the ground, have failed to readopt a balanced cadence, water walking can be very helpful. They appear to rapidly recover and re-establish balance and normal limb sequence.

The Sea Walker

The sea walker brings the benefits of the sea to the rehabilitation yard. Rather than walking on rubber or matted surface, as on the normal walker, horses walk in a trough filled with a filtered, chilled, saline solution. Depth and speed can be adjusted in order to create varied recruitment of muscle, e.g. fetlock deep does not radically change normal limb action, but 19 inches (48 cm) of depth does, the limb movement adopted increasing activation of back and abdominal musculature; thus, if the point of the exercise is to strengthen the back, an increase in water depth will achieve this.

The Water Treadmill

The rehabilitation unit's water treadmill is a modified version of the standard treadmill originally designed for respiratory research. The addition of the water increases the amount of work that has to be done in order to ambulate at the required speed. The horse on a treadmill does not recruit its musculature exactly as it does when walking over the ground, because the moving belt repositions the weight-bearing limb/limbs to some extent: the frontlimb is taken back under the body and the hindlimb is carried behind the horse immediately the foot has been placed under the body mass. In the water treadmill, the tank is usually filled to mid-chest level, so, in order to move individual limbs, each is required to be lifted up rather than swung normally due to the resistance of the water. In the forelimb this is achieved by recruiting trapezius, normally acting in a pivotal rather than a lifting manner. The different usage eventually makes the horse appear thick through the withers, due to muscle overbuild; this has also demonstrated an apparent reduced stride length.

In the hindlimb (also required to be lifted) muscle recruitment occurs primarily in the loins, the horse reversing the normal function of a part of longissimus. When in deep water the horse must lift the hindquarter of the advancing hindlimb, then use the hip flexors, not required normally as a strong muscle group, to bring the leg forward under the body. Over ground, this positioning occurs just before the hindquarter musculature creates the tremendous backward thrust, delivered as the limb straightens, to push the body mass over the planted forelimb. On the treadmill there is no need for this thrust – the leg is taken backwards by the moving belt.

It is difficult to build the muscles of the back when the horse is being ridden because, in order to carry rider's weight, the back muscles need to achieve considerable tension, functioning in a holding or static, rather than active, manner; the static hold is necessary to resist a weight-induced downward curve. Static work does not build muscle, so, for a horse with a weak back, active recruitment of the back musculature in the water treadmill is very beneficial.

With the device and programme carefully chosen, the use of water to increase resistance can be of great benefit within a rehabilitation programme and may be utilised by the rider following an initial rehabilitation programme given by the RT.

Conclusion

A request for rehabilitation should follow accurate diagnosis by a veterinary surgeon. The diagnosis should result in the appropriate medical or surgical intervention, followed by treatment from an appropriate para-practitioner, osteopath, chiropractor, physiotherapist or masseur.

As previously stated, rehabilitation is directed at restoration of pre-injury function and is effected by selecting appropriate active exercise regimes; these are designed, first, to target the muscle groups compromised as a result of accident, injury or disease, and then to restore normal biomechanics.

Following any disruption from normal, multifactorial dysfunction occurs; all body components are affected to a greater or lesser degree: bone, joints, ligament, tendon, nerve, muscle, the circulatory and lymphatic systems.

The person undertaking rehabilitation requires an understanding of the muscular skeletal system, healing mechanisms and possible restrictions precluding the restoration of full function, and the programme should include ridden work only when appropriate in order to achieve the best possible outcome rather than starting too early.

References

Back, W. Development of equine locomotion from foal to adult. PhD Thesis, University of Utrecht, 1994.

Back, W. and Clayton, H.M. *Equine Locomotion.* Philadelphia, PA: Saunders Co., 2000.

Becher, R. *Schooling by the Natural Method.* London: J.A. Allen & Co Ltd, 1963.

Belasik, P. *Exploring Dressage Technique: Journeys into the Art of Classical Riding.* London: J.A. Allen & Co. Ltd, 1994.

Budras, K.-D., Rock, S. and Sack, W.O. *Anatomy of the Horse: An Illustrated Text,* 4th edn. Hannover: Schlütersche, 2003.

Comas, A.J. *Skeletal Muscle: Form and Function.* Champaign, IL: Human Kinetics Publishers, 1996.

Decarpentry, A.E. *Academic Equitation: A Preparation for International Dressage Tests.* Tonbridge: J.A. Allen & Co. Ltd, 1971.

De Lahunta, A. *Veterinary Neuroanatomy and Clinical Neurology,* 3rd edn. Philadelphia, PA: W.B. Saunders Co., 2008.

Delforge, G. *Musculoskeletal Trauma: Implications for Sports Injury Management.* Champaign, IL: Human Kinetics Publishers, 2003.

Edwards, E.H. *Training Aids in Theory and Practice.* Tonbridge: J.A. Allen & Co. Ltd, 1990.

Fonesca, B.P.A., Alves, A.L.G., Nicoletti, J.L.M. et al. Thermography and ultrasonography in back pain diagnosis of equine athletes. *Journal of Equine Veterinary Science* 2006; **26**:507–516.

Goody, P.C. *Horse Anatomy: A Pictorial Approach to Equine Structure.* Tonbridge: J.A. Allen & Co. Ltd, 1976.

Harris, S.E. *Horse Gaits, Balance and Movement.* Toronto: John Wiley & Sons Ltd, 1993.

Hinchcliff, K.W., Kaneps, A.J. and Geor, R.J. *Equine Sports Medicine and Surgery.* Philadelphia, PA: W.B. Saunders, 2004.

Jones, W.E. *Equine Sports Medicine.* Philadelphia, PA: Lea & Febiger, 1989.

Klimke, R. *Cavalletti.* Canaan, NY: Sydney R. Smith, 1995.

Oliviera, N. *Reflections on Equestrian Art.* Tonbridge: J.A. Allen & Co. Ltd, 1976.

Olivera, N. *Classical Principles of the Art of Training Horses.* Tonbridge: J.A. Allen & Co. Ltd, 1983.

Podhajsky, A. *The Complete Training of Horse and Rider.* Chatsworth, CA: Wilshire Book Co., 1965.

Rooney, J.R. *Mechanics of the Horse.* Malabar, FL: Krieger Publishing Co., 1980.

Schoen, A.M. and Wynn, S.G. *Complementary and Alternative Veterinary Medicine.* Philadelphia, PA: Mosby, 1998.

Short, C.E. and Van Poznak, A. *Animal Pain.* New York: Churchill Livingstone, 1992.

Sissons, S. and Grossman, J.D. *The Anatomy of the Domestic Animals.* Philadelphia, PA: W.B. Saunders Co., 1975.

Stanier, S. *The Art of Long Reining.* Tonbridge: J.A. Allen & Co. Ltd, 1975.

Stodulka, R. *Medizinische Reitlehre.* Stuttgart: Parey Bei Mvs, 2006.

Index

Equine Neck and Back Pathology: Diagnosis and Treatment, Second Edition. Edited by Frances M.D. Henson.
© 2018 John Wiley & Sons, Ltd. Published 2018 by John Wiley & Sons, Ltd.